I0072218

Clinical Handbook of Gastroenterology

Clinical Handbook of Gastroenterology

Editor: Calvin Bush

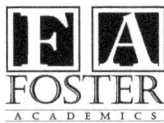

FA
FOSTER
ACADEMICS

www.fosteracademics.com

www.fosteracademics.com

FA
FOSTER
ACADEMICS

Cataloging-in-Publication Data

Clinical handbook of gastroenterology / edited by Calvin Bush.
    p. cm.
Includes bibliographical references and index.
ISBN 978-1-63242-533-1
1. Gastroenterology. 2. Digestive organs--Diseases. 3. Internal medicine. I. Bush, Calvin.
RC801 .C55 2018
616.33--dc23

© Foster Academics, 2018

Foster Academics,
118-35 Queens Blvd., Suite 400,
Forest Hills, NY 11375, USA

ISBN 978-1-63242-533-1 (Hardback)

This book contains information obtained from authentic and highly regarded sources. Copyright for all individual chapters remain with the respective authors as indicated. All chapters are published with permission under the Creative Commons Attribution License or equivalent. A wide variety of references are listed. Permission and sources are indicated; for detailed attributions, please refer to the permissions page and list of contributors. Reasonable efforts have been made to publish reliable data and information, but the authors, editors and publisher cannot assume any responsibility for the validity of all materials or the consequences of their use.

Trademark Notice: Registered trademark of products or corporate names are used only for explanation and identification without intent to infringe.

Contents

Preface

Every book is a source of knowledge and this one is no exception. The idea that led to the conceptualization of this book was the fact that the world is advancing rapidly; which makes it crucial to document the progress in every field. I am aware that a lot of data is already available, yet, there is a lot more to learn. Hence, I accepted the responsibility of editing this book and contributing my knowledge to the community.

This book provides comprehensive insights into the field of gastroenterology. Gastroenterology is a branch of medical science that deals with the study and prevention of diseases affecting the digestive system, that is, organs from mouth to anus and also the alimentary canal. Gastroenterology as a science includes various processes namely endoscopic retrograde cholangiancreatography (ERCP), endoscopy, liver biopsy, colonoscopy, etc. This book includes some of the vital pieces of work being conducted across the world, on various topics related to this field. It aims to shed light on some of the unexplored aspects of the subject and the recent researches in this area. The extensive content of this book provides the readers with a thorough understanding of gastroenterology.

While editing this book, I had multiple visions for it. Then I finally narrowed down to make every chapter a sole standing text explaining a particular topic, so that they can be used independently. However, the umbrella subject sinews them into a common theme. This makes the book a unique platform of knowledge.

I would like to give the major credit of this book to the experts from every corner of the world, who took the time to share their expertise with us. Also, I owe the completion of this book to the never-ending support of my family, who supported me throughout the project.

Editor

Accuracy of Colon Capsule Endoscopy in Detecting Colorectal Polyps in Individuals with Familial Colorectal Cancer: Could We Avoid Colonoscopies?

Cristina Alvarez-Urturi,[1] Gloria Fernández-Esparrach,[2] Inés Ana Ibáñez,[1] Cristina Rodríguez De Miguel,[2] Josep Maria Dedeu,[1] Xavier Bessa,[1] Henry Córdova,[2] Maria Pellisé,[2] Francesc Balaguer,[2] Angels Ginés,[2] Luis Barranco,[1] Isis K. Araujo,[2] Montserrat Andreu,[1] Josep Llach,[2] Antoni Castells,[2] and Begoña González-Suarez[2]

[1]*Department of Gastroenterology, Hospital del Mar, UAB, Parc de Salut Mar, Barcelona, Catalonia, Spain*
[2]*Gastroenterology Department, Endoscopy Unit, ICMDiM, Hospital Clinic, CIBEREHD, IDIBAPS, University of Barcelona, Catalonia, Spain*

Correspondence should be addressed to Begoña González-Suarez; bgonzals@clinic.ub.es

Academic Editor: Rami Eliakim

Background. Individuals with a family history of colorectal cancer (CRC) have an increased risk of CRC. We evaluated the diagnostic yield of CCE in the detection of lesions and also two different colon preparations. *Methods.* A prospective multicenter study was designed to assess CCE diagnostic yield in a cohort of asymptomatic individuals with a family history of CRC. CCE and colonoscopy were performed on the same day by 2 endoscopists who were blinded to the results of the other procedure. *Results.* Fifty-three participants were enrolled. The sensitivity, specificity, PPV, and NPV of CCE for detecting advanced adenomas were 100%, 98%, 67%, and 100%. Sensitivity, specificity, PPV, and NPV of CCE for the diagnosis of individuals with polyps were 87%, 97%, 93%, and 88%, respectively. CCE identify 100% of individuals with significant or advanced lesions. Overall cleanliness was adequate by 60.7% of them. The PEG-ascorbic boost seems to improve colon cleanliness, with similar colonic transit time. *Conclusion.* CCE is a promising tool, but it has to be considered as an alternative technique in this population in order to reduce the number of colonoscopies performed. More studies are needed to understand appropriate screening follow-up intervals and optimize the bowel preparation regimen.

1. Introduction

Most colorectal cancer (CRC) cases are sporadic but familial clustering is found in 25%. It is well known that the risk of developing CRC is 2 to 4-fold higher in individuals with a family history of CRC than in the general population, depending on the number of cases of CRC in the family and how closely the individuals are related [1]. A recent Chinese study [2] has also shown that the prevalence of advanced neoplasm (defined as CRC or adenoma of at least 10 mm with high-grade dysplasia or villous component in histology) is higher in the siblings of patients with CRC than in controls (7.5% *versus* 2.9%, odds ratio [OR] 3.07,

$P < 0.05$). Thus, in this group of high-risk individuals, it is recommended that screening begin at an earlier age and be conducted with increased frequency [2]. For instance, screening in individuals with a first-degree relative diagnosed with CRC before the age of 60 years or in persons with 2 or more cases in the family diagnosed at any age should begin at the age of 40 years or 10 years before the age at diagnosis of the relative. The current recommendation for this group is to perform CRC screening with colonoscopy every 5 years [2–4].

However, colonoscopy, which is considered the gold standard, has some limitations that may affect compliance. One of them is perception of the test, which varies by country,

TABLE 1: Study protocol: colon preparation.

Clear liquid diet	
Day 1	
12:00 p.m.	200 g carbohydrates + water
17:00 p.m.	200 g carbohydrates + water
19–21:00 p.m.	1 liter PEG + ascorbic + water
Day 0	
7:00 a.m.	1 liter PEG + ascorbic + water
9:00 a.m.	10 mg metoclopramide
9:30 a.m.	*Capsule ingestion*
10:00 a.m.	1° boost- 2/3 l. PEG + ascorbic + water or Sodium Phosphate[*]
13:00 p.m.	2° boost- 1/3 l. PEG + ascorbic + water or sodium phosphate (3 hours after first boost).[Ψ]
	Suppository
17:00 PM p.m.	*Colonoscopy*

[*] (30 minutes after pylorus pass checked by RAPID real-time viewer).
[Ψ] If capsule was not excreted.

ethnicity, and socioeconomic status. Recent published data from a multicenter study showed that colonoscopy participation rate in a population screening program was only 24.6% [5]. The risk of potential complications is another limitation. Rate of perforation after a diagnostic colonoscopy is very low (1/1000 patients) but exists [6].

Another important drawback of colonoscopy is the risk of missed lesions, which, according to a recent study, occurs in 2% to 26% cases [7]. Studies also suggest that colonoscopy may not be as sensitive in the right colon as it is in the left colon [8, 9]. Then other alternatives have been explored [10].

Colon capsule endoscopy (CCE) allows visualization of the colon mucosa without the need for sedation and insufflation. Since its introduction in 2006, this procedure has demonstrated to be safe and well-tolerated [10–17]. CCE has emerged as a potential cost-effective alternative to colonoscopy because it may improve adherence to CRC screening programs, although this has not been demonstrated yet [18]. Therefore, the objective of this study was to assess the diagnostic yield of CCE in the detection of significant colonic lesions (polyps and cancer) in individuals with a family history of CRC and to compare the efficacy of two different colon preparations.

2. Patients and Methods

2.1. Study Group. Individuals with CRC familial history were recruited from colonoscopy screening schedules. The protocol was approved by the Ethics Committee of Hospital Clinic and participants gave informed consent.

Participants were prospectively enrolled from January 2009 to January 2011 in 2 tertiary hospitals in Barcelona. CCE and colonoscopy were performed on the same day by 2 different endoscopists who were blinded to the results of the other examination.

Inclusion criteria included asymptomatic individuals with a first-degree relative diagnosed with CRC before the age of 60 years or with 2 or more relatives diagnosed with CRC at any age. Exclusion criteria were previous history of colonic lesions (polyps and/or neoplasia, inflammatory bowel disease, polyposis syndromes, or Lynch syndrome), severe heart failure or renal failure, dysphagia, suspicion of intestinal obstruction, or pregnancy.

2.2. CCE. CCE was performed using the first-generation Pillcam® Colon capsule (Given Imaging, Israel) which measures 31 × 11 mm and acquires images at a rate of 4 frames per second. All capsule videos were read by 2 physicians with expertise in this technique. A dissolvable capsule (Agile® Patency Capsule, Given Imaging) was administered prior to the procedure in case of major previous intestinal surgery, chronic use of nonsteroidal anti-inflammatory drugs, or abdominal pain to rule out stenosis. Exploration was considered complete when hemorrhoids plexus were seen or capsule was excreted before colonoscopy.

2.3. Colon Preparation. Preparation started the day before with a diet consisting of liquids and carbohydrates (plain noodles cooked in salt water) at lunch time in order to increase motility. At night and the next morning, participants ingested a low-volume preparation containing polyethylene glycol (PEG) plus ascorbic acid in split dose (Moviprep) (Table 1). As boosters they took PEG + ascorbic (group 1) or sodium phosphate (group 2) in order to compare colon cleanliness and transit time.

Similarly to previous studies, a 4-point scale grading system for the evaluation of colon preparation was used [11]. Colon cleanliness was scored as excellent (no more than small pieces of adherent feces), good (small amount of feces or dark fluid but not enough to interfere with the examination), fair (enough feces or dark fluid present to preclude a completely reliable examination), or poor (large amount of faecal residue) in 5 segments (cecum, ascending, transverse, descending-sigmoid, and rectum). An overall colon cleansing grade was also evaluated by using the same grading system. It was considered an adequate preparation when excellent or good and inadequate if fair or poor.

2.4. Colonoscopy (Gold Standard). Colonoscopy was performed in the afternoon, between 8 and 10 hours after capsule ingestion, under sedation (midazolam or propofol at the physician's discretion). Cleansing was graded upon colon withdrawal for each segment after completion of washing with the Boston Bowel Preparation [19]. Polyps detected during colonoscopy were removed and sent for histological assessment. If the capsule was seen during colonoscopy, it was retrieved.

Significant polyps were considered as those with size ≥6 mm. Advanced adenomas were considered those ≥10 mm, with villous histology or high-grade dysplasia. When a polyp was identified by CCE but not in colonoscopy, the patient was rescheduled for a second colonoscopy. False positives were defined as lesions detected only by CCE, after 2 consecutive colonoscopies.

2.5. Satisfaction Level. A patient satisfaction questionnaire consisting of 3 questions was done telephonically one month later. Patients were asked to evaluate their degree of satisfaction with the CCE and colonoscopy procedures using a 5-point subjective scale (from poor to excellent).

2.6. Statistical Analysis. Sample size was calculated assuming that CCE would detect the same number of lesions than colonoscopy, giving a total of 51 patients, with a significance level of 5%, statistical power of 80% assuming 10% of dropout rate.

Performance characteristics and 95% CI were calculated for any-sized polyps and for polyps 6 mm or larger. Descriptive statistics for continuous variables are expressed as mean and standard error and categorical variables as percentage. A two-sided Student's t-test was used to compare continuous variables, and the χ^2 test was applied to compare categorical variables. Statistical analysis was performed with SPSS software, version 19.0.

3. Results

A total of 53 participants were eligible for inclusion but two were excluded because of technical CCE failure and incomplete colonoscopy, respectively. Therefore, 51 participants were included and data analyzed: 27 in group 1 (boosters with ascorbic) and 24 in group 2 (boosters with sodium phosphate). Eighteen individuals (35.2%) had a total of 51 polyps. Demographic characteristics of the participants are shown in Table 2. Characteristics of the lesions detected by colonoscopy and CCE are shown in Table 3.

Capsule Agile Patency was administered to 4 patients confirming intestinal permeability and CCE was ingested without problem.

3.1. Per Individuals Analysis. CCE detected polyps in 15 individuals (29.4%). In four patients in whom CCE was normal and colonoscopy detected lesions, all of them were nonsignificant lesions. One of them had poor preparation and 5 polyps were missed and the other 3 subjects had good preparation and 4 polyps were missed. Histological analysis

TABLE 2: Demographic characteristics of the population.

Sex (M/F), n (%)	23 (43.1%)/28 (56.9%)
Age (years), mean (SD)	48.6 (8.9)
NSAIDs or anticoagulant therapy, n (%)	7 (13.7%)
Relatives with CRC, mean (SD)	1.42 (0.54)
First degree relative, n (%)	33 (64.7%)
Two or more relatives with CRC, n (%)	18 (39.6%)
Age at diagnosis of CRC (years), mean (SD)	56.8 (1.8)

of these lesions was tubular adenoma ($n = 3$) and hyperplastic polyps ($n = 6$).

Sensitivity, specificity, PPV, and NPV of CCE for the detection of individuals with polyps of any size were 87%, 97%, 93%, and 88% respectively. Remarkably, when we analyzed only subjects with significant or advanced lesions, CCE identified all of them.

3.2. Per Polyps Analysis. CCE detected 38 polyps and colonoscopy 51 polyps. Four polyps were seen by CCE and not in the first colonoscopy. However, the second colonoscopy found a 4 mm polyp that was removed and the other 3 were considered false positives. Therefore, 17 polyps in 8 individuals were missed by CCE. All of them were nonsignificant lesions. 14 of these polyps were hyperplastic and 3 were tubular adenoma. None of the missed polyps showed a villous component or high-grade dysplasia.

The diagnostic yield, sensitivity, specificity, PPV, and NPV of CCE are shown in Table 4. No cases of CRC were diagnosed.

Potential factors associated with missed polyps including complete examination with CCE, CCE cleanliness, type of booster, or location of polyps were included in an univariate analysis. Only location was a significant risk *factor* from univariate and was included in a multivariate analysis. Finally, the only independent predictor for missed polyps in our study was location in the left colon, rectum essentially (OR 0.4; $p < 0.001$).

3.3. Excretion Rate and Colon Cleanliness. The mean transit time from mouth to the anus was 251.0 ± 17.9 min.

CCE was excreted within 10 hours of ingestion in 84.3% of the participants. Patients of group one had a shorter colonic transit time (128,5 ± 95.6 versus 166.8 ± 121 minutes, pNS). CCE examination was complete in 44 individuals (87%) and incomplete in 7 cases (13%; 6 in group 1 and only 1 in group 2); in these cases capsule was retrieved during colonoscopy in the rectosigmoid area in 5 participants and in the cecum in 2 of them.

Overall cleanliness was excellent or good in 60.7% of CCE examinations (70.3% in group 1 and 50% in group 2, $p = 0.1$) (Figure 1). Colon cleanliness was graded better in the group of PEG + ascorbic boost compared to the cleanliness in the sodium phosphate boost group but this difference was not statistically achieved.

TABLE 3: Characteristics of the polyps found in CCE and colonoscopy.

Individuals	Booster	Cleanness in colon segments	CCE polyps	Colonoscopy polyps	Histology
(1)	PEG-Asc	Good	10 mm sigmoid	10 mm sigmoid	Tub-vell
(2)	NaP	Good	8 mm descending colon 3 mm sigmoid	8 mm descending colon 3 mm sigmoid	Tubular adenoma
(3)	NaP	Excellent Good	10 mm cecum 5 mm sigmoid	12 mm cecum 5 mm sigmoid	Tubular adenoma
(4)	PEG.Asc	Fair Fair Poor Fair Fair	8 mm descending colon 5 mm descending colon 8 mm sigmoid 10 mm sigmoid 4 mm recto 3 mm recto	7 mm transverse colon 5 mm sigmoid 4 mm rectum 7 mm recto 4 mm recto 4 mm recto	Tubular adenoma
(5)	PEG.Asc	Excellent	3 mm recto	4 mm recto	Tubular adenoma
(6)	PEG Asc	Fair	— 3 mm sigmoid —	5 mm transverse 3 mm recto 3 mm recto	Tubular adenoma
(7)	NaP	Excellent	3 mm sigmoid 3 mm sigmoid 3 mm sigmoid 4 mm sigmoid 2 mm recto 3 mm recto	3 mm sigmoid 3 mm sigmoid 2 mm sigmoid 3 mm recto 3 mm recto 2 mm recto	Hyperplastic
(8)	*NaP*	*Good*	*3 mm recto* — —	2 mm recto 2 mm recto 2 mm recto	Hyperplastic
(9)	*NaP*	Good	6 mm descending 5 mm descending 3 mm recto	— — 3 mm sigmoid	Hyperplastic
(10)	*NaP*	Good	2 mm recto	2 mm recto	Hyperplastic
(11)	*NaP*	Good	3 mm descending — — 2 mm recto	2 mm descending 2 mm descending 2 mm descending 2 mm recto	Hyperplastic
(12)	NaP	Good	4 mm sigma	5 mm sigma	Tubular adenoma
(13)	PEG Asc	Poor	5 mm descending 2 mm descending	— —	
(14)	PEG Asc	Good	2 mm transverse 2 mm descending 2 mm descending 7 mm sigmoid	3 mm ascending 3 mm transverse 2 mm sigmoid 5 mm sigmoid	Tubular adenoma Tubular adenoma Hyperplastic Tubular adenoma
(15)	NaP	Fair	5 mm ascending 4 mm descending — —	3 mm ascending 5 mm sigmoid 4 mm sigmoid 2 mm sigmoid	Tubular adenoma
(16)	PEG Asc	Good	—	3 mm sigmoid	Tubular adenoma
(17)	NaP	Poor	— — — —	5 mm transverse 2 mm recto 3 mm recto 2 mm recto	Tubular adenoma Hyperplastic

TABLE 3: Continued.

Individuals	Booster	Cleanness in colon segments	CCE polyps	Colonoscopy polyps	Histology
(18)	NaP	Excellent	— —	3 mm recto 3 mm recto	*
(19)	PEG Asc	Good	—	3 mm sigmoid	Hyperplastic

* Unrecovered polyps.

TABLE 4: Diagnostic yield of colon capsule endoscopy for detection polyps.

		Prevalence (%)	Sensitivity% (95% IC)	Specificity% (95% IC)	PPV% (95% IC)	NPV% (95% IC)
Polyps	Any size	51 (74%)	66 (61–97)	100	100	89 (79–99)
	≥6 mm	4 (7.8)	100	96 (90–100)	67 (29–100)	100
	≥10 mm	2 (3.9)	100	98 (94–100)	67 (29–100)	100
Adenoma	Any size	12 (23.5)	83 (62–100)	100	100	95 (89–100)
	≥6 mm	4 (7.8)	100	98 (94–100)	67 (29–100)	100
	≥10 mm	2 (3)	100	98 (94–100)	67 (29–100)	100
Advanced adenoma	Any size	2 (3.8)	100	98 (94–100)	67 (29–100)	100
	≥6 mm	2 (3.8)	100	98 (94–100)	67 (29–100)	100
	≥10 mm	2 (3.8)	100	98 (94–100)	67 (29–100)	100
CRC		0				

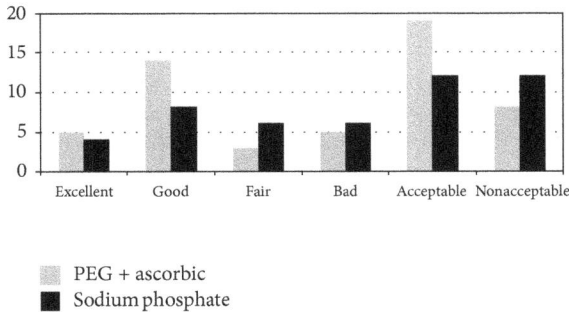

FIGURE 1: Number of patients with acceptable preparation in capsule endoscopy with different boosters ($p = 0.1$).

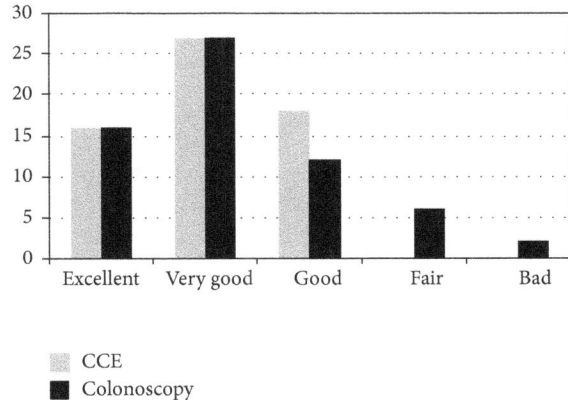

FIGURE 2: Patients satisfaction level (%) with colon capsule and colonoscopy.

3.4. Safety and Tolerability. There were no adverse effects related to CCE, colonoscopy or bowel preparation. Only 31 out of 51 subjects answered the satisfaction questionnaire. CCE was evaluated as excellent, very good, or good in 100% of participants, while 16% of them evaluated colonoscopy as fair-bad. Overall, 70.9% of participants submitted to the questionnaire preferred CCE, while 29% preferred colonoscopy (Figure 2).

4. Discussion

In this prospective, multicenter study specifically designed to assess CCE diagnostic yield in asymptomatic subjects with a family history of CRC, we can conclude that CCE is an accurate, feasible, well-tolerated, and safe alternative for this CRC high-risk population. CCE was able to identify all the individuals with significant polyps, using a low-volume preparation regimen with very good tolerance and acceptable cleanliness level. Most important target is to identify patients

to be submitted to colonoscopy (with any significant polyp), with a noninvasive test. This strategy could be accepted for a higher number of subjects.

Sacher-Huvelin et al. analyzed a cohort of 545 patients at average risk ($n = 163$) or increased risk of CRC ($n = 376$) and described a low overall sensitivity for polyp detection, probably due to poor colon cleanliness [17]. Gay et al. also analyzed 128 individuals with any indication for colonoscopy (76% with excellent or good preparation) and showed sensitivity for CCE of 87.5% [16]. Our results are in line with more recent studies that have shown that CCE is as effective as colonoscopy for detecting significant lesions [20–23].

The role of colon capsule endoscopy is still unclear and it seems a contradiction to use an alternative technique in a high-risk population because colonoscopy is our gold standard. However, most of these colonoscopies, about 70%, will be negative and we could use other noninvasive alternatives in order to select individuals with polyps for a therapeutic colonoscopy. With this strategy we would perform colonoscopy only in patients with significant lesions and avoid a lot of unnecessary explorations. Otherwise, in our study from 51 subjects included, 18 (35%) had lesions in colonoscopy and only 4 (7%) had significant lesions. CCE identified all of these patients with significant lesions. This could have a positive impact on waiting colonoscopy lists and reduce the care burden of the endoscopy units. On the other hand, less colonoscopy implies less complication. We think that all of these can make the CCE a cost-effective alternative. A great option in CCE will be a same-day CCE and colonoscopy if the patient has polyps, avoiding two colon preparations, but this is logistically difficult for the moment as Adrián-de-Ganzo et al. hypothesize recently [18].

CCE is a well-tolerated exploration and probably its use could increase colorectal cancer screening adherence although this has not yet been demonstrated [23]. Satisfaction level is another key feature in adherence to screening programs. In our study 70% of subjects preferred CCE for screening method. The results of the subjective assessment questionnaire showed that CCE was rated higher than colonoscopy and was perceived as good, very good, or excellent by all patients. In addition, we found that individuals would prefer to repeat CCE rather than colonoscopy for surveillance purposes. Again, we have data about a small number of patients and more studies have to be done.

Colon cleanliness is a crucial aspect related to sensitivity of CCE. Colon preparation usually consists in the administration of a clear liquid diet and a combination of laxatives and prokinetic agents [24]. We used a new low-volume solution consisting of PEG associated with ascorbic acid. This preparation has recently been evaluated with adequate results, achieving excellent or good cleanliness in >80% of patients [25]. In our study, however, overall excellent or good cleanliness was achieved in 60.7% of the patients (70.3% in patients in group 1, MoviPrep booster). Patient tolerance of this preparation was good and the procedure was classified as easier for the participants since a low volume of liquid was ingested. Also we found that PEG + ascorbic boost seems to improve overall colon cleanliness compared to sodium phosphate boost but we have a small size of patients need more studies in order to optimize colon capsule preparation.

More studies are needed to investigate the long-term follow-up of these individuals, as they are at higher risk of CRC and small polyps can be missed. It is unknown whether persons with familial risk might have faster growth and progression of polyps. Only one study has evaluated the cost-effectiveness of CCE in these persons, using a computer model, and concluded that cost-effectiveness depends mainly on the ability of the procedure to improve adherence to CRC screening [24].

The limitation of this study is that it was performed with a first-generation capsule endoscopy. Recently, a second-generation capsule, Pillcam Colon 2, has been developed, which has higher sensitivity and obtains better results in the detection of colonic lesions [21]. The main studies published with first-generation CCE [10, 12, 13] reported sensitivities of 63–88% and specificities of 64–94% in the detection of colonic lesions with high NPVs. Two recent meta-analyses with 626 patients and 837 patients, respectively, found sensitivities for significant polyps of 69–76%, with specificities of 86% and 82% [20, 22]. In our study, CCE detected 4 polyps that were missed on colonoscopy and repeat colonoscopy confirmed only 1 of them as a true positive result. The remainder was confirmed as false positives of CCE. Assessment of polyp size can also lead to confusion. In this respect, the second-generation capsule is an important new advance that allows measurement of polyp size, which will probably decrease the number of false-positive results but not make them disappear completely [26].

In conclusion, CCE is a promising tool that should be considered as an alternative technique in the screening of patients with familial colorectal cancer in order to reduce the number of colonoscopies performed. More studies are needed to understand appropriate screening follow-up intervals and optimize the bowel preparation regimen.

Competing Interests

The authors declare that they have no competing interests.

References

[1] A. S. Butterworth, J. P. T. Higgins, and P. Pharoah, "Relative and absolute risk of colorectal cancer for individuals with a family history: a meta-analysis," *European Journal of Cancer*, vol. 42, no. 2, pp. 216–227, 2006.

[2] S. C. Ng, J. Y. W. Lau, F. K. L. Chan et al., "Increased risk of advanced neoplasms among asymptomatic siblings of patients with colorectal cancer," *Gastroenterology*, vol. 144, no. 3, pp. 544–550, 2013.

[3] A. Castells, M. Marzo, B. Bellas et al., "Clinical guidelines for the prevention of colorectal cancer," *Gastroenterologia y Hepatologia*, vol. 27, no. 10, pp. 573–634, 2004.

[4] V. Piñol, M. Andreu, A. Castells, A. Payá, X. Bessa, and R. Jover, "Frequency of hereditary non-polyposis colorectal cancer and other colorectal cancer familial forms in Spain: A Multicentre, Prospective, Nationwide Study," *European Journal of Gastroenterology and Hepatology*, vol. 16, no. 1, pp. 39–45, 2004.

[5] I. Dove-Edwin, P. Sasieni, J. Adams, and H. J. W. Thomas, "Prevention of colorectal cancer by colonoscopic surveillance in individuals with a family history of colorectal cancer: 16 year, prospective, follow-up study," *British Medical Journal*, vol. 331, no. 7524, pp. 1047–1049, 2005.

[6] D. Saraste, A. Martling, P. J. Nilsson et al., "Complications after colonoscopy and surgery in a population-based colorectal cancer screening programme," *Journal of Medical Screening*, vol. 23, no. 3, pp. 135–140, 2016.

[7] J. C. Van Rijn, J. B. Reitsma, J. Stoker, P. M. Bossuyt, S. J. Van Deventer, and E. Dekker, "Polyp miss rate determined by tandem colonoscopy: a systematic review," *American Journal of Gastroenterology*, vol. 101, no. 2, pp. 343–350, 2006.

[8] N. N. Baxter, M. A. Goldwasser, L. F. Paszat, R. Saskin, D. R. Urbach, and L. Rabeneck, "Association of colonoscopy and death from colorectal cancer," *Annals of Internal Medicine*, vol. 150, no. 1, pp. 1–8, 2009.

[9] H. Brenner, M. Hoffmeister, V. Arndt, C. Stegmaier, L. Altenhofen, and U. Haug, "Protection from right-and left-sided colorectal neoplasms after colonoscopy: Population-Based Study," *Journal of the National Cancer Institute*, vol. 102, no. 2, pp. 89–95, 2010.

[10] R. Eliakim, Z. Fireman, I. M. Gralnek et al., "Evaluation of the PillCam Colon capsule in the detection of colonic pathology: results of the first multicenter, prospective, comparative study," *Endoscopy*, vol. 38, no. 10, pp. 963–970, 2006.

[11] J. A. Leighton and D. K. Rex, "A grading scale to evaluate colon cleansing for the PillCam COLON capsule: a reliability study," *Endoscopy*, vol. 43, no. 2, pp. 123–127, 2011.

[12] A. Van Gossum, M. M. Navas, I. Fernandez-Urien et al., "Capsule endoscopy versus colonoscopy for the detection of polyps and cancer," *New England Journal of Medicine*, vol. 361, no. 3, pp. 264–270, 2009.

[13] A. Sieg, K. Friedrich, and U. Sieg, "Is PillCam COLON capsule endoscopy ready for colorectal cancer screening? A prospective feasibility study in a community gastroenterology practice," *American Journal of Gastroenterology*, vol. 104, no. 4, pp. 848–854, 2009.

[14] C. Spada, M. E. Riccioni, C. Hassan, L. Petruzziello, P. Cesaro, and G. Costamagna, "Pillcam colon capsule endoscopy: a prospective, randomized trial comparing two regimens of preparation," *Journal of Clinical Gastroenterology*, vol. 45, no. 2, pp. 119–124, 2011.

[15] J. B. Pilz, S. Portmann, S. Peter, C. Beglinger, and L. Degen, "Colon capsule endoscopy compared to conventional colonoscopy under routine screening conditions," *BMC Gastroenterology*, vol. 10, article 66, 2010.

[16] G. Gay, M. Delvaux, M. Frederic, and I. Fassler, "Could the colonic capsule pillcam colon be clinically useful for selecting patients who deserve a complete colonoscopy? results of clinical comparison with colonoscopy in the perspective of colorectal cancer screening," *American Journal of Gastroenterology*, vol. 105, no. 5, pp. 1076–1086, 2010.

[17] S. Sacher-Huvelin, E. Coron, M. Gaudric et al., "Colon capsule endoscopy vs. colonoscopy in patients at average or increased risk of colorectal cancer," *Alimentary Pharmacology and Therapeutics*, vol. 32, no. 9, pp. 1145–1153, 2010.

[18] Z. Adrián-de-Ganzo, O. Alarcón-Fernández, L. Ramos et al., "Uptake of colon capsule endoscopy vs colonoscopy for screening relatives of patients with colorectal cancer," *Clinical Gastroenterology and Hepatology*, vol. 13, no. 13, pp. 2293.e1–2301.e1, 2015.

[19] E. J. Lai, A. H. Calderwood, G. Doros, O. K. Fix, and B. C. Jacobson, "The Boston bowel preparation scale: a valid and reliable instrument for colonoscopy-oriented research," *Gastrointestinal Endoscopy*, vol. 69, no. 3, pp. 620–625, 2009.

[20] C. Spada, C. Hassan, R. Marmo et al., "Meta-analysis shows colon capsule endoscopy is effective in detecting colorectal polyps," *Clinical Gastroenterology and Hepatology*, vol. 8, no. 6, pp. 516.e8–522.e8, 2010.

[21] R. Eliakim, K. Yassin, Y. Niv et al., "Prospective multicenter performance evaluation of the second-generation colon capsule compared with colonoscopy," *Endoscopy*, vol. 41, no. 12, pp. 1026–1031, 2009.

[22] T. Rokkas, K. Papaxoinis, K. Triantafyllou, and S. D. Ladas, "A meta-analysis evaluating the accuracy of colon capsule endoscopy in detecting colon polyps," *Gastrointestinal Endoscopy*, vol. 71, no. 4, pp. 792–798, 2010.

[23] D. K. Rex, S. N. Adler, J. Aisenberg et al., "Accuracy of capsule colonoscopy in detecting colorectal polyps in a screening population," *Gastroenterology*, vol. 148, no. 5, pp. 948–957.e2, 2015.

[24] C. Hassan, A. Zullo, S. Winn, and S. Morini, "Cost-effectiveness of capsule endoscopy in screening for colorectal cancer," *Endoscopy*, vol. 40, no. 5, pp. 414–421, 2008.

[25] D. Hartmann, M. Keuchel, M. Philipper et al., "A pilot study evaluating a new low-volume colon cleansing procedure for capsule colonoscopy," *Endoscopy*, vol. 44, no. 5, pp. 482–486, 2012.

[26] C. Spada, C. Hassan, B. Barbaro et al., "Colon capsule versus CT colonography in patients with incomplete colonoscopy: a prospective, comparative trial," *Gut*, vol. 64, no. 2, pp. 272–281, 2015.

A Review of the Role of Neurotensin and Its Receptors in Colorectal Cancer

Shengyang Qiu,[1] Gianluca Pellino,[2] Francesca Fiorentino,[1] Shahnawaz Rasheed,[2] Ara Darzi,[2] Paris Tekkis,[1,2] and Christos Kontovounisios[1,2]

[1]*Department of Surgery and Cancer, Imperial College London, Chelsea & Westminster Hospital Campus, London, UK*
[2]*Department of Colorectal Surgery, The Royal Marsden Hospital, Chelsea, London, UK*

Correspondence should be addressed to Christos Kontovounisios; c.kontovounisios@imperial.ac.uk

Academic Editor: Wenhao Weng

Neurotensin (NTS) is a physiologically occurring hormone which affects the function of the gastrointestinal (GI) tract. In recent years, NTS, acting through its cellular receptors (NTSR), has been implicated in the carcinogenesis of several cancers. In colorectal cancer (CRC), a significant body of evidence, from in vitro and in vivo studies, is available which elucidates the molecular biology of NTS/NTSR signalling and the resultant growth of CRC cells. There is growing clinical data from human studies which corroborate the role NTS/NTSR plays in the development of human CRC. Furthermore, blockade and modulation of the NTS/NTSR signalling pathways appears to reduce CRC growth in cell cultures and animal studies. Lastly, NTS/NTSR also shows potential of being utilised as a diagnostic biomarker for cancers as well as targets for functional imaging. We summarise the existing evidence and understanding of the role of NTS and its receptors in CRC.

1. Introduction

The hormone dependence of certain human cancers (e.g., breast and prostate cancers) is well described. As a result, hormonal modulation has become a cornerstone of therapy in these conditions. There is increasing recognition that cancers of the gastrointestinal (GI) tract, pancreas, and other organs express receptors for various endogenous host hormones. This raises the possibility of hormones' role in the proliferation of these cancers and therefore highlights the potential of these hormonal signalling pathways as targets for novel cancer diagnostic and therapeutic strategies. One of these promising candidates in GI cancers such as colorectal cancers (CRC) is the tridecapeptide neurotensin (NTS) [1–3].

NTS was first isolated in 1973 from the bovine hypothalamus and the digestive tract [4]. Its pharmacological and biochemical properties suggested its physiological functions are those of a neurotransmitter in the central nervous system (CNS) and a hormone peripherally. Centrally, it affects sensory and motor functions, temperature regulation, neuroendocrine control of the pituitary, and control of blood flow and blood pressure. In the gut, it is released by endocrine N cells in the jejunum and released after a meal, particularly those containing high lipid levels [5]. It has a range of paracrine and endocrine functions modulating vascular smooth muscle activity, gastrointestinal motility, and pancreaticobiliary secretions [6, 7]. Its action in the periphery is mediated by a G-protein-coupled receptor, neurotensin receptor 1 (NTSR1), whilst a second subtype, neurotensin receptor 2 (NTSR2), has mainly been identified in the central nervous system [8]. The third NTS receptor, NTSR3, is identical to sortilin, a 100 kDa protein with a single transmembrane domain [9]. Whilst NTSR1 and NTSR3 are found in a series of human cancer cell lines, the role of NTSR2 is much less studied in CRC [10].

NTS and its receptors have been implicated in the progression of a broad range of human cancers. These include cancers of the breast, prostate, lung, liver, and pancreas amongst others [11–15]. For example, Dupouy et al. reported that the upregulation of NTSR1 is associated with increased tumour size, number of metastatic lymph nodes, and Scarff-Bloom-Richardson grade of invasive ductal cell

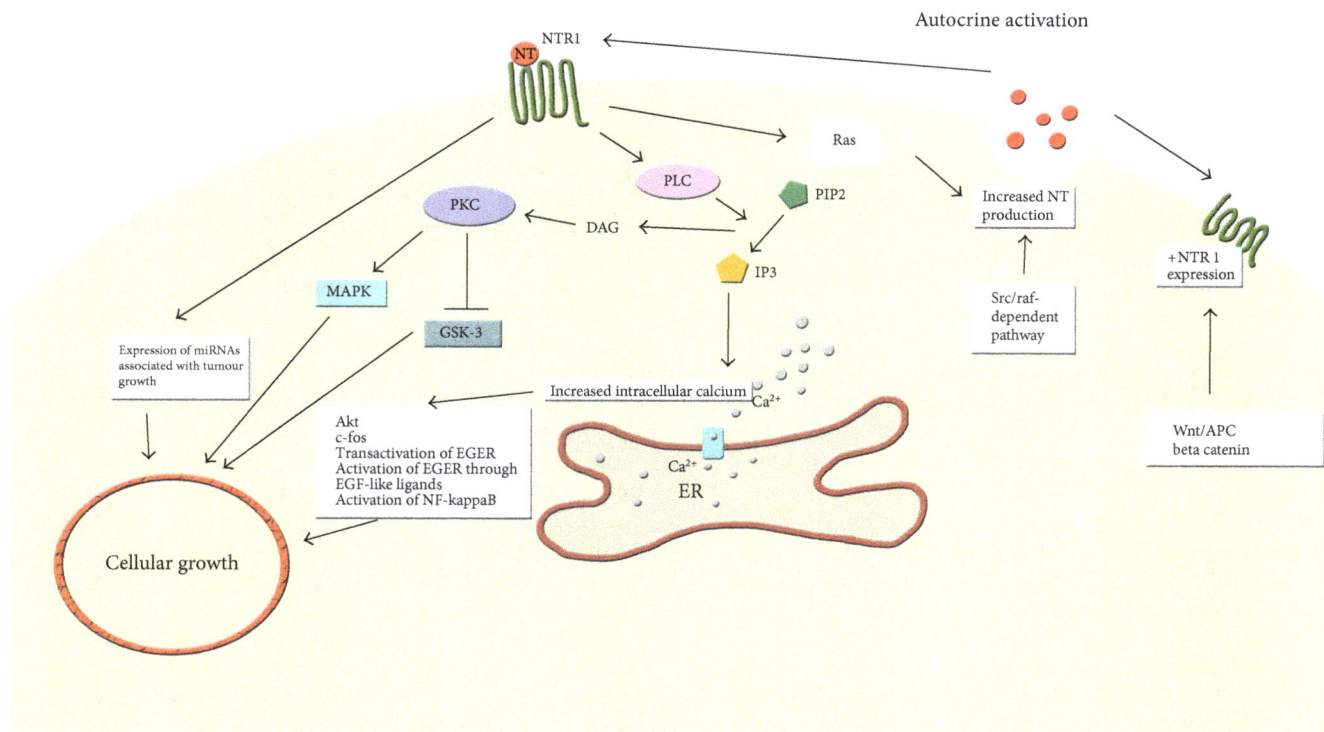

FIGURE 1: Neurotensin signalling in colorectal cancer cells. NTS: neurotensin, NTSR1: neurotensin receptor 1, PLC: protein lipase C, PKC: protein kinase C, MAPK: mitogen-activated protein kinase, GSK-3: glycogen synthase kinase-3, DAG: diacylglycerol, PIP2: phosphatidylinositol 4,5-bisphosphate, IP3: inositol trisphosphate, ER: endoplasmic reticulum, EGFR: epidermal growth factor receptor, APC: adenomatous polyposis coli.

carcinomas of the breast [11]. Expression of NTSR1 was also increased in gastrointestinal stromal tumours [16]. The mechanism of action responsible for these effects is increasingly well understood, and NTS signalling has been shown to interact with multiple important oncogenic pathways [17]. Concurrently, there is increasing evidence of the roles NTS play in CRC.

This review consolidates the current evidence for the role NTS and its receptors play in the oncogenesis of CRC and identifies areas of translational research required to allow NTS to be used in the diagnosis and treatment of this prevalent cancer.

2. Material and Method

A search of the original published work was done by use of PUBMED, MEDLINE, and EMBASE databases. The following search terms used were "colorectal neoplasms" [MeSH Terms] OR colorectal cancer [Text Word] and ("neurotensin" or "neurotensin receptor"). Lists of references were obtained, and potentially relevant papers were retrieved. Reference lists in every paper were scrutinised to identify other possible relevant studies. All studies relevant to CRC were included.

3. Results

3.1. Neurotensin Signalling Pathways in Colorectal Cancer Cells. Whilst prohormone convertase 1 has been implicated

in the activation of NTS from its precursors in the GI tract, NTS appears to be derived from its precursor proneurotensin/neuromedian N via prohormone convertase 5 in CRC cell lines [18, 19]. Some colonic tumours synthesise and release NTS, resulting in autocrine control and cellular proliferation [20]. In cell cultures, physiological levels of NTS appear to stimulate the growth of many human colon cancer cell lines (SW480, SW620, HT29, HCT116, and Cl.19A) expressing NTSR1 [21]. The signalling pathways identified in NTSR1 are summarised in Figure 1.

Although NTSR1 was not normally detectable on human colonic epithelial cells, it appeared to be expressed as ectopic receptors in human colon cancer cells. Concurrently, neurotensin receptor-binding proteins and mRNA were undetectable on normal epithelial cells of the human colon. NTS receptors were found in 40% of human colon cancer cell lines in culture [22]. Moreover, NTSR1 expression on colon cancer cells appears to be upregulated by the Wnt/APC (adenomatous polyposis coli) signalling pathway, a well-known carcinogenesis pathway in CRC [23]. This may result in CRC cells which not only produce NTS, but also have increased sensitivity to its oncogenic effects, and contribute to their escape from the normal cell cycle.

In inflammatory bowel disease- (IBD-) related colon cancers, NTSR1 appears to be a β-catenin inducible gene. Precancerous and cancerous colonic lesions coexpressed NTSR1 and β-catenin, in the absence of NTS. Therefore, NTSR1 overexpression, during IBD-related oncogenesis at least, may be associated with an activation of the APC/ β-catenin pathway [24].

With regard to downstream signalling, NTS was found to have little effect on cyclic nucleotide (cAMP and cGMP) levels in HT29 colonic cancer cell lines but strongly stimulates phosphatidylinositol turnover [25]. In one study, NTS stimulated inositol trisphosphate-mediated calcium mobilisation but not protein kinase C (PKC) activation in HT29 cells [26]. NTS receptors in HT29 cells appear to be coupled to phospholipase C (PLC). Activation of PLC leads to an increase in inositol phosphate levels, and this in turn resulted in Ca^{2+} release [26]. Calcium signalling is a key regulator of processes important in differentiation in CRC. Chowdhury et al. found that differentiation of HT29 colon cancer cells is associated with a remodelling of NTS-mediated Ca^{2+} signalling, a key stage in CRC cell transformation [27]. Confirmatory studies demonstrated that addition of NTS to human colon cancer cell lines resulted in calcium mobilisation as well as activation of the mitogen-activated extracellular signal-regulated kinase (MAPK/ERK) pathway and induction of c-fos expression [28–30].

NTS also has been shown to induce the phosphorylation of glycogen synthase kinase- (GSK-) 3 in HCT116 human colon cancer cell line via protein kinase C (PKC) [31]. GSK-3 is a regulator of a diverse range of cellular processes including cell growth. In HT29 cells, NTS induced DNA synthesis through phosphorylation of ERK and Akt via transactivation of epidermal growth factor receptors (EGFR). Similarly, in the HCT116 cell line, both PKC and EGFR pathways are implicated. In other cancers, NTS induces the autocrine activation of EGFR mediated through EGF "like" ligands [32]. However, Massa et al. found that, in HT29 and HCT116 cell lines, NTS-stimulated MAP kinase phosphorylation did not appear to involve EGFR and blocking EGFR alone may not be able to inhibit NTS-induced cancer proliferation in these cell lines [33]. These mechanisms of activation and transactivation need to be investigated further in CRC.

Further downstream, NTS was found to stimulate differential expression of 38 microRNAs, including miR-21 and miR-155, which have been associated with tumour growth and include nuclear factor kappa-light-chain-enhancer of activated B cells- (NF-κB-) binding sites. NTS expression increased colony formation by HCT116 cells [34]. The NF-κB pathways have also been implicated in NTS-induced inflammation and mitogenesis in colonocytes [35].

In addition to the activation of potentially oncogenic pathways in CRC cells, NTS production is increased within some CRC cells, resulting in autocrine control of cellular growth and proliferation. NTS promoter activity is increased by Src in Caco-2 human colon cancer cells, partly through a proximal AP-1/CRE promoter element. Additionally, Src regulation of the NTS promoter appears to be mediated through a Raf-dependent pathway [36]. Moreover, Ras, downstream of the NTSR1 signalling cascade, also targets the NTS promoter region resulting in increased NTS release [37, 38].

Clearly, the effects of NTS/NTSR1 signalling involve multiple signalling pathways and are cell line-dependent. Although many intermediary steps need to be clarified, the common end-effect of these pathways is colon cancer cell growth and proliferation [39].

Whereas the mitogenic effects of NTS were mediated through NTSR1, the role of the third NTS receptor, NTSR3, is less clearly defined. NTSR3 is not a G-protein-coupled receptor but appears to be a sortilin receptor. They were found not only predominantly in endoplasmic reticulum-Golgi compartments but also in the cell membrane of colonic cancer cells [40]. NTSR1 and NTSR3 exist as a heterodimer on the cell surface of HT29 human colon cancer cells. Upon stimulation with NTS, the receptor complex is internalised. This heterodimeric assembly appeared to modify the intracellular response to NTS [41]. Indeed, two forms of NTSR3 have been found on the HT29 cell line, a high molecular weight, membrane-associated form responsible for NTS endocytosis from the cell surface, and a lower molecular weight, intracellular form responsible for the sorting of internalised NTS to the trans-Golgi network, to its onward destinations, for example, the cell nuclei to carry out its mitogenic effects [42].

3.2. The Presence of Neurotensin in Colorectal Cancers In Vivo. Ulich et al. first described large numbers of neuroendocrine cells within well-differentiated colonic adenocarcinoma [43]. NTS mRNA, peptide, and receptor were found in resected human colon cancer specimens as well as in 4 well-known human colon cancer cell lines in vitro. In surgical specimens where NTS was identified in cancer cells, none was identified in adjacent normal bowel mucosa [20]. This suggested that the CRC cells had developed the propensity for NTS expression. The role of NTS in CRC was further highlighted by its detection in 13 human colon cancer cell lines and confirmation of its presence in numerous other colorectal cancer tissue specimens [18]. At the same time, NTSR expression in stromal versus epithelial cells was 35% and 12%, respectively, in CRC [44]. In a study of 30 patients with inflammatory bowel disease-related large bowel adenocarcinomas, dysplasias, and inflammation, the percentage of NTSR1-positive epithelial cells progressively increased from the inflammatory condition to adenocarcinoma and was significantly higher in adenocarcinomas than in inflammation [24]. Based on this evidence, it is possible that although NTS and NTSR may not play an active role in every case of colorectal cancer, it appears to play an important role in the growth of the cancer in which they are present. This theory is further supported by the work of Gui et al. who measured NTSR1 mRNA expression in normal colonic mucosa, adenomas, and colonic adenocarcinoma tissue specimens. Whilst NTSR1 mRNA expression was undetectable in differentiated epithelial cells of normal colonic epithelium, it was expressed at a moderate level in adenomas and adenocarcinomas. Higher level of expression was seen in adenocarcinomas' infiltrating margins. Tissue from lymphovascular invasion showed even higher intensity of expression of NTSR1 than the rest of the tumour. This further supports that increased NTSR1 expression may be an early event during colonic tumourigenesis and also contributes to tumour progression and aggressive behaviour in colonic adenocarcinomas [45].

Exogenous NTS causes significant proliferation of normal small bowel mucosa. In the colon, high doses and duration of NTS exposure (300 milligrams kg^{-1} administered three times daily for 10 days) stimulate the proliferation of colonic mucosa in rat models. Whereas there was an increase in cell volume in adult rats, the cell number was drastically increased in younger subjects [20]. NTS, at high doses, appeared to be able to stimulate cellular division and growth. NTS was found to accelerate colonic cancer carcinogenesis in animals. Rats injected with a colonic cancer carcinogen azoxymethane and NTS (200 micrograms kg^{-1} every other day for 40 weeks) significantly increased the number, size, and invasiveness of colon tumours [46]. Administration of NTS alone (300 and 600 micrograms kg^{-1}) significantly stimulated growth in both murine colon tumours as well as human colon cancers xenografted into mice. Administration of NTS also resulted in significantly decreased survival of mice with CRC compared with the control group given saline injections [47]. A study compared sporadic and inflammation-induced colon cancers in which mice were exposed to either the carcinogens azoxymethane or azoxymethane with dextran sulfate sodium. NTSR1 stimulation appeared to significantly increase the development of sporadic cancers although not inflammatory cancers. Cancer rates were also significantly reduced in NTSR1-deficient mice compared to wild-type mice [48].

Growth of colon cancer cell lines xenografted into athymic mice was stimulated by NTS whilst the NTS receptor antagonist SR 48692 inhibited tumour growth [21]. Similarly, intraperitoneal administration of NTS increased the growth rate of HCT116 xenograft tumours in mice. Blocking miR-21 and/or miR-155 appeared to slow tumour growth [34]. Therefore, NTS/NTSR1 may be a potential target for preventive or therapeutic strategies in colon cancer. Kamimae et al. found that epigenetic silencing of NTSR1 was associated with reduction of invasive growth of colorectal tumours. They found that whereas noninvasive colorectal tumours tended to express high levels of hypermethylated NTSR1, invasive CRC tended to have unmethylated NTSR1. It is possible that methylation of specific CpG islands of the NTSR1 gene may result in gene silencing in CRC cells. The authors validated these findings against data sets from The Cancer Genome Atlas and observed an inverse relationship between the methylation levels on multiple probe sets of an Infinium BeadChip and levels of NTSR1 expression in CRC tissue [49]. However, the impact of methylation on any gene is dependent on the CpG islands studied. Therefore, more evidence is required to substantiate the expression or suppression of NTSR1 and NTS by methylation before it can be used as a reliable clinical prognostic marker.

The human tissue studies as well as the animal models above demonstrated, in observational studies at least, that NTS plays a role in carcinogenesis in some CRC subtypes. When it is involved, it played a significant role in the growth and aggressiveness of the cancer, affecting the survival outcome of subjects. Moreover, blockade of NTSR signalling attenuated CRC growth. This evidence raises the possibility for NTS and NTSR to be used as prognostic indicators in CRC, similar to the established use of oestrogen (ER) and Herceptin (HER) receptors in breast cancers. Like ER and HER receptors, this evidence also raises the tantalising possibility for NTSR to be a target for cancer therapy.

3.3. Clinical Applications of Neurotensin in Colorectal Cancer. Several groups have explored the potential use of the NTS pathway as target for functional imaging for the detection of cancers [50–53]. Furthermore, a fluorescence-based yeast biosensor has been developed that can monitor the activation of human NTSR1 by its agonist [54].

In a study evaluating blood NTS levels in colorectal cancer using 56 colorectal cancer patients and 15 controls, blood NTS and IL-8 levels differed between healthy and colorectal cancer patients. NTS values appeared to differentiate the control group from the cancer group. The value of plasma NTS $\geq$ 54.47 pg/ml at enrollment demonstrated a sensitivity of 77% and specificity of 90%, in predicting colorectal cancer confirmed by colonoscopy. This raises the possibility of using NTS as a diagnostic biomarker for colorectal cancer. Larger prospective studies are awaited [55].

3.4. Role of Neurotensin in Colorectal Cancer Treatment. Treatments which target the NTS/NTSR signalling pathway have been tested in cell culture and animal models. Sodium butyrate (NaBT), a potent histone deacetylase inhibitor (HDACi), dramatically decreased endogenous NTSR1 mRNA, protein, and NTSR1 promoter activity. HDACis are known to induce growth arrest, differentiation, and apoptosis of CRC cells. Therefore, the inhibitory effects of HDACi on CRC cells may in part be due to the suppression of the NTS/NTSR signalling pathway [56].

More directly, Iwase et al. found that NTS receptor antagonist SR48692 abolished the stimulatory effect of exogenous NTS administration on tumour growth in mice xenografted with human colon cancers. Interestingly, this is despite the lack of expression of NTSR in either tumour cells or xenografted tumours. They hypothesised that the trophic effect of NTS may be an indirect one [57].

Levy et al. treated both cultured human colon cancer cell line and mice colon cancers with combination of NTS and vasoactive intestinal peptide antagonists. The antagonist effectively inhibited cell growth in culture at nanomolar concentrations. Furthermore, colonic cancers harvested from mice treated with the antagonist showed reduced tumour volume, staging, lymphocyte infiltrate, and number of dysplastic crypts [58].

Other isolated studies have reported on the effect of dietary supplements and antioxidants on the effect of NTS on CRC cells. The natural dietary product, curcumin, appeared to inhibit NTS-mediated IL-8 protein secretion and colon cancer cell migration in culture [59]. Briviba et al. show that NTS and epidermal growth factor (EGF) caused a strong rise in the intracellular Ca^{2+} concentration, induced phosphorylation of ERK1 and ERK2, and stimulated growth of human carcinoma cells. The dietary antioxidant cyanidin found in fruits and vegetables appeared to inhibit the NTS- and EGF-induced cancer cell metabolism [29].

Another area of investigation is the use of NTSR1 over-expression in cancer cells as the target to deliver therapeutic molecules. This approach is made possible by NTSR1 endocytosis which resulted in delivery of molecules of interest inside the targeted cell. An example trialed in CRC cells was the targeted delivery of liposomes filled with doxorubicin and functionalised on the external surface with a branched moiety containing four copies of the 8–13 neurotensin (8–13 NTS) peptide. It dramatically increased the cytotoxic effects of this nanotherapeutic agent on HT29 cell lines [60]. Hernandez et al. and Hernandez-Chan et al. developed a NTS-based polyplex gene nanocarrier which has the potential nanomedicine-based application in the treatment of cancers which express NTSRs as well as diseases of the CNS-like Parkinson's disease [61, 62]. The prospect of NTS-based nanomedicine is an exciting one and awaits validation and translation into the clinical setting.

4. Discussion

Similar to other cancers, there is a convincing, albeit predominantly experimental, body of evidence to implicate NTS and its receptors in the carcinogenesis of human CRC. Human research on this subject remains sparse and lacking in strength. To date, only retrospective series have been reported in colorectal cancers. Prospective studies have been carried on in other cancers, for example, glioma, which demonstrated that increased NTS and NTSR1 expression is associated with significantly decreased 3-year survival [63]. The potential for NTS/NTSR pathway as novel targets for cancer therapies has been advocated in CRC as well as other cancers such as non-small-cell lung cancers [64]. NTS as a diagnostic and therapeutic target is being explored in numerous other cancers, for example, cancers in the pancreas, prostate, and breast [65]. In breast cancer, NTSR1-induced activation of EGFR and HER2 receptors rendered these cancers aggressive, yet highly responsive to lapatinib and metformin in mice [66]. However, translational studies into clinical settings are awaited in all of these cancers.

NTS and NTSR expression appear to be related to increased aggressiveness and invasiveness of colon cancers highlighting its potential role as a prognostic marker in CRC. Furthermore, NTS and NTSR can be easily quantified in resection specimens as a part of routine histopathological diagnosis. The NTS/NTSR status of a cancer, much like Herceptin and oestrogen receptor status in breast carcinoma, could be used to stratify patients for adjuvant chemotherapy agents. However, there has only been small retrospective case series reported thus far. The validity of NTS/NTSR as a prognostic factor requires improved understanding of the prevalence of human CRC which expresses them at a genetic and protein level. Cancer genetic databases may hold the answer. Prospective cohort studies are required to establish the effect of NTS or NTSR expression on disease aggressiveness, recurrence, and survival.

Functional imaging targeting NTS/NTSR is in the experimental stages but is fast approaching clinical validation. Targeting of cancer cells which express NTSR1 ectopically is a useful strategy for both detection and therapy of NTSR1 expressing cancers. The rapidly expanding fields of nanotherapeutics and immune therapeutics may be able to take advantage of NTS and NTSR to advance the treatment of CRC and other cancers. The technological aspects await validation in the clinical setting.

Antagonists of NTSRs, much like tamoxifen in breast cancer, may be a hitherto unexplored endocrine modulatory chemotherapy in patients with CRC expressing NTS/NTSR. The efficacy and safety of these antagonists require future clinical studies to assess both its safety and efficacy before it can be used in the treatment of cancers.

The road to developing a new cancer drug is long and arduous. For example, in the case of breast cancer, the role oestrogen played was described as early as 1896. George Beatson found that the lives of breast cancer patients were extended by bilateral oophorectomies. It took eight decades of work for tamoxifen, the oestrogen receptor antagonist, to be used in the treatment of breast cancer. Even more recently, almost 20 years separated the discovery of the HER2 receptor and the licensing of Herceptin (trastuzumab). It is clear that significant future work and investment is required if NTS pathways are to be exploited for the benefit of patients with cancer. The increasing body of evidence should propel ongoing research and be built upon by robust prospective studies to achieve this goal.

Competing Interests

The authors state there are no existing or potential conflicts of interest.

References

[1] B. M. Evers and C. M. Townsend Jr., "Growth factors, hormones and receptors in GI cancers," in *Molecular Mechanisms in Gastrointestinal Cancer*, pp. 1–196, R.G. Landes Company, 1999.

[2] L. E. Heasley, "Autocrine and paracrine signaling through neuropeptide receptors in human cancer," *Oncogene*, vol. 20, no. 13, pp. 1563–1569, 2001.

[3] R. P. Thomas, M. R. Hellmich, C. M. Townsend Jr., and B. M. Evers, "Role of gastrointestinal hormones in the proliferation of normal and neoplastic tissues," *Endocrine Reviews*, vol. 24, no. 5, pp. 571–599, 2003.

[4] R. Carraway and S. E. Leeman, "The isolation of a new hypotensive peptide, neurotensin, from bovine hypothalami," *The Journal of Biological Chemistry*, vol. 248, no. 19, pp. 6854–6861, 1973.

[5] C. F. Ferris, R. E. Carraway, R. A. Hammer, and S. E. Leeman, "Release and degradation of neurotensin during perfusion of rat small intestine with lipid," *Regulatory Peptides*, vol. 12, no. 2, pp. 101–111, 1985.

[6] C. F. Ferris, "Neurotensin," in *Comprehensive Physiology*, pp. 559–586, Wiley & Sons, Inc., 2011.

[7] D. Zhao and C. Pothoulakis, "Effects of NT on gastrointestinal motility and secretion, and role in intestinal inflammation," *Peptides*, vol. 27, no. 10, pp. 2434–2444, 2006.

[8] P. Chalon, N. Vita, M. Kaghad et al., "Molecular cloning of a levocabastine-sensitive neurotensin binding site," *FEBS Letters*, vol. 386, no. 2–3, pp. 91–94, 1996.

[9] J. Mazella, N. Zsurger, V. Navarro et al., "The 100-kDa neurotensin receptor is gp95/sortilin, a non-G-protein-coupled receptor," *The Journal of Biological Chemistry*, vol. 273, no. 41, pp. 26273–26276, 1998.

[10] C. Dal Farra, P. Sarret, V. Navarro, J. M. Botto, J. Mazella, and J. P. Vincent, "Involvement of the neurotensin receptor subtype NTSR3 in the growth effect of neurotensin on cancer cell lines," *International Journal of Cancer*, vol. 92, no. 4, pp. 503–509, 2001.

[11] S. Dupouy, V. Viardot-Foucault, M. Alifano et al., "The neurotensin receptor-1 pathway contributes to human ductal breast cancer progression," *PLoS One*, vol. 4, no. 1, article e4223, 2009.

[12] F. Souaze, S. Dupouy, V. Viardot-Foucault et al., "Expression of neurotensin and NT1 receptor in human breast cancer: a potential role in tumor progression," *Cancer Research*, vol. 66, no. 12, pp. 6243–6249, 2006.

[13] M. Alifano, F. Souaze, S. Dupouy et al., "Neurotensin receptor 1 determines the outcome of non-small cell lung cancer," *Clinical Cancer Research*, vol. 16, no. 17, pp. 4401–4410, 2010.

[14] J. G. Wang, N. N. Li, H. N. Li, L. Cui, and P. Wang, "Pancreatic cancer bears overexpression of neurotensin and neurotensin receptor subtype-1 and SR 48692 counteracts neurotensin induced cell proliferation in human pancreatic ductal carcinoma cell line PANC-1," *Neuropeptides*, vol. 45, no. 2, pp. 151–156, 2011.

[15] A. E. Allen, D. N. Carney, and T. W. Moody, "Neurotensin binds with high affinity to small cell lung cancer cells," *Peptides*, vol. 9, Supplement 1, pp. 57–61, 1988.

[16] P. Gromova, B. P. Rubin, A. Thys, C. Erneux, and J. M. Vanderwinden, "Neurotensin receptor 1 is expressed in gastrointestinal stromal tumors but not in interstitial cells of Cajal," *PLoS One*, vol. 6, no. 2, article e14710, 2011.

[17] R. M. Myers, J. W. Shearman, M. O. Kitching, A. Ramos-Montoya, D. E. Neal, and S. V. Ley, "Cancer, chemistry, and the cell: molecules that interact with the neurotensin receptors," *ACS Chemical Biology*, vol. 4, no. 7, pp. 503–525, 2009.

[18] C. Rovere, P. Barbero, J. J. Maoret, M. Laburthe, and P. Kitabgi, "Pro-neurotensin/neuromedin N expression and processing in human colon cancer cell lines," *Biochemical and Biophysical Research Communications*, vol. 246, no. 1, pp. 155–159, 1998.

[19] C. Rovere, P. Barbero, and P. Kitabgi, "Evidence that PC2 is the endogenous pro-neurotensin convertase in rMTC 6-23 cells and that PC1- and PC2-transfected PC12 cells differentially process pro-neurotensin," *The Journal of Biological Chemistry*, vol. 271, no. 19, pp. 11368–11375, 1996.

[20] B. M. Evers, J. Ishizuka, D. H. Chung, C. M. Townsend Jr., and J. C. Thompson, "Neurotensin expression and release in human colon cancers," *Annals of Surgery*, vol. 216, no. 4, pp. 421–430, 1992.

[21] J. J. Maoret, Y. Anini, C. Rouyer-Fessard, D. Gully, and M. Laburthe, "Neurotensin and a non-peptide neurotensin receptor antagonist control human colon cancer cell growth in cell culture and in cells xenografted into nude mice," *International Journal of Cancer*, vol. 80, no. 3, pp. 448–454, 1999.

[22] J. J. Maoret, D. Pospai, C. Rouyer-Fessard et al., "Neurotensin receptor and its mRNA are expressed in many human colon cancer cell lines but not in normal colonic epithelium: binding studies and RT-PCR experiments," *Biochemical and Biophysical Research Communications*, vol. 203, no. 1, pp. 465–471, 1994.

[23] F. Souaze, V. Viardot-Foucault, N. Roullet et al., "Neurotensin receptor 1 gene activation by the Tcf/beta-catenin pathway is an early event in human colonic adenomas," *Carcinogenesis*, vol. 27, no. 4, pp. 708–716, 2006.

[24] C. Bossard, F. Souaze, A. Jarry et al., "Over-expression of neurotensin high-affinity receptor 1 (NTS1) in relation with its ligand neurotensin (NT) and nuclear beta-catenin in inflammatory bowel disease-related oncogenesis," *Peptides*, vol. 28, no. 10, pp. 2030–2035, 2007.

[25] S. Amar, P. Kitabgi, and J. P. Vincent, "Activation of phosphatidylinositol turnover by neurotensin receptors in the human colonic adenocarcinoma cell line HT29," *FEBS Letters*, vol. 201, no. 1, pp. 31–36, 1986.

[26] J. C. Bozou, N. Rochet, I. Magnaldo, J. P. Vincent, and P. Kitabgi, "Neurotensin stimulates inositol trisphosphate-mediated calcium mobilization but not protein kinase C activation in HT29 cells. Involvement of a G-protein," *The Biochemical Journal*, vol. 264, no. 3, pp. 871–878, 1989.

[27] M. A. Chowdhury, A. A. Peters, S. J. Roberts-Thomson, and G. R. Monteith, "Effects of differentiation on purinergic and neurotensin-mediated calcium signaling in human HT-29 colon cancer cells," *Biochemical and Biophysical Research Communications*, vol. 439, no. 1, pp. 35–39, 2013.

[28] R. A. Ehlers 2nd, R. M. Bonnor, X. Wang, M. R. Hellmich, and B. M. Evers, "Signal transduction mechanisms in neurotensin-mediated cellular regulation," *Surgery*, vol. 124, no. 2, pp. 237–246, 1998.

[29] K. Briviba, S. L. Abrahamse, B. L. Pool-Zobel, and G. Rechkemmer, "Neurotensin-and EGF-induced metabolic activation of colon carcinoma cells is diminished by dietary flavonoid cyanidin but not by its glycosides," *Nutrition and Cancer*, vol. 41, no. 1–2, pp. 172–179, 2001.

[30] V. Navarro, S. Martin, and J. Mazella, "Internalization-dependent regulation of HT29 cell proliferation by neurotensin," *Peptides*, vol. 27, no. 10, pp. 2502–2507, 2006.

[31] Q. Wang, Y. Zhou, and B. M. Evers, "Neurotensin phosphorylates GSK-3alpha/beta through the activation of PKC in human colon cancer cells," *Neoplasia*, vol. 8, no. 9, pp. 781–787, 2006.

[32] M. Younes, Z. Wu, S. Dupouy et al., "Neurotensin (NTS) and its receptor (NTSR1) causes EGFR, HER2 and HER3 over-expression and their autocrine/paracrine activation in lung tumors, confirming responsiveness to erlotinib," *Oncotarget*, vol. 5, no. 18, pp. 8252–8269, 2014.

[33] F. Massa, A. Tormo, S. Beraud-Dufour, T. Coppola, and J. Mazella, "Neurotensin-induced Erk1/2 phosphorylation and growth of human colonic cancer cells are independent from growth factors receptors activation," *Biochemical and Biophysical Research Communications*, vol. 414, no. 1, pp. 118–122, 2011.

[34] K. Bakirtzi, M. Hatziapostolou, I. Karagiannides et al., "Neurotensin signaling activates microRNAs-21 and -155 and Akt, promotes tumor growth in mice, and is increased in human colon tumors," *Gastroenterology*, vol. 141, no. 5, pp. 1749–1761.e1, 2011.

[35] D. Zhao, S. Kuhnt-Moore, H. Zeng, J. S. Wu, M. P. Moyer, and C. Pothoulakis, "Neurotensin stimulates IL-8 expression in human colonic epithelial cells through rho GTPase-mediated NF-kappa B pathways," *American Journal of*

Physiology. Cell Physiology, vol. 284, no. 6, pp. C1397–C1404, 2003.

[36] N. A. Banker, M. R. Hellmich, H. J. Kim, C. M. Townsend Jr., and B. M. Evers, "Src-mediated activation of the human neurotensin/neuromedin N promoter," *Surgery*, vol. 122, no. 2, pp. 180–186, 1997.

[37] D. Zhao, Y. Zhan, H. W. Koon et al., "Metalloproteinase-dependent transforming growth factor-alpha release mediates neurotensin-stimulated MAP kinase activation in human colonic epithelial cells," *The Journal of Biological Chemistry*, vol. 279, no. 42, pp. 43547–43554, 2004.

[38] B. M. Evers, Z. Zhou, P. Celano, and J. Li, "The neurotensin gene is a downstream target for Ras activation," *The Journal of Clinical Investigation*, vol. 95, no. 6, pp. 2822–2830, 1995.

[39] K. M. Muller, I. H. Tveteraas, M. Aasrum et al., "Role of protein kinase C and epidermal growth factor receptor signalling in growth stimulation by neurotensin in colon carcinoma cells," *BMC Cancer*, vol. 11, no. 1, p. 421, 2011.

[40] C. Munck Petersen, M. S. Nielsen, C. Jacobsen et al., "Propeptide cleavage conditions sortilin/neurotensin receptor-3 for ligand binding," *The EMBO Journal*, vol. 18, no. 3, pp. 595–604, 1999.

[41] S. Martin, V. Navarro, J. P. Vincent, and J. Mazella, "Neurotensin receptor-1 and -3 complex modulates the cellular signaling of neurotensin in the HT29 cell line," *Gastroenterology*, vol. 123, no. 4, pp. 1135–1143, 2002.

[42] A. Morinville, S. Martin, M. Lavallee, J. P. Vincent, A. Beaudet, and J. Mazella, "Internalization and trafficking of neurotensin via NTS3 receptors in HT29 cells," *The International Journal of Biochemistry & Cell Biology*, vol. 36, no. 11, pp. 2153–2168, 2004.

[43] T. R. Ulich, L. Cheng, H. Glover, K. Yang, and K. J. Lewin, "A colonic adenocarcinoma with argentaffin cells. An immunoperoxidase study demonstrating the presence of numerous neuroendocrine products," *Cancer*, vol. 51, no. 8, pp. 1483–1489, 1983.

[44] C. Chao, M. L. Tallman, K. L. Ives, C. M. Townsend Jr., and M. R. Hellmich, "Gastrointestinal hormone receptors in primary human colorectal carcinomas," *The Journal of Surgical Research*, vol. 129, no. 2, pp. 313–321, 2005.

[45] X. Gui, G. Guzman, P. R. Dobner, and S. S. Kadkol, "Increased neurotensin receptor-1 expression during progression of colonic adenocarcinoma," *Peptides*, vol. 29, no. 9, pp. 1609–1615, 2008.

[46] M. Tasuta, H. Iishi, M. Baba, and H. Taniguchi, "Enhancement by neurotensin of experimental carcinogenesis induced in rat colon by azoxymethane," *British Journal of Cancer*, vol. 62, no. 3, pp. 368–371, 1990.

[47] K. Yoshinaga, B. M. Evers, M. Izukura et al., "Neurotensin stimulates growth of colon cancer," *Surgical Oncology*, vol. 1, no. 2, pp. 127–134, 1992.

[48] J. M. Bugni, L. A. Rabadi, K. Jubbal, I. Karagiannides, G. Lawson, and C. Pothoulakis, "The neurotensin receptor-1 promotes tumor development in a sporadic but not an inflammation-associated mouse model of colon cancer," *International Journal of Cancer*, vol. 130, no. 8, pp. 1798–1805, 2012.

[49] S. Kamimae, E. Yamamoto, M. Kai et al., "Epigenetic silencing of NTSR1 is associated with lateral and noninvasive growth of colorectal tumors," *Oncotarget*, vol. 6, no. 30, pp. 29975–29990, 2015.

[50] F. Alshoukr, C. Rosant, V. Maes et al., "Novel neurotensin analogues for radioisotope targeting to neurotensin receptor-positive tumors," *Bioconjugate Chemistry*, vol. 20, no. 8, pp. 1602–1610, 2009.

[51] P. J. Janssen, M. de Visser, S. M. Verwijnen et al., "Five stabilized 111In-labeled neurotensin analogs in nude mice bearing HT29 tumors," *Cancer Biotherapy & Radiopharmaceuticals*, vol. 22, no. 3, pp. 374–381, 2007.

[52] Z. Wu, L. Li, S. Liu et al., "Facile preparation of a thiol-reactive (18)F-labeling agent and synthesis of (18)F-DEG-VS-NT for PET imaging of a neurotensin receptor-positive tumor," *Journal of Nuclear Medicine*, vol. 55, no. 7, pp. 1178–1184, 2014.

[53] E. Garcia-Garayoa, P. Blauenstein, A. Blanc, V. Maes, D. Tourwe, and P. A. Schubiger, "A stable neurotensin-basedradiopharmaceutical for targeted imaging and therapy of neurotensin receptor-positive tumours," *European Journal of Nuclear Medicine and Molecular Imaging*, vol. 36, no. 1, pp. 37–47, 2009.

[54] J. Ishii, A. Oda, S. Togawa et al., "Microbial fluorescence sensing for human neurotensin receptor type 1 using Galpha-engineered yeast cells," *Analytical Biochemistry*, vol. 446, pp. 37–43, 2014.

[55] G. Sgourakis, A. Papapanagiotou, C. Kontovounisios et al., "The combined use of serum neurotensin and IL-8 as screening markers for colorectal cancer," *Tumour Biology*, vol. 35, no. 6, pp. 5993–6002, 2014.

[56] X. Wang, L. N. Jackson, S. M. Johnson, Q. Wang, and B. M. Evers, "Suppression of neurotensin receptor type 1 expression and function by histone deacetylase inhibitors in human colorectal cancers," *Molecular Cancer Therapeutics*, vol. 9, no. 8, pp. 2389–2398, 2010.

[57] K. Iwase, B. M. Evers, M. R. Hellmich et al., "Indirect inhibitory effect of a neurotensin receptor antagonist on human colon cancer (LoVo) growth," *Surgical Oncology*, vol. 5, no. 5–6, pp. 245–251, 1996.

[58] A. Levy, R. Gal, R. Granoth, Z. Dreznik, M. Fridkin, and I. Gozes, "In vitro and in vivo treatment of colon cancer by VIP antagonists," *Regulatory Peptides*, vol. 109, no. 1–3, pp. 127–133, 2002.

[59] X. Wang, Q. Wang, K. L. Ives, and B. M. Evers, "Curcumin inhibits neurotensin-mediated interleukin-8 production and migration of HCT116 human colon cancer cells," *Clinical Cancer Research*, vol. 12, no. 18, pp. 5346–5355, 2006.

[60] C. Falciani, A. Accardo, J. Brunetti et al., "Target-selective drug delivery through liposomes labeled with oligobranched neurotensin peptides," *ChemMedChem*, vol. 6, no. 4, pp. 678–685, 2011.

[61] M. E. Hernandez, J. D. Rembao, D. Hernandez-Baltazar et al., "Safety of the intravenous administration of neurotensin-polyplex nanoparticles in BALB/c mice," *Nanomedicine*, vol. 10, no. 4, pp. 745–754, 2014.

[62] N. G. Hernandez-Chan, M. J. Bannon, C. E. Orozco-Barrios et al., "Neurotensin-polyplex-mediated brain-derived neurotrophic factor gene delivery into nigral dopamine neurons prevents nigrostriatal degeneration in a rat model of early Parkinson's disease," *Journal of Biomedical Science*, vol. 22, no. 1, p. 59, 2015.

[63] Q. Ouyang, X. Gong, H. Xiao et al., "Neurotensin promotes the progression of malignant glioma through NTSR1 and impacts the prognosis of glioma patients," *Molecular Cancer*, vol. 14, no. 1, p. 21, 2015.

[64] K. Takahashi, C. Furukawa, A. Takano et al., "The neuromedin U-growth hormone secretagogue receptor 1b/neurotensin receptor 1 oncogenic signaling pathway as a therapeutic target for lung cancer," *Cancer Research*, vol. 66, no. 19, pp. 9408–9419, 2006.

[65] Z. Wu, D. Martinez-Fong, J. Tredaniel, and P. Forgez, "Neurotensin and its high affinity receptor 1 as a potential pharmacological target in cancer therapy," *Frontiers in Endocrinology*, vol. 3, p. 184, 2012.

[66] S. Dupouy, V. K. Doan, Z. Wu et al., "Activation of EGFR, HER2 and HER3 by neurotensin/neurotensin receptor 1 renders breast tumors aggressive yet highly responsive to lapatinib and metformin in mice," *Oncotarget*, vol. 5, no. 18, pp. 8235–8251, 2014.

3

Albumin Binding Function: The Potential Earliest Indicator for Liver Function Damage

Penglei Ge,[1] Huayu Yang,[1] Jingfen Lu,[2] Wenjun Liao,[1]
Shunda Du,[1] Yingli Xu,[2] Haifeng Xu,[1] Haitao Zhao,[1] Xin Lu,[1] Xinting Sang,[1]
Shouxian Zhong,[1] Jiefu Huang,[1] and Yilei Mao[1]

[1]*Department of Liver Surgery, Peking Union Medical College (PUMC) Hospital, Chinese Academy of Medical Sciences and PUMC, Beijing, China*
[2]*State Key Laboratory of Natural and Biomimetic Drugs, School of Pharmaceutical Sciences, Peking University, Beijing, China*

Correspondence should be addressed to Yilei Mao; pumch-liver@hotmail.com

Academic Editor: Amosy M'Koma

Background. Currently there is no indicator that can evaluate actual liver lesion for early stages of viral hepatitis, nonalcoholic fatty liver disease (NAFLD), and cirrhosis. Aim of this study was to investigate if albumin binding function could better reflect liver function in these liver diseases. *Methods.* An observational study was performed on 193 patients with early NAFLD, viral hepatitis, and cirrhosis. Cirrhosis patients were separated according to Child-Pugh score into A, B, and C subgroup. Albumin metal ion binding capacity (Ischemia-modified albumin transformed, IMAT) and fatty acid binding capacity (total binding sites, TBS) were detected. *Results.* Both IMAT and TBS were significantly decreased in patients with NAFLD and early hepatitis. In hepatitis group, they declined prior to changes of liver enzymes. IMAT was significantly higher in cirrhosis Child-Pugh class A group than hepatitis patients and decreased in Child-Pugh class B and class C patients. Both IMAT/albumin and TBS/albumin decreased significantly in hepatitis and NAFLD group patients. *Conclusions.* This is the first study to discover changes of albumin metal ion and fatty acid binding capacities prior to conventional biomarkers for liver damage in early stage of liver diseases. They may become potential earliest sensitive indicators for liver function evaluation.

1. Introduction

Viral hepatitis in some countries, especially Asian countries, has an incidence rate that is 8% or higher [1]. It is recognized as an important contributive factor for cirrhosis and hepatocellular carcinoma [2, 3]. The currently conventional biochemical markers for liver function, such as bilirubin, albumin, and liver enzymatic assays, often do not exhibit detectable changes at early stage of viral hepatitis [4]. This makes early detection, assessment, and timely treatment of this disease very difficult. In most cases, liver fibrosis or cirrhosis has already occurred when these indicators become abnormal. NAFLD is becoming a common chronic disease in both developed and developing countries with increasing incidence [5–7]. Nonalcoholic steatohepatitis (NASH) may also cause cirrhosis and eventually lead to hepatocyte carcinoma [8, 9]. Conventional liver function tests are not able

to assess the liver damages at the early stages of the diseases; effective markers for early liver damages are needed.

Serum albumin, the most abundant circulating proteins in the body, plays a very important role in maintaining the osmotic pressure in blood vessels. In addition, it has binding and transportation functions [10, 11]. However, most of the studies focused on the importance of serum albumin levels instead of its binding functions. Albumin binding functions include its metal ion binding and fatty acid binding. Metal ion binding function reflects the binding capacity of the N-terminal metal ion binding site to metal ions. Fatty acid binding function is the binding capacity for long-chain fatty acids that can be detected with electron paramagnetic resonance (EPR) technique [12, 13].

In recent years, some studies have been published related to the significance of albumin binding functions. Jalan et al. [14] found that albumin fatty acid binding ability and metal

TABLE 1: Inclusion and exclusion criteria for NAFLD, hepatitis, and cirrhosis patients.

NAFLD	Inclusion criteria	No alcohol history or consuming of alcohol < 210 g/week for male and < 140 g/week for female
		Ultrasound, CT, MRI, or liver biopsy prompted fatty liver
NAFLD	Exclusion criteria	Viral hepatitis, drug-induced hepatitis, alcoholic fatty liver, autoimmune liver disease, liver degeneration
		Diagnosis of cirrhosis by ultrasound, CT, MRI, or liver biopsy pathology; neoplasm in liver or other organs
		With myocardial ischemia, hepatorenal syndrome, diabetes, infections, intestinal ischemia, cerebrovascular accident
		Albumin infusion within a month
Hepatitis	Inclusion criteria	Viral hepatitis over six months
		HBsAg and/or HBeAg positive
		Ultrasound, CT, MRI, or liver biopsy prompted no liver cirrhosis; AST, ALT < 40 U/L
Hepatitis	Exclusion criteria	Neoplasm in liver or other organs
		With myocardial ischemia, hepatorenal syndrome, diabetes, infections, intestinal ischemia, cerebrovascular accident
		Albumin infusion within a month
Cirrhosis	Inclusion criteria	Diagnosis of cirrhosis by ultrasound, CT, MRI, liver biopsy pathology, or operation
Cirrhosis	Exclusion criteria	Neoplasm in liver or other organs
		With myocardial ischemia, hepatorenal syndrome, diabetes, infections, intestinal ischemia, cerebrovascular accident
		Alcoholic, nonalcoholic, drug-induced, primary biliary cirrhosis, and unexplained hepatic cirrhosis albumin infusion within a month

ion binding capacity were significantly lower in advanced cirrhosis, which can be used to predict prognosis of acute on chronic liver failures. Oettl et al. [15] reported that in patients with advanced liver disease, the reduction of binding capacity at albumin binding site II that binds to aromatic carboxylic compounds is related to impaired liver function. However, there were no reports about the changes in albumin binding activities in the early stages of viral hepatitis or nonalcoholic fatty liver disease (NAFLD). In the present observational study, we observed for the first time that albumin cobalt binding capacity and albumin fatty acid binding capacity changed prior to any changes observed in other conventional liver function assays; and the extents of the changes were associated with the degrees of liver damage. Therefore, these may become new markers for early hepatic dysfunction.

2. Materials and Methods

2.1. Patients. Patients were enrolled from January 2014 to February 2015 at this hospital, among whom are NAFLD (n = 23), viral hepatitis (n = 37), and cirrhosis (n = 133) [6, 8, 16] (Table 1). Cirrhosis patients were further divided according to Child-Pugh score [17] into three subgroups, Child-Pugh class A had 81 patients, Child-Pugh class B had 30 patients, and Child-Pugh class C had 22 patients. Another 60 healthy volunteers were also enrolled as control. The study was approved by the ethics committee of Peking Union Medical College Hospital. All subjects were provided with written informed consent in accordance with the Declaration of Helsinki prior to their inclusion in the study.

2.2. Serum Sample Collection. Peripheral venous blood was collected after at least 12 hours of fasting. Blood samples were collected into the additive-free vacuum tube and allowed 30–60 minutes for coagulation. The samples were then centrifuged at 3000 revolutions per minute for 10 minutes, and serum was stored at −80°C before analysis.

2.3. Routine Serological Tests. Routine tests included total bilirubin, aspartate aminotransferase (AST), alanine aminotransferase (ALT), creatinine, prothrombin time (PT), and international normalized ratio (INR). Child-Pugh score and model for end stage liver disease (MELD) score were also computed [17].

2.4. Albumin Binding Activity Assay

2.4.1. Albumin Cobalt Binding Capacity. The procedure was based on prior description by Bar-Or et al. [18]. In short, 100 μL of serum was mixed with 25 μL cobalt chloride ($CoCl_2$, 1 mg/mL) (Sigma-Aldrich, USA) in a 96-well plate and incubated at room temperature for 10 minutes. 25 μL dithiothreitol (DTT, 1.5 mg/mL) (Sigma-Aldrich, USA) was added, followed by 2-minute incubation to allow the reaction with free cobalt salt. Finally 150 μL saline was added to terminate the reaction. Absorbance was measured by a spectrophotometer Synergy H1 (BioTek, USA) at 470 nm. The IMA was expressed as absorbance unit, which equaled the absorbance of the testing well minus the absorbance of control well with no DTT added. High absorbance value indicated more free cobalt salt reacting with DTT; therefore fewer cobalt salt was bound to albumin.

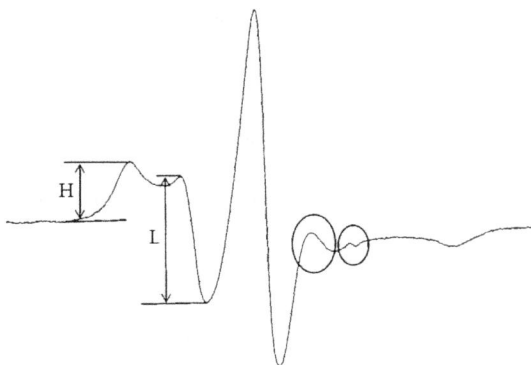

FIGURE 1: EPR spectrum of the 16-DS bound to albumin and with some unbounded 16-DS in serum. Spin labels bounded at albumin binding sites could be released free to the serum when albumin structure was impaired. The large circle part represents the low affinity binding sites to fatty acid in albumin at $I = +1$. The small circle part represents the free label in serum at $I = +1$. The area of the two circles should be deducted when calculating TBS. H and L, respectively, represent the number of 16-DS bounded to high and low affinity fatty acid binding sites. H/L reflects the fatty acid binding affinity of albumin.

2.4.2. Albumin Fatty Acid Binding Capacity. Serum (100 μL) was transferred into 0.5 mL of an Eppendorf tube and 3.0 mmol/L of spin label, 16-doxyl stearic acid (Sigma-Aldrich, USA), was added. The mixture was gently stirred with a 2 mm diameter glass rod for 3 minutes at 4°C. The Eppendorf tube was then sealed and placed in a water bath at 37°C and incubated for 20 minutes. 10 μL of the mixture was then transferred with a quartz capillary onto an electron paramagnetic resonance instrument (Bruker EMX A200, Bruker BioSpin GmbH, German), operated with center field of 3427.4 G, sweep width of 100 G, microwave frequency of 9.6 GHz, microwave power of 6.5 MW, and modulation frequency of 100 KHz with modulation amplitude 2.5 G.

The obtained data was analyzed with the Origin 8 image processing software (OriginLab, USA) to construct a spectral diagram (Figure 1). This was a spectral diagram constructed from the data generated on the electron paramagnetic resonance spectrometer of the spin label and albumin complex. Total area under the spectrum represented the sum of the serum albumin bound spin label and the free label [12], which was calculated by integration.

The spin label, 16-doxyl stearic acid, had very high binding constant to albumin [12]. Thus, normally there were very few free labels present in the serum. However, when albumin structure was impaired, spin labels that were albumin bound at their binding sites had been released free and, therefore, could be detected and recorded on the spectrum. The effect of free spin label in serum on the total fatty acid binding sites of albumin was determined through simulation experiments. Then, TBS, the sum of the binding sites on albumin molecules that were capable of fatty acid binding, was calculated by deducting the free spin labels in serum from the total amount of labels. This also reflected the total amount of functional albumin.

Meanwhile, the ratio between the number of fatty acid binding sites with high-affinity and that with low affinity could also be measured and calculated from the spectrum (H/L). H/L reflected not only the binding strength of albumin to fatty acid, but also the changes in its conformation.

2.5. Statistical Analysis. Continuous variables were expressed as mean ± standard deviation, or median and interquartile. Statistical analysis was performed with SPSS 13.0 statistical software (SPSS Inc., USA). Nonparametric Kruskal-Wallis test was used for paired comparisons between data sets with different sample sizes. Two-way test was used for all analysis. $P < 0.01$ was considered statistically significant.

Correlation analysis between groups of data was done with Pearson product-moment correlation coefficient if both variables followed a normal distribution, or with Spearman's rank-order correlation coefficient if one of them did not follow a normal distribution, or between the ranked variables.

3. Results

All hepatitis patients were infected with either hepatitis B or C virus, where 78.4% (29/37) of them were hepatitis B patients. Hepatitis B or hepatitis C virus infection was the cause for all cirrhosis, in which hepatitis B accounted for 91.0% (121/133). All patients infected with hepatitis B virus in hepatitis group and cirrhosis group received antiviral therapy. The ratios of patients receiving continuous interferon and nucleos(t)ide analogue therapies for at least six months to that receiving irregular antiviral therapy less than six months in hepatitis, Child-Pugh classes A, B, and C groups were, respectively, 20 : 9, 54 : 21, 19 : 9, and 10 : 8.

No differences were observed in albumin levels among the healthy control and NAFLD and hepatitis patients ($P = 0.36$). However, the albumin levels of cirrhotic patients were significantly lower than those of the noncirrhotic patients ($P < 0.001$). Furthermore, the albumin levels continued to decrease as the liver lost more function. At the same time, clinical Child-Pugh scores and MELD scores of Child-Pugh class B and class C group patients are higher than those of Child-Pugh class A group patients ($P < 0.01$). PT gradually increased, from patients with viral hepatitis to cirrhosis, indicating the decline of liver synthetic function (Table 2).

3.1. Albumin Cobalt Binding Capacity. The direct reading of IMA assay reflected the serum albumin that had lost metal ion binding ability. To simplify the presentation, we converted it into IMAT (IMA transformed), which is 1-IMA. Thus, the higher value of IMAT indicated that the tested albumin had higher metal ion binding capacity. There were no differences in serum albumin levels in noncirrhotic patients (NAFLD or viral hepatitis) and control healthy volunteers. However, IMAT values in NAFLD as well as hepatitis patients were lower than the healthy people ($P < 0.001$). There was no difference in IMAT values between the NAFLD and hepatitis patients ($P = 0.48$). In cirrhotic patients, however, higher IMAT values were found in patients in Child-Pugh class A comparing to the NAFLD or hepatitis patients. As the

TABLE 2: Baseline characteristics of the participants in different subjects groups.

Parameters	Control (n = 60)	NAFLD (n = 23)	Hepatitis (n = 37)	Cirrhosis Child-Pugh class A (n = 81)	Cirrhosis Child-Pugh class B (n = 30)	Cirrhosis Child-Pugh class C (n = 22)
Age (yr)	47.4 ± 9.7	43.5 ± 11.4	47.0 ± 10.6	49.0 ± 12.8	50.7 ± 11.7	56.1 ± 9.2
Sex (M/F)	32/28	17/6	22/15	75/6	21/9	16/6
Viral hepatitis (hbv/hcv)	No	No	29/8	75/6	28/2	18/4
Albumin (g/L)	46.7 ± 3.6	48.0 ± 2.6	47.0 ± 3.1	$41.3 \pm 5.2^{*\#\Delta}$	$33.1 \pm 4.1^{*\#\Delta\dagger}$	$30.0 \pm 5.2^{*\#\Delta\dagger}$
Bilirubin (μmol/L)						
Median	11.7	12.5	12.4	15.6^*	$21.1^{*\#\Delta}$	$114.1^{*\#\Delta\dagger\S}$
Interquartile range	9.0–15.2	8.0–17.3	10.9–16.3	11.6–21.7	12.3–29.7	52.0–308.6
AST (U/L)						
Median	17.5	40.0^*	$24.0^{\#}$	$25.9^{*\#}$	$37.5^{*\Delta}$	$47.3^{*\Delta\dagger}$
Interquartile range	14.0–20.8	36.0–57.0	20.0–26.0	21.0–40.0	29.0–62.3	38.0–120.0
ALT (U/L)						
Median	17.5	66.0^*	$20.0^{\#}$	$26.0^{*\#\Delta}$	$34.5^{*\Delta}$	$24.7^{\#}$
Interquartile range	12.5–24.0	58.0–95.0	15.0–25.0	17.5–39.5	26.8–43.0	18.0–75.2
Creatinine (μmol/L)	68.5 ± 12.1	70.1 ± 17.9	72.0 ± 12.3	74.1 ± 14.1	73.9 ± 17.4	$84.1 \pm 13.8^{*\Delta}$
PT (s)	11.5 ± 0.6	11.5 ± 0.7	11.6 ± 0.6	$12.3 \pm 1.3^*$	$13.5 \pm 1.4^{*\#\Delta\dagger}$	$19.4 \pm 5.5^{*\#\Delta\dagger}$
INR	1.0 ± 0.1	1.0 ± 0.1	1.0 ± 0.1	$1.1 \pm 0.2^{*\#\Delta}$	$1.2 \pm 0.1^{*\#\Delta\dagger}$	$1.7 \pm 0.5^{*\#\Delta\dagger}$
Child-Pugh score	n.a.	n.a.	n.a.	5.2 ± 0.4	$7.5 \pm 0.7^\dagger$	$11.0 \pm 1.2^\dagger$
MELD score	n.a.	n.a.	n.a.	7.9 ± 1.9	$10.5 \pm 3.1^\dagger$	$21.3 \pm 12.7^\dagger$

Continuous variables are expressed as means $\pm$ standard deviation, or median and interquartile. M: male; F: female; hbv: hepatitis B virus; hcv: hepatitis C virus; n.a.: not available; MELD: model for end stage liver disease.
$^*P < 0.01$ compared with control group; $^{\#}P < 0.01$ compared with NAFLD group.
$^{\Delta}P < 0.01$ compared with hepatitis group; $^{\dagger}P < 0.01$ compared with Child-Pugh class A group.
$^{\S}P < 0.01$ compared with Child-Pugh class B group.

TABLE 3: Functional albumin parameters in different subjects groups.

Parameters	Control (n = 60)	NAFLD (n = 23)	Hepatitis (n = 37)	Cirrhosis Child-Pugh class A (n = 81)	Cirrhosis Child-Pugh class B (n = 30)	Cirrhosis Child-Pugh class C (n = 22)
IMAT	0.59 ± 0.06	$0.42 \pm 0.16^*$	$0.41 \pm 0.12^*$	$0.51 \pm 0.13^{*\Delta}$	$0.38 \pm 0.12^{*\dagger}$	$0.22 \pm 0.06^{*\#\Delta}$
IMAT/albumin (10^{-2})	1.27 ± 0.15	$0.88 \pm 0.32^*$	$0.87 \pm 0.24^*$	$1.25 \pm 0.32^{\#\Delta}$	$1.15 \pm 0.35^{\Delta}$	$0.77 \pm 0.22^{*\dagger\S}$
TBS (10^8)	6.03 ± 0.36	5.69 ± 0.31	$5.42 \pm 0.22^*$	$5.34 \pm 0.32^{*\#}$	$5.97 \pm 0.58^{\Delta\dagger}$	$5.48 \pm 0.46^{*\S}$
TBS/albumin (10^7)	1.30 ± 0.14	$1.19 \pm 0.09^*$	$1.18 \pm 0.12^*$	1.29 ± 0.15	$1.86 \pm 0.29^{*\#\Delta\dagger}$	$1.88 \pm 0.32^{*\#\Delta\dagger}$
H/L	0.76 ± 0.08	0.73 ± 0.03	$0.69 \pm 0.04^{*\#}$	0.72 ± 0.02	$0.68 \pm 0.04^{*\#}$	$0.59 \pm 0.10^{*\#\dagger}$

Continuous variables are expressed as means $\pm$ standard deviation.
$^*P < 0.01$ compared with control group; $^{\#}P < 0.01$ compared with NAFLD group.
$^{\Delta}P < 0.01$ compared with hepatitis group; $^{\dagger}P < 0.01$ compared with Child-Pugh class A group.
$^{\S}P < 0.01$ compared with Child-Pugh class B group.

condition of liver becomes further deteriorated, the levels of serum albumin decreased as well as the IMAT values (Table 3).

Since the serum albumin levels changed during disease progression, it is perceivable that it may influence the IMAT value tested. To avoid this, we normalized the IMAT against albumin concentration and expressed it as IMAT/albumin. After normalization, similar results were found in which IMAT/albumin levels in NAFLD or hepatitis patients were significantly lower than the healthy volunteers ($P < 0.001$);

there were no differences between these two groups of patients ($P = 0.70$). Due to the significant decreases in serum albumin levels seen in cirrhosis patients, the IMAT/albumin values were greatly increased in patients of Child-Pugh classes A and B comparing to that of the hepatitis patients. Their IMAT/albumin values were not different than the healthy control ($P = 0.07$). However, patients of Child-Pugh class C had significant lower IMAT/albumin values comparing to that of the healthy control ($P < 0.001$) (Table 3).

3.2. Albumin Fatty Acid Binding Capacity. The ability of albumin in binding fatty acids was assessed by EPR and expressed as TBS. Even though none of the NAFLD or hepatitis patients had yet developed cirrhosis and there were no significant changes in their serum albumin levels in comparison to the healthy people, their TBS values had already shown various degrees of decline. Among them, hepatitis patients had a more significant decline over the healthy control ($P < 0.001$) than the NAFLD patients ($P = 0.11$). The observations in cirrhosis patients were more complicated. Although the serum albumin levels in patients of Child-Pugh class A were significantly lower than that of the hepatitis patients ($P < 0.001$), there were no differences in their TBS values ($P = 0.31$). Increased TBS values were seen in the patients of Child-Pugh class B compared to that in the patients of Child-Pugh class A ($P < 0.001$) (Table 3).

Similarly, we normalized TBS value against the serum albumin concentration. Both NAFLD and hepatitis patients showed significantly decreased TBS/albumin values compared to that of the healthy volunteers ($P < 0.001$). Liver became more dysfunctional during cirrhosis; instead, TBS/albumin values of these patients increased. We observed a minimum increase in Child-Pugh class A patients and a significant increase in Child-Pugh class B and class C patients ($P < 0.01$). There were no statistical differences between class B and class C patients ($P = 0.89$) (Table 3).

3.3. Fatty Acid Binding Affinity of Albumin. The binding affinity of each fatty acid binding sites is also part of the binding capacity of albumin, which can be demonstrated as the ratio between high and low affinity binding sites (H/L). To certain extend, this ratio can also imply the changes in albumin protein structure. The results shown in Table 3 indicated that all patients had various declines in H/L compared to that of healthy volunteers. Hepatitis patients as well as cirrhosis patients of Child-Pugh class B and class C all showed significant decrease in H/L compared to healthy control ($P < 0.001$). Patients of Child-Pugh class A did not have significantly different H/L as hepatitis patients ($P = 0.16$). However, as cirrhosis progressed, H/L gradually declined.

3.4. Correlation Analysis. Correlation analysis showed that a moderate positive correlation could be found between albumin levels and IMAT, $r = 0.41$ ($P < 0.001$). There was a weak correlation between the H/L and IMAT, $r = 0.34$ ($P < 0.001$), but no correlation between TBS and albumin levels ($P = 0.13$).

4. Discussion

Viral hepatitis is one of the main causes for liver cirrhosis and cancer. In addition, the incidents of NAFLD are on the rise in recent years, while the patients suffering from liver cirrhosis and even cancers due to NASH are also increased [8, 19]. The accurate evaluation of liver function and the extent of the damage in the early disease course can help the physicians to devise a reasonable treatment plan promptly to better control the disease development. Thus, it is very important to assess liver damage in the beginning stages of the disease even before the changes in liver enzyme activities become detectable. However, there are limitations in the conventional detection indexes used to assess early liver lesions [4].

The level of serum albumin is one of the indicators for liver synthetic function [17, 20]. However, albumin level itself does not reflect its binding activities, which may be the more sensitive indication for functionality. This study revealed for the first time that there were changes in the albumin binding activities in NAFLD, viral hepatitis, and liver cirrhosis patients; and our findings suggested that albumin binding activity may be an early marker for liver function during disease development comparing to other liver parameters.

Higher value of IMAT indicates greater metal ion binding capacity of albumin. Our results showed that, in NAFLD and viral hepatitis patients, even before their albumin levels, total bilirubin, and prothrombin time became abnormal, their IMAT value decreased significantly comparing to the healthy volunteers ($P < 0.001$). This suggested that IMAT was an earlier and more sensitive indicator for liver dysfunction than the conventional liver biomarkers. In the liver cirrhosis patients, however, we had a more interesting observation. The IMAT values increased in Child-Pugh class A patients comparing to the viral hepatitis patients ($P < 0.01$) but decreased in class B patients and further more in class C patients. It is possible that the Child-Pugh class A patients were in the stage that their livers were trying to compensate the lost function; thus, although the albumin levels decreased in these patients, their ion binding activities increased. This suggested that, during this stage, the albumin levels did not correlate to their binding capacities. However, as the liver function continued to deteriorate, the compensatory increase in binding capacity became lost and the IMAT value started to decrease from patients in Child-Pugh class B to class C.

We used the normalized IMAT/albumin, representing the ion binding capacity in unit albumin molecule, to minimize the influence of fluctuations in serum albumin levels. Results showed that albumin binding capacity per unit albumin in patients of NAFLD and hepatitis decreased significantly compared to normal control ($P < 0.001$). During the liver functional compensation period in patients of cirrhosis, IMAT/albumin also has a short compensation period and then declined progressively with the deterioration of liver function.

The reason that the binding capacity of albumin changes in the early stage of liver damage is still unclear. It is possible that during hepatocytes steatosis, inflammation response, or viral infection, the three-dimensional structure of the albumin molecule is altered, leading to the structural changes on its metal ion binding site and the reduction of its ion binding capacity. In the early cirrhosis, there is limited compensation for albumin ion binding capacity.

The fatty acid binding ability of albumin is directly associated with the correct structure at its fatty acid binding sites. Therefore, the normal fatty acid binding capacity can only be maintained in structurally normal albumin. Studies have found that there are seven fatty acid binding sites on albumin, in which three are high-affinity and four are low affinity binding sites [12]. The spin labeling electron paramagnetic resonance spectroscopy enabled us to detect not only the number of total binding sites but also the binding affinity of albumin to fatty acid. We found that, in the early stages of NAFLD and hepatitis, there were already various extents of damage to albumin's fatty acid binding capacity, in which hepatitis patients suffered more severe damages. Normalized TBS/albumin represented the number of binding sites per unit of albumin. Our results showed that TBS/albumin value decreased significantly in NAFLD and hepatitis patients over the healthy volunteers ($P < 0.01$). Compared to conventional biochemical markers, TBS may be a more effective early indicator for liver damage. In the later stage of cirrhosis, when albumin levels had shown significant decline, their fatty acid binding capacity was still in a compensation stage. TBS/albumin values showed a compensatory increase in patients with further declined liver function. TBS/albumin values were both higher in patients in Child-Pugh class B and class C compared to that of the patients in class A ($P < 0.001$). As cirrhosis became more severe, the fatty acid binding capacity of albumin gradually declined. The patients in Child-Pugh class C lost the compensatory increase of fatty acid binding capacity of their albumins.

We try to explain the possible reasons for this outcome in light of three-dimensional structural changes in albumin. The ratio between high-affinity and low affinity binding sites (H/L) also indicates the albumin conformational changes in addition to albumin binding ability. Our results showed that albumin conformation was damaged in NAFLD and hepatitis patients, while the damage was more severe in hepatitis patients. Accordingly, the TBS values of hepatitis patients were lower than that of NAFLD patients. As disease progressed to cirrhosis, compensatory increases of TBS/albumin were seen to overcome the adverse effect of decreased albumin levels. Once the structural damage of albumin became more severe, the values of TBS/albumin stopped to increase and TBS started to decline.

Both metal ion binding and fatty acid binding capacities of albumin reflected liver damage earlier than the changes in albumin levels. There is no correlation between the changes of IMAT and TBS, suggesting that there were differential effects on various ligand-binding sites of albumin in different diseases that impaired liver functions. The exact mechanism of compensatory binding function increase seen in albumin remains unclear. In addition, it is complex for the changing of albumin binding function in patients with cirrhosis, so further studies are needed to probe the internal mechanism.

5. Conclusions

Currently, there are no effective markers for detecting liver damages in the early stages of viral hepatitis and NAFLD. In conclusion, this study is the first to discover that the metal ion binding and fatty acid binding capacities of albumin had undergone significant change at this early stage. They may potentially become earliest sensitive indicators to suggest liver dysfunction, which could have positive impacts on evaluation and treatment of early stage liver diseases.

One limitation of the study is the small sample size. Furthermore, because antiviral treatment can give a significant effect on liver function in patients with hepatitis and reduce the cirrhosis decompensation, treatment protocols may affect the results of albumin binding function.

Abbreviations

NAFLD: Nonalcoholic fatty liver disease
IMA: Ischemia-modified albumin
IMAT: Ischemia-modified albumin transformed
TBS: Total binding sites
NASH: Nonalcoholic steatohepatitis
EPR: Electron paramagnetic resonance
AST: Aspartate aminotransferase
ALT: Alanine aminotransferase
PT: Prothrombin time
INR: International normalized ratio
MELD: Model for end stage liver disease
DTT: Dithiothreitol.

Consent

All study participants provided informed written consent prior to study enrollment.

Competing Interests

The authors declare that they have no conflict of interests in any form with respect to this article.

Authors' Contributions

Penglei Ge and Yilei Mao designed the study; Huayu Yang, Jingfen Lu, Wenjun Liao, and Yingli Xu helped to analyze data; Shunda Du, Haifeng Xu, Haitao Zhao, Xin Lu, Xinting Sang, Shouxian Zhong, and Jiefu Huang helped to collect data; Penglei Ge drafted the manuscript; Yilei Mao provided revision, edited the manuscript, and was the supervisor. All authors read and approved the final manuscript.

Acknowledgments

The authors thank Yanan Wang for the valuable advice on test technique and Zixing Wang for the help on statistical analysis. This study was sponsored by the funding from National Natural Science Foundation of China (81201566) and National Key Technology Research and Development Program of China (2012BA I06B01).

References

[1] C. M. N. Croagh and J. S. Lubel, "Natural history of chronic hepatitis B: phases in a complex relationship," *World Journal of Gastroenterology*, vol. 20, no. 30, pp. 10395–10404, 2014.

[2] T. T. Cheung and C. M. Lo, "Laparoscopic liver resection for hepatocellular carcinoma in patients with cirrhosis," *Hepatobiliary Surgery and Nutrition*, vol. 4, pp. 406–410, 2015.

[3] J. H. Kao, P. J. Chen, and D. S. Chen, "Recent advances in the research of hepatitis B virus-related hepatocellular carcinoma: epidemiologic and molecular biological aspects," *Advances in Cancer Research*, vol. 108, pp. 21–72, 2010.

[4] K. M. Field, C. Dow, and M. Michael, "Part I: liver function in oncology: biochemistry and beyond," *The Lancet Oncology*, vol. 9, no. 11, pp. 1092–1101, 2008.

[5] J.-G. Fan and G. C. Farrell, "Epidemiology of non-alcoholic fatty liver disease in China," *Journal of Hepatology*, vol. 50, no. 1, pp. 204–210, 2009.

[6] N. N. Than and P. N. Newsome, "A concise review of non-alcoholic fatty liver disease," *Atherosclerosis*, vol. 239, no. 1, pp. 192–202, 2015.

[7] P. Zezos and E. L. Renner, "Liver transplantation and non-alcoholic fatty liver disease," *World Journal of Gastroenterology*, vol. 20, no. 42, pp. 15532–15538, 2014.

[8] S. Watanabe, E. Hashimoto, K. Ikejima et al., "Evidence-based clinical practice guidelines for nonalcoholic fatty liver disease/nonalcoholic steatohepatitis," *Journal of Gastroenterology*, vol. 50, no. 4, pp. 364–377, 2015.

[9] K. B. Linhart, K. Glassen, T. Peccerella et al., "The generation of carcinogenic etheno-DNA adducts in the liver of patients with nonalcoholic fatty liver disease," *Hepatobiliary Surgery and Nutrition*, vol. 4, no. 2, pp. 117–123, 2015.

[10] European Association for the Study of the Liver, "EASL clinical practice guidelines on the management of ascites, spontaneous bacterial peritonitis, and hepatorenal syndrome in cirrhosis," *Journal of Hepatology*, vol. 53, no. 3, pp. 397–417, 2010.

[11] R. Garcia-Martinez, P. Caraceni, M. Bernardi, P. Gines, V. Arroyo, and R. Jalan, "Albumin: pathophysiologic basis of its role in the treatment of cirrhosis and its complications," *Hepatology*, vol. 58, no. 5, pp. 1836–1846, 2013.

[12] S. C. Kazmierczak, A. Gurachevsky, G. Matthes, and V. Muravsky, "Electron spin resonance spectroscopy of serum albumin: a novel new test for cancer diagnosis and monitoring," *Clinical Chemistry*, vol. 52, no. 11, pp. 2129–2134, 2006.

[13] M. J. N. Junk, H. W. Spiess, and D. Hinderberger, "The distribution of fatty acids reveals the functional structure of human serum albumin," *Angewandte Chemie—International Edition*, vol. 49, no. 46, pp. 8755–8759, 2010.

[14] R. Jalan, K. Schnurr, R. P. Mookerjee et al., "Alterations in the functional capacity of albumin in patients with decompensated cirrhosis is associated with increased mortality," *Hepatology*, vol. 50, no. 2, pp. 555–564, 2009.

[15] K. Oettl, R. Birner-Gruenberger, W. Spindelboeck et al., "Oxidative albumin damage in chronic liver failure: relation to albumin binding capacity, liver dysfunction and survival," *Journal of Hepatology*, vol. 59, no. 5, pp. 978–983, 2013.

[16] N. Chalasani, Z. Younossi, J. E. Lavine et al., "The diagnosis and management of non-alcoholic fatty liver disease: practice Guideline by the American Association for the Study of Liver Diseases, American College of Gastroenterology, and the American Gastroenterological Association," *Hepatology*, vol. 55, no. 6, pp. 2005–2023, 2012.

[17] P.-L. Ge, S.-D. Du, and Y.-L. Mao, "Advances in preoperative assessment of liver function," *Hepatobiliary and Pancreatic Diseases International*, vol. 13, no. 4, pp. 361–370, 2014.

[18] D. Bar-Or, E. Lau, and J. V. Winkler, "A novel assay for cobalt-albumin binding and its potential as a marker for myocardial ischemia—a preliminary report," *The Journal of Emergency Medicine*, vol. 19, no. 4, pp. 311–315, 2000.

[19] G. Vernon, A. Baranova, and Z. M. Younossi, "Systematic review: the epidemiology and natural history of non-alcoholic fatty liver disease and non-alcoholic steatohepatitis in adults," *Alimentary Pharmacology and Therapeutics*, vol. 34, no. 3, pp. 274–285, 2011.

[20] L. T. Hoekstra, W. De Graaf, G. A. A. Nibourg et al., "Physiological and biochemical basis of clinical liver function tests: a review," *Annals of Surgery*, vol. 257, no. 1, pp. 27–36, 2013.

4

Prevalence and Risk Factors of Gastric Adenoma and Gastric Cancer in Colorectal Cancer Patients

Dae Hyun Tak, Hee Seok Moon, Sun Hyung Kang, Jae Kyu Sung, and Hyun Yong Jeong

Division of Gastroenterology, Departments of Internal Medicine, Chungnam National University School of Medicine, Daejeon, Republic of Korea

Correspondence should be addressed to Hee Seok Moon; mhs1357@cnuh.co.kr

Academic Editor: Daniele Marrelli

Background/Aims. To evaluate the incidence of gastric adenoma and gastric cancer in colorectal cancer patients, as well as the clinicopathological features that affect their incidence. *Methods.* Among patients who underwent surgery after being diagnosed with colorectal cancer between January 2004 and December 2013 at Chungnam National University Hospital, 142 patients who underwent follow-up upper gastrointestinal endoscopy were assigned to the patient group. The control group included 426 subjects randomly selected. The patient group was subdivided into two: one that developed gastric adenoma or cancer and one that did not. Clinicopathological characteristics were compared between these groups. *Results.* In total, 35 (24.6%) colorectal cancer patients developed a gastric adenoma or gastric cancer, which was higher than the number in the control group (20 [4.7%] patients; $p <$ 0.001). Age, alcohol history, and differentiation of colorectal cancer were associated with higher risks of gastric adenoma or gastric cancer, with odds ratios of 1.062, 6.506, and 5.901, respectively. *Conclusions.* In colorectal cancer patients, screening with upper gastrointestinal endoscopy is important, even if no lesions are noted in the upper gastrointestinal tract at colorectal cancer diagnosis. Endoscopic screening is particularly important with increasing age, history of alcohol consumption, and poor cancer differentiation.

1. Introduction

Based on the National Cancer Registration Annual Report 2010, in Korea, gastric cancer and colorectal cancer are the second and third most common cancers, respectively, nationwide. The incidence of colorectal cancer, in particular, is dramatically increasing owing to its association with environmental factors such as the Westernized eating habits and genetic predispositions [1]. The molecular biological pathogenesis of sporadic colorectal carcinoma, which includes most cases of colorectal cancer, involves activation of APC/β-catenin pathway, chromosomal instability of various oncogenes such as *p53, DCC,* and *SMAD2/4,* and microsatellite instability due to defective DNA mismatch repair gene and serrated pathways [2]. However, the pathogenesis of gastric cancer differs from that of colorectal cancer in that it is affected by racial, regional, and environmental factors and that its molecular biological pathogenesis involves genetic and epigenetic alteration and histological differentiation; all this leads to various findings within tumors or tumor heterogeneity, suggesting biologically and/or genetically heterogeneous complexity [3]. Considering the various pathogenetic mechanisms underlying colorectal and gastric cancer, it is challenging to identify the mechanism of association between the two cancers. According to some studies, among patients with positive stool occult blood test but negative of any lesions during colonoscopy, some had upper gastric lesions during upper gastrointestinal (GI) endoscopy [4–6]. Some reports have found a high correlation between upper GI lesions in patients with colorectal cancer and colon polyp [7]. These studies have classified upper GI lesions such as gastric ulcer, duodenal ulcers, gastric polyp, and gastric cancer as meaningful findings. However, only a few studies detail the frequency of precancerous lesions such as gastric adenomas or gastric cancer in colorectal cancer patients. Furthermore, the subgroup of patients who would benefit from follow-up upper GI endoscopy is not defined. Therefore, the authors investigated the difference in the frequency of occurrence of gastric adenomas or gastric cancer and the

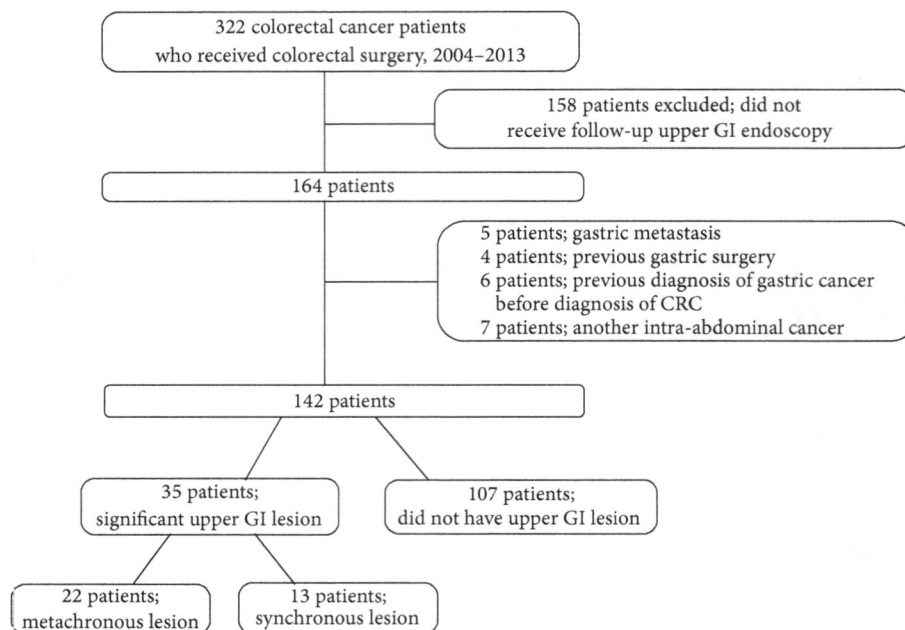

FIGURE 1: Study design and enrollment of patients. GI, gastrointestinal; CRC, colorectal cancer.

clinicopathological characteristics that affect their incidence in colorectal cancer patients.

2. Materials and Method

2.1. Materials. Between January 2004 and December 2013, 322 patients underwent colorectal surgery at Chungnam National University Hospital. Of these, the following patients were excluded: 158 patients who did not undergo follow-up upper GI endoscopy; 5 patients with gastric metastasis; 4 patients with previous gastric surgery, 6 patients diagnosed with gastric cancer before the diagnosis of colorectal cancer, and 7 patients with intra-abdominal cancer other than of gastric or colorectal origin. The remaining 142 patients were retrospectively studied (Figure 1). Patients with genetic diseases such as hereditary nonpolyposis colorectal cancer (HNPCC) and familial adenomatous polyposis (FAP) were also excluded for their strong association with the development of gastric cancer. We selected age, sex-matched controls from among those who were negative of colorectal cancer and rectal polyp during health screening. All patients in the matched cohort underwent follow-up upper GI endoscopy. Control group were 3:1 matched to patient group, and 426 patients were selected for matched control group. Colonoscopy was performed in patients who were tested from the rectum to cecum and were found to be free of rectal cancer or rectal polyp.

2.2. Method. Patients who were diagnosed with colorectal cancer and had undergone surgical treatment underwent upper GI endoscopy regardless of their upper GI symptoms. Precancerous lesions such as gastric adenomas or gastric cancer were regarded as significant lesions: their incidence was analyzed and their clinicopathological correlation was investigated by comparing with colorectal cancer patients negative for upper GI lesions. The colorectal cancer group was subdivided into two groups according to the presence of associated significant upper GI lesions, and the clinical characteristics were compared between the groups. In addition, among the patients with significant upper GI lesions, those whose upper GI lesions were diagnosed 6 months after the initial diagnosis of colorectal cancer (metachronous) were compared with patients without associated lesions. Demographic data included age; sex; body weight; body mass index (BMI); hypertension; diabetes; smoking history; alcohol history; family history of solid tumors; size, location, stage, histological differentiation, vessel invasion, and lymph node invasion of colorectal cancer; and carcinoembryonic antigen (CEA) levels. And, the cumulative incidence of gastric adenoma and gastric cancer was compared between the control group and colorectal cancer group. Furthermore, incidences of other upper GI lesions were compared between the two groups both at the time of diagnosis and follow-up evaluation.

2.3. Definition. Significant lesions were defined as precancerous lesions such as gastric adenomas or gastric cancer, and TNM stage was determined according to the American Joint Committee on Cancer (AJCC) cancer staging, seventh edition. Family history of solid tumors was defined as solid tumors occurring in the same family for two generations. Solid tumors included cancer of the colorectum, stomach, pancreas, biliary tree, esophagus, lung, larynx, and brain. Hepatocellular cancer and head and neck cancer were excluded because they are mostly of viral origin. Follow-up period was defined from the time of diagnosis of colorectal cancer in colorectal cancer group and from the time of initial health screening upper GI endoscopy for the control group, up to the end of the last upper GI endoscopy for both groups. For colorectal cancer patients, alcohol and smoking history were based upon admission records and nurse records, whereas for the control group, patients were asked to fill in a questionnaire. Both current and ex-smokers were counted as patients with smoking experience. Synchronous and metachronous lesions were classified based on the time the upper GI lesions were detected. If gastric cancer and colorectal cancer were diagnosed at the same time or within 6 months of follow-up, these lesions were defined as synchronous lesions. If the diagnosis was made after 6 months, they were defined as metachronous lesion.

2.4. Statistical Analysis. Based on the development of upper GI lesions in the colorectal cancer group, clinical and pathological continuous variables were analyzed using independent t-test, whereas categorical data analysis was conducted using a chi-square test. Multivariate analysis was done using binary logistic regression analysis. Only age was divided into five categories (under 40, 40–49, 50–59, 60–69, and over 70) and analyzed after assigning a serial number. When comparing the occurrence rate of upper GI lesions and other variables between the colorectal cancer group and the control group, independent t-test and chi-square test were used. The time-dependent cumulative incidence of gastric adenoma and gastric cancer between the two groups was analyzed using the Kaplan-Meyer survival analysis. Statistical calculation was performed with PASW Statistics version 18.0 (IBM Co., Armonk, NY, USA), and $p < 0.05$ was regarded as statistically significant.

3. Results

3.1. Factors Significantly Related to the Development of Upper GI Lesions in Colorectal Cancer Patients. Clinical and pathological variables were compared between 35 patients who developed significant upper GI lesions, which were detected during follow-up upper GI endoscopy after colorectal cancer surgery (13 synchronous lesions and 22 metachronous lesions), and 107 patients who did not develop such lesions. Age; sex; body weight; BMI; hypertension; diabetes; smoking, drinking, and family history of solid tumors; size, location, stage, histological differentiation, vessel invasion, and lymph node invasion of cancer; and CEA levels were the variables analyzed. Factors that were statistically significantly different between the groups were age, drinking, and lymph node invasion. When we compared the group with metachronous lesions and the group without lesions, drinking was the only factor to show statistical significance (Table 1). Multivariate analysis was performed to exclude the confounder effect: comparison of the group with both synchronous and metachronous lesions and the group with only metachronous lesions showed that age, drinking, and histological differentiation were statistically significant. Drinking and histological differentiation increased cancer risks up to approximately 6.5 and 5.9 times, respectively (Table 2).

3.2. Upper GI Endoscopy Findings and Their Relation to Diagnosis of Colorectal Cancer in the Colorectal Cancer Group and Control Group. The occurrence rate of gastric adenoma and

gastric cancer during upper GI endoscopy at the diagnosis of colorectal cancer in the colorectal cancer group was 9.1% (13 patients) and 2.1% (9 patients) higher than that in the control group. There was no between-group significant difference in other endoscopic findings, including chronic atrophic gastritis (56.3% versus 62.7%, $p = 0.180$), gastric ulcer (1.4% versus 0.9%, $p = 0.636$), duodenal ulcer (2.1% versus 1.9%, $p = 0.860$), and hyperplastic polyp (1.4% versus 4.7%, $p = 0.079$). We however found an increased incidence of intestinal metaplasia in the colorectal cancer group when compared with the control group (10.6% versus 5.6%, $p = 0.044$; Table 3).

3.3. Follow-Up of Upper GI Endoscopy Findings in the Colorectal Cancer Group and Control Group. Excluded from the study were 13 patients who were diagnosed with upper GI lesions within 6 months of colorectal cancer diagnosis in colorectal cancer group and 9 patients who were diagnosed with upper GI lesions within 6 months of their first health inspection in the control group. The remaining 129 patients and 417 patients were compared for the occurrence rate of gastric adenoma and gastric cancer: the colorectal cancer group showed a higher rate, with 22 patients (17.1%) and 11 patients (2.6%), respectively ($p < 0.001$; Table 4). So, among the 35 patients who developed significant upper GI lesions in the colorectal cancer group, 13 patients (9.1%) had synchronous lesions and 22 patients (15.5%) had metachronous lesions. We also found a trend toward increased incidence of intestinal metaplasia in the colorectal cancer group when compared with the control group over time (24.8% versus 13.4%, $p = 0.002$).

3.4. Cumulative Occurrence of Gastric Adenoma and Gastric Cancer according to Time in Colorectal Cancer Patients. Precancerous lesions such as gastric adenoma or gastric cancer were diagnosed through follow-up upper GI endoscopy mostly within 2 years of colorectal cancer diagnosis and up to 4 years after diagnosis (Figure 2). Also, the patient group showed a significantly high accumulative incidence rate when compared with the control group ($p < 0.001$).

4. Discussion

Geller et al., in their study, showed that patients with colon polyp and positive stool occult blood test had a higher incidence of upper GI lesions [5]. Shin et al. showed that patients with colorectal cancer or colon polyp had a higher incidence of upper GI lesions [7]. Our results are similar to these reports in that the colorectal cancer group showed a statistically significant higher incidence of upper GI lesions when compared with the control group. It must be noted that previous studies did not restrict study patients to those with colorectal cancer; these studies included patients with benign lesions (gastric ulcer and duodenal ulcer), precancerous lesions such as gastric adenoma, and gastric cancer [4–7]. However, we studied only colorectal cancer patients and focused on the development of precancerous lesions such as gastric adenoma and gastric cancer at the time of colorectal cancer diagnosis or during follow-up.

TABLE 1: Comparison of clinicopathologic features in the subjects with or without UGI lesion in colorectal cancer patients.

Variables	Patients without UGI lesion ($n = 107$)	Patients with synchronous and metachronous UGI[a] lesion ($n = 35$)	p value	Patients with metachronous UGI[a] lesion ($n = 22$)	p value
Sex			0.078		0.060
Male	65 (60.7%)	27 (77.1%)		18 (81.8%)	
Female	42 (39.3%)	8 (22.9%)		4 (18.2%)	
Age (yrs)	64.76 ± 11.72	68.29 ± 7.90	0.048	68.36 ± 8.01	0.128
Body weight (kg)	58.50 ± 9.26	60.78 ± 9.09	0.918	61.91 ± 9.95	0.650
BMI (body mass index, kg/m^2)	22.60 ± 3.05	23.01 ± 2.97	0.723	23.44 ± 3.13	0.931
Hypertension	33 (30.8%)	12 (34.3%)	0.704	8 (36.4%)	0.612
Diabetes	19 (17.8%)	10 (40.0%)	0.168	6 (27.3%)	0.304
Smoking	21 (19.6%)	12 (34.3%)	0.075	7 (31.8%)	0.206
Alcohol	25 (26.4%)	20 (57.1%)	<0.001	12 (54.5%)	0.003
Family history (solid tumor)	10 (9.35%)	6 (17.1%)	0.205	4 (18.2%)	0.225
Tumor size (cm)[b]	5.06 ± 2.39	4.49 ± 3.02	0.504	4.57 ± 3.46	0.271
CRC location[c]			0.828		0.844
Rt.colon	62 (57.9%)	21 (60.0%)		14 (63.6%)	
Transverse colon	4 (3.7%)	2 (5.7%)		1 (4.6%)	
Lt.colon	41 (38.3%)	12 (34.3%)		7 (31.8%)	
Cancer staging			0.749		0.907
I	22 (20.6%)	10 (28.6%)		6 (27.3%)	
II	42 (39.3%)	11 (31.4%)		8 (36.4%)	
III	36 (33.6%)	12 (34.3%)		7 (31.8%)	
IV	7 (6.5%)	2 (5.7%)		1 (4.5%)	
Vascular invasion	84 (78.5%)	22 (62.9%)	0.065	15 (68.2%)	0.297
Lymphatic invasion	86 (80.4%)	21 (60.0%)	0.015	14 (63.6%)	0.087
Differentiation			0.077		0.147
Well differentiated	2 (1.9%)	1 (2.86%)		0 (0%)	
Moderate differentiated	101 (94.4%)	29 (82.9%)		19 (86.4%)	
Poorly differentiated	4 (3.7%)	5 (14.3%)		3 (13.6%)	
CEA level (ng/mL)	8.20 ± 18.71	6.22 ± 12.31	0.530	5.58 ± 11.20	0.417
Follow-up duration (month)	25.57 ± 23.75	36.69 ± 27.55	0.581	29.77 ± 22.4	0.417

[a]Upper GI lesion includes gastric adenoma or cancer.
[b]Length of the long axis of the tumor.
[c]Tumors located in the cecum and ascending colon were categorized as Rt.colon and those located in descending colon and S-colon, rectum, were categorized as Lt.colon.

TABLE 2: Multivariate analysis for the clinicopathologic factors associated with gastric adenoma or gastric cancer in colorectal cancer patients.

Variables	Group with both synchronous and metachronous lesions			Group with only metachronous lesions		
	Odds ratio	p value	95% CI	Odds ratio	p value	95% CI
Age	1.062	0.015	1.012–1.116	1.885	0.048	1.005–3.534
BMI	1.066	0.417	0.913–1.244	1.124	0.209	0.936–1.351
Smoking	1.521	0.442	0.523–4.425	1.427	0.577	0.409–4.972
Alcohol	6.506	<0.001	2.388–17.728	6.314	0.002	1.952–20.430
Family history (solid tumor)	3.201	0.065	0.930–11.020	3.797	0.076	0.870–16.578
Differentiation	5.901	0.029	1.202–28.970	9.748	0.022	1.390–68.366
Vascular invasion	1.027	0.965	0.303–3.484	1.252	0.759	0.299–5.236
Lymphatic invasion	0.424	0.174	0.123–1.461	0.528	0.385	0.125–2.228

TABLE 3: Comparison of baseline characteristics and endoscopic findings in the subjects with colorectal cancer patients and control group.

Variables	Colorectal cancer patients ($n = 142$)	Control group ($n = 426$)	p value
Sex			0.105
Male	91 (64.1%)	240 (56.3%)	
Female	51 (35.9%)	186 (43.7%)	
Age (yrs)	65.63 ± 10.98	61.87 ± 9.99	0.184
Body weight (kg)	59.06 ± 9.23	64.67 ± 11.02	0.023
BMI (body mass index, kg/m^2)	22.71 ± 3.03	23.97 ± 3.29	0.583
Hypertension	45 (31.7%)	110 (25.8%)	0.174
Diabetes	29 (20.4%)	55 (12.9%)	0.029
Smoking	33 (23.2%)	71 (16.7%)	0.079
Alcohol	45 (31.7%)	162 (38.0%)	0.174
Family history (solid tumor)	16 (11.3%)	103 (24.2%)	0.001
Follow-up period (months)	28.3 ± 25.11	44.4 ± 25.37	0.577
Baseline endoscopic findings			
Chronic atrophic gastritis	80 (56.3%)	267 (62.7%)	0.180
Intestinal metaplasia	15 (10.6%)	24 (5.6%)	0.044
Gastric ulcer	2 (1.4%)	4 (0.9%)	0.636
Duodenal ulcer	3 (2.1%)	8 (1.9%)	0.860
Hyperplastic polyp	2 (1.4%)	20 (4.7%)	0.079
Gastric adenoma	3 (2.1%)	7 (1.6%)	0.713
Gastric cancer	10 (7.0%)	2 (0.5%)	<0.001
Subepithelial tumor (SET)	3 (2.1%)	0 (0%)	0.003

TABLE 4: Follow-up endoscopic findings in colorectal cancer group and control group.

Endoscopic findings	Colorectal cancer patients ($n = 129$)	Control group ($n = 417$)	p value
Chronic atrophic gastritis	86 (66.7%)	289 (69.3%)	0.572
Intestinal metaplasia	32 (24.8%)	56 (13.4%)	0.002
Gastric ulcer	7 (5.4%)	11 (2.6%)	0.121
Duodenal ulcer	7 (5.4%)	11 (2.6%)	0.121
Hyperplastic polyp	5 (3.9%)	35 (8.4%)	0.085
Gastric adenoma	9 (7.0%)	9 (2.2%)	0.007
Gastric cancer	13 (10.0%)	2 (0.5%)	<0.001
Subepithelial tumor (SET)	3 (2.3%)	0 (0%)	0.002

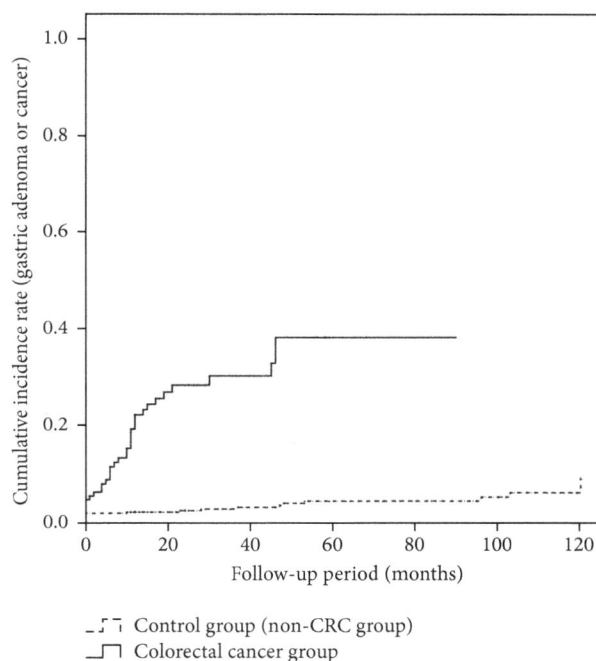

_ ⌐ ⌐ Control group (non-CRC group)
_ ⌐ Colorectal cancer group

FIGURE 2: Cumulative Incidence Rate of Gastric Adenoma or Cancer in Colorectal Cancer Patients Group and Control Group. The cumulative incidence rate was higher in the colorectal cancer patients group than in the control group over the follow-up period ($p < 0.001$). Gastric adenoma or cancer mostly developed during the first 2 years of follow-up and as late as 4 years after diagnosis.

To compare the incidence of gastric adenoma and gastric cancer between the colorectal cancer group and control group, we first compared baseline clinical characteristics and endoscopic findings. Underlying characteristics associated with the development of gastric cancer, such as age and smoking history, were not significantly different between the two groups. Body weight and diabetes were statistically significantly different between the two groups, but these factors are not known risk factors of gastric cancer. Therefore, it is difficult to say that these factors contribute to gastric cancer and gastric adenoma in the patient group. Our study, however, did not include the known risk factors of gastric cancer, such as *Helicobacter pylori* infection, patients' socioeconomic status, and blood type A, thereby limiting statistical results. Furthermore, cases of family history of solid tumors were more in the control group; this observation can be attributed solely to the data collection method: from past medical nurses' records for the patient group

and survey before health inspection for the control group. Another important finding during upper GI endoscopy, other than gastric adenoma or gastric cancer, is the prevalence of intestinal metaplasia, which was higher in the colorectal cancer group than in the control group [8]. This finding is in line with the results that gastric adenoma and gastric cancer frequently occur in intestinal metaplasia, probably through a morphological factor.

Bok et al. compared the clinical and pathological characteristics of colorectal cancer accompanied with gastric cancer and of colorectal cancer alone; they found that increased age, low BMI, and peritoneal seeding of metastatic colorectal cancer were highly related [9]. However, among patients with concomitant gastric cancer and colon cancer, as 67% of patients had gastric cancer before colon cancer, most cases of colon cancer were diagnosed at follow-up examinations for gastric cancer. Also, a previous study assessed the development of colon adenoma or colorectal cancer in patients with gastric cancer. Some studies have investigated the need for screening colonoscopy in gastric cancer patients, but there is no concrete evidence favoring follow-up upper GI endoscopy in colorectal cancer patients. However, in the present study, we assessed the incidence of precancerous lesions such as gastric adenoma or gastric cancer through follow-up upper GI endoscopy in colorectal cancer patients and analyzed the contributing factors.

For colon cancer patients who had synchronous or metachronous lesion at follow-up upper GI endoscopy, we conducted multivariate analysis using two methods. First, we included all patients with synchronous and metachronous lesion, and, second, we only included patients with metachronous lesion. In both the analyses, patients with a significant upper GI lesion were older, had a history of alcohol drinking, and had poor histological differentiation of colorectal cancer when compared with patients without lesions. In this study we did not evaluate the linear association between amount of alcohol intake and significant upper GI lesion incidence. However, previous metaanalysis study shows that there is a positive association between heavy alcohol drinking (>4 drinks per day) and gastric cancer [10]. But, heavy alcohol drinking is commonly associated with poor nutrition and this could increase the risk in heavy drinkers. So, a confounding effect due to dietary habits cannot be ruled out. And, it was not factors such as staging, vascular invasion, lymphatic infiltration of colorectal cancer, and CEA levels, but histological differentiation that affected the occurrence of gastric adenoma and gastric cancer in colorectal cancer patients. In 2010, Yoon et al. studied factors related to the occurrence of synchronous or metachronous gastric cancer in colorectal cancer patients through multivariate analysis; they found that old age, male sex, family history of solid tumors, and loss of *MSH2* expression were significantly related. On the other hand, multivariate analysis showed no statistical significance of histological differentiation, a finding different from ours [11]. This difference is possibly due to the elimination of precancerous lesions such as gastric adenoma and sole inclusion of gastric cancer.

In the colorectal cancer group, when comparing the time-dependent cumulative occurrence of gastric adenoma or gastric cancer, most lesions developed within 2 years and up to 4 years. Previous studies reported similar results in that most gastric cancer and colorectal cancer appeared within 3 years [12, 13]. Also, compared with the control group, the cumulative occurrence rate was continuously high at the time of colorectal cancer diagnosis and even during the entire follow-up period after colorectal cancer surgery [14–19]. This shows that genetic factors are also as important as

morphological factors in the pathogenesis of gastric cancer and colorectal cancer. Gastric cancer and colorectal cancer possess identical genetic changes in *p53*, *APC*, *DCC*, and *K-ras* [14–17]. Genes such as *hMLH1* and *hMSH2*, which play an important role in HNPCC, appear in 10% to 15% of sporadic gastric cancer and colorectal cancer cases [18]. Microsatellite instability (MSI) is reported to appear in 18% of solitary gastric cancer cases, and in 13% to 17% of solitary colorectal cancer cases [19], suggesting, though partially, a genetic causality.

Our study has several limitations. First, this is a retrospective analysis of past medical records of a single center. Second, data on alcohol consumption was collected solely from past medical records; therefore, exact amount or duration of alcohol consumption remains uncertain. Lastly, not all patients underwent annual follow-up upper GI endoscopy during the study period.

Our results show higher occurrence rates of precancerous lesions such as gastric adenoma and gastric cancer in colorectal patients than in the general population group. In patients with colorectal cancer, increased age, alcohol history, and poor histologic differentiation were associated with higher incidence of gastric adenoma and gastric cancer in overall patients with significant upper GI lesions, and such clinical correlation is also observed in the patients with metachronous lesions alone. Also, follow-up upper GI endoscopy revealed that most lesions appeared within 2 years and up to 4 years.

5. Conclusions

In comparison to previous studies, our results suggest that screening with upper GI endoscopy at the time of colorectal cancer diagnosis is very important, especially with factors such as increased age, history of drinking, and poor histological differentiation. It is also important to note that even if lesions such as gastric adenoma or gastric cancer are not present at the time of diagnosis in colorectal cancer patients with these risk factors, there is a high possibility of its development in the future. Therefore, it is important to perform follow-up upper GI endoscopy screening, even 4 to 5 years after colorectal cancer surgery.

Finally, further research is needed to reveal the interactive association between the development of colorectal cancer and gastric cancer, and studies on molecular biologic interactive mechanisms and larger prospective studies are needed.

Competing Interests

The authors declare that they have no competing interests regarding the publishing of this paper.

References

[1] National Cancer Center, *Annual Report of Cancer Statistics in Korea in 2010*, National Cancer Center, Goyang, Korea, 2012.

[2] C. N. Arnold, A. Goel, H. E. Blum, and C. R. Boland, "Molecular pathogenesis of colorectal cancer: implications for molecular diagnosis," *Cancer*, vol. 104, no. 10, pp. 2035–2047, 2005.

[3] W. S. Park, "Molecular pathogenesis of gastric cancer," *Journal of the Korean Medical Association*, vol. 53, no. 4, pp. 270–282, 2010.

[4] P. C. Hsia and F. H. Al-Kawas, "Yield of upper endoscopy in the evaluation of asymptomatic patients with hemoccult-positive stool after a negative colonoscopy," *American Journal of Gastroenterology*, vol. 87, no. 11, pp. 1571–1574, 1992.

[5] A. J. Geller, B. E. Kolts, S. R. Achem, and R. Wears, "The high frequency of upper gastrointestinal pathology in patients with fecal occult blood and colon polyps," *The American Journal of Gastroenterology*, vol. 88, no. 8, pp. 1184–1187, 1993.

[6] E. Joosten, B. Ghesquiere, H. Linthoudt et al., "Upper and lower gastrointestinal evaluation of elderly inpatients who are iron deficient," *American Journal of Medicine*, vol. 107, no. 1, pp. 24–29, 1999.

[7] W. G. Shin, H. Y. Kim, P. S. Heo et al., "Prevalence of upper gastrointestinal lesions in patients with or without colon polyp and cancer," *The Korean Journal of Gastroenterology*, vol. 62, pp. 27–32, 2013.

[8] P. Correa, "Human gastric carcinogenesis: a multistep and multifactorial process—first American Cancer Society award lecture on cancer epidemiology and prevention," *Cancer Research*, vol. 52, no. 24, pp. 6735–6740, 1992.

[9] H. J. Bok, J. H. Lee, J. K. Shin et al., "Clinicopathologic features of colorectal cancer combined with synchronous and metachronous gastric cancer," *The Korean Journal of Gastroenterology*, vol. 62, no. 1, pp. 27–32, 2013.

[10] I. Tramacere, E. Negri, C. Pelucchi et al., "A meta-analysis on alcohol drinking and gastric cancer risk," *Annals of Oncology*, vol. 23, no. 1, pp. 28–36, 2012.

[11] S. N. Yoon, S. T. Oh, S.-B. Lim et al., "Clinicopathologic characteristics of colorectal cancer patients with synchronous and metachronous gastric cancer," *World Journal of Surgery*, vol. 34, no. 9, pp. 2168–2176, 2010.

[12] M. Ueno, T. Muto, M. Oya, H. Ota, K. Azekura, and T. Yamaguchi, "Multiple primary cancer: an experience at the Cancer Institute Hospital with special reference to colorectal cancer," *International Journal of Clinical Oncology*, vol. 8, no. 3, pp. 162–167, 2003.

[13] H. R. Yun, L. J. Yi, Y. K. Cho et al., "Double primary malignancy in colorectal cancer patients—MSI is the useful marker for predicting double primary tumors," *International Journal of Colorectal Disease*, vol. 24, no. 4, pp. 369–375, 2009.

[14] S. Uchino, M. Noguchi, A. Ochiai, T. Saito, M. Kobayashi, and S. Hirohashi, "p53 mutation in gastric cancer: a genetic model for carcinogenesis is common to gastric and colorectal cancer," *International Journal of Cancer*, vol. 54, no. 5, pp. 759–764, 1993.

[15] S. Nakatsuru, A. Yanagisawa, S. Ichii et al., "Somatic mutation of the APC gene in gastric cancer: frequent mutations in very well differentiated adenocarcinoma and signet-ring cell carcinoma," *Human Molecular Genetics*, vol. 1, no. 8, pp. 559–563, 1992.

[16] S. Uchino, H. Tsuda, M. Noguchi et al., "Frequent loss of heterozygosity at the DCC locus in gastric cancer," *Cancer Research*, vol. 52, no. 11, pp. 3099–3102, 1992.

[17] J. Isogaki, K. Shinmura, W. Yin et al., "Microsatellite instability and K-ras mutations in gastric adenomas, with reference to associated gastric cancers," *Cancer Detection and Prevention*, vol. 23, no. 3, pp. 204–214, 1999.

[18] D. C. Chung and A. K. Rustgi, "DNA mismatch repair and cancer," *Gastroenterology*, vol. 109, no. 5, pp. 1685–1699, 1995.

[19] H. Ohtani, M. Yashiro, N. Onoda et al., "Synchronous multiple primary gastrointestinal cancer exhibits frequent microsatellite instability," *International Journal of Cancer*, vol. 86, no. 5, pp. 678–683, 2000.

5

The Application of Hemospray in Gastrointestinal Bleeding during Emergency Endoscopy

Alexander F. Hagel,[1] **Heinz Albrecht,**[1] **Andreas Nägel,**[1] **Francesco Vitali,**[1] **Marcel Vetter,**[1] **Christine Dauth,**[2] **Markus F. Neurath,**[1] **and Martin Raithel**[3]

[1]*Department of Gastroenterology, University of Erlangen, Ulmenweg 18, 91054 Erlangen, Germany*
[2]*Institute for Employment Research, Regensburger Straße 104, 90478 Nuremberg, Germany*
[3]*Department of Gastroenterology, Waldkrankenhaus St. Marien, Rathsberger Str. 57, 91054 Erlangen, Germany*

Correspondence should be addressed to Alexander F. Hagel; alexander.hagel@uk-erlangen.de

Academic Editor: Eiji Sakai

Introduction. Gastrointestinal bleeding represents the main indication for emergency endoscopy (EE). Lately, several hemostatic powders have been released to facilitate EE. *Methods.* We evaluated all EE in which Hemospray was used as primary or salvage therapy, with regard to short- and long-term hemostasis and complications. *Results.* We conducted 677 EE in 474 patients (488 examinations in 344 patients were upper GI endoscopies). Hemospray was applied during 35 examinations in 27 patients (19 males), 33 during upper and 2 during lower endoscopy. It was used after previous treatment in 21 examinations (60%) and in 14 (40%) as salvage therapy. Short-term success was reached in 34 of 35 applications (97.1%), while long-term success occurred in 23 applications (65.7%). Similar long-term results were found after primary application (64,3%) or salvage therapy (66,7%). Rebleeding was found in malignant and extended ulcers. One major adverse event (2.8%) occurred with gastric perforation after Hemospray application. *Discussion.* Hemospray achieved short-term hemostasis in virtually all cases. The long-term effect is mainly determined by the type of bleeding source, but not whether it was applied as first line or salvage therapy. But, even in the failures, patients had benefit from hemodynamic stabilization and consecutive interventions in optimized conditions.

1. Introduction

Gastrointestinal bleeding (GIB) represents a potentially life-threatening condition and is a main indication for gastrointestinal endoscopy. Its incidence is given with roughly 150 patients per 100000 population and year, with a mortality rate of still 10% [1, 2]. Various bleeding sources may be identified and they may be induced either because of an underlying morbidity with ulcerative and nonulcerative lesions, respectively (e.g., ulcers, esophageal varices, and gastrointestinal vascular malformations), and malignancy or as a consequence of iatrogenic interventions (e.g., postpolypectomy bleeding) [3]. In addition, GIB becomes an emerging issue in the light of increasing numbers of disease entities requiring strict anticoagulant therapy with increasing use of new direct oral anticoagulants (DOAC) [4].

Hemostasis can be achieved according to the type of lesion and extent of bleeding by injection of saline, diluted epinephrine solution, macrogollaurylether (e.g., aethoxysklerol), the application of various types of through-the-scope (TTS) or over-the-scope clips (OTSC), or using argon-plasma-coagulation and other thermic coagulation procedures [5]. Despite these possibilities, 10–30% of all patients remain in which an endoscopic hemostasis cannot be obtained, or in which a prompt recurrence of the bleeding occurs [2, 6–8].

Recently, sprayable powders for induction of immediate bleeding stop were introduced in gastrointestinal endoscopy. The latest innovative system introduced into clinical use is the EndoClot system (EndoClot Plus Inc., Santa Clara, CA, USA) which consists of starch, while the Hemospray (Cook Medical, Winston-Salem, NC, USA) consisting of an inorganic powder is the most widely used chemical in this regard [5]. It exerts multimodal mechanisms to achieve hemostasis, becoming cohesive and adhesive after coming in contact with moisture hence forming a stable mechanical barrier, sealing the bleeding site. Due to its composition, it is neither absorbed nor metabolized within the mucosa, hence minimizing the risk of systemic toxicity [6].

Previous studies described Hemospray as a feasible and possible new option to obtain rapid hemostasis during gastrointestinal endoscopy either as primary treatment option [9–14] or as a salvage indication, when refractory bleeding persists despite application of other conventional methods (e.g., injection therapy and clips) [11, 14]. In these studies with defined inclusion and exclusion criteria, a high initial success of up to 100% is reported. However, rebleeding rates, depending on the bleeding source of up to 38.9%, are noted in literature [5]. The aim of this paper is to report the indications, experience, results, and adverse events from the use of Hemospray between August 2013 and November 2014 from a high-volume endoscopy university center investigating unselected consecutive emergency patients.

2. Material and Methods

2.1. Patient Collective. In this study, we included all consecutive patients in whom the use of Hemospray was deemed necessary for achieving successful hemostasis. Between August 2013 and November 2014 all emergency endoscopies (EE) for the indication of GIB were analyzed. Endoscopies were defined as EE when patients presented with signs of acute bleeding (e.g., coffee-ground or fresh blood vomit, melena, and perianal bleeding) and/or anemia (hemoglobin < 10 g/dL) and/or compromised cardiovascular parameters (hypotonia, tachycardia). Emergency endoscopies fulfilling above listed criteria were routinely conducted within 6 hours after initial presentation.

Depending on the suspected bleeding source, either gastroscopy, colonoscopy, or both were performed within the emergency examination.

All patients resulted from daily routine or emergency schedule and represented nonselected patients arising from real-life conditions. In 27 patients, Hemospray was applied and they were thus enrolled for further detailed analysis.

Hemospray is not the first possible intervention during EE in our department when coagulation parameters are normal or moderately altered. In patients without severely disturbed coagulation, Hemospray was generally used as salvage therapy. In patients under therapeutic anticoagulation or with severely disturbed coagulation, Hemospray was also used as a primary therapeutic modality.

The data obtained was prospectively entered in a database and retrospectively evaluated. Approval for this study was obtained from the local ethics committee.

2.2. Indications and Performance of Emergency Endoscopy (EE). EE was performed in standard manner with Olympus gastroduodenoscopes (GIF 1T160, GIFH180) and Pentax colonoscopes (FC-38M) in the case of acute GIB (hematemesis, hematochezia, and melena) and/or suspected

GIB because of anemia and hypovolemic shock or deterioration of physical status in patients with known underlying GIB source. EE was performed during pethidine and midazolam or pethidine and propofol analgosedation, respectively. Erythromycin before EE was given to some patients after decision of the endoscopists on duty. Standard examination of gastroscopy or colonoscopy was performed with cleansing of each segment to identify the bleeding source(s).

Usually, conventional bleeding treatment was applied with a stepwise treatment approach, for example, (i) first injection techniques (epinephrine 1 : 100000, fibrin glue (Baxter, Unterschleißheim, Germany)); or (ii) in case of visible vessels, perforating or gapping lesions through-the-scope (TTS) or over-the-scope clips (OTSC) were tried (Olympus, Hamburg, or Ovesco, Tübingen, Germany); (iii) in variceal bleeding band ligation technique (6 Shooter Saeed Multi-Band-Ligator, Cook Medical, Bloomington, IN, USA) or injection of Histoacryl (n-butyl-2-cyanoacrylat/lipiodol mixture), respectively, was used; (iv) diffuse tumor bleeding or angiectasias were treated by argon-plasma-coagulation (BOWA Electronics Arc 400, Gomaringen, Germany, or ERBE VIO 200, Tübingen, Germany).

Following this stepwise endoscopic treatment approach using these modalities (i–iv), Hemospray was not intentionally used as the primary treatment option in most patients. Only in patients with diffuse mucosal bleeding combined with a severe coagulopathy (e.g., due to liver cirrhosis) or with therapeutic anticoagulation (e.g., intake of vitamin K antagonists (VKA) or direct oral anticoagulants (DOAC)) Hemospray was held as a possible option for primary bleeding treatment to avoid any risky tissue manipulation (table indications).

2.3. Hemospray Application. Hemospray was applied using the standard 10 French catheter which is supplied by the manufacturer (Cook Medical, Bloomington, Indiana, USA) [9]. Normally, Hemospray is applied in bursts, which release 1–5 g of powder each. In order to prevent sticking of the catheter tip in moisture and hence clotting of the catheter, release of powder was normally started with the tip being 2-3 cm away from the bleeding source.

2.4. Study Parameters, Definitions, and Statistics. The primary aim of this study was to assess whether Hemospray application resulted in successful bleeding treatment (short-term and long-term hemostasis) with stop of bleeding from the causal lesion at least for 5 minutes under direct visual endoscopic observation. These findings were each documented in the Viewpoint files and the clinical data register.

Secondary aims were recurrence rate, side effects, and outcome parameters in the patients treated with Hemospray.

Short-term success of bleeding treatment was defined as direct hemostasis, achieved during EE and no further bleeding signs within the next 24 hours.

Long-term success of bleeding treatment was defined as no further bleeding event and/or treatment for at least 30 days after the index EE.

However, another bleeding source than the originally treated one which may have occurred after or independently from the index EE did not affect registration of the long-term success related to the treated lesion.

3. Results

3.1. Frequency of Hemospray Requirement in Emergency Endoscopy (EE). During the study period of 15 months 488 upper GI EE in 345 patients were registered. Twenty-seven of 345 patients with emergency GIB (7,8%) received at least one Hemospray application. In total, in these 25 patients 33 applications of Hemospray were recorded (1.2 Hemospray applications per patient).

In 344 of these 488 upper GI endoscopies, a bleeding source could be identified. In 158 examinations, ulcers have been found as bleeding source (Forrest Ia: 31, Ib 61, IIa 27, IIb 39). Variceal ligature was performed in 23 patients.

We conducted further 189 emergency colonoscopies in 130 patients. During two of these examinations (1.05%), Hemospray was applied.

In three patients, previous EE were conducted, with Hemospray being applied in a follow-up endoscopy. In one patient, an endoscopic intervention was conducted previously (ligature of esophageal varices with consecutive bleeding of the ligature ulcer). In two further examinations, diffuse gastral erosions in one patient and an erythematous anastomosis following gastrectomy were recorded, without initial bleeding signs. In follow-up endoscopies, diffuse bleeding instances in these areas were found and a primary Hemospray application was conducted.

3.2. Bleeding Sources, Patient Characteristics, Hemostasis, and Recurrence Rate. The characteristics of all patients in whom Hemospray was applied are listed in Table 1 according to their main indications and bleeding sources. Next to a plethora of GIB sources during upper GI endoscopy, two anastomotic ulcers in the colon were treated with a Hemospray application, which was performed as an off-label use. The different bleeding sources have been subdivided according to the following therapy in Table 2.

Hemostasis rates are listed in Table 3 and assigned to upper or lower GIB. Short-term success with hemostasis (24 h) was high with 97.1% and was recorded in nearly all applications except for one fatal bleeding case. However, long-term success decreased to 65.7% after 30 days of observation.

Recurrent bleeding was found after treatment with Hemospray after 11 examinations (31.4%) in 10 patients (37.0%).

3.3. Use of Hemospray as Salvage Treatment. Previous bleeding treatment was performed in 21 of 35 examinations (60.0%). Here, Hemospray was used as salvage therapy because of failure of conventional bleeding treatment. Thus, among all EE performed during this time period 4,3% (21/488 EE) presented as real refractory emergency bleeding.

Previous bleeding treatment was conducted in bleeding esophageal varices by ligature but did not achieve the defined bleeding stop; thus the ligatures were combined with Hemospray for definitive hemostasis. In bleeding ulcers, injection of epinephrine with/without fibrin glue with/without the

TABLE 1: Patient characteristics and frequency distribution of the treatment indications. In several patients suffering from upper GI bleeding, more than one endoscopy involving hemostatic measures and the application of Hemospray was necessary. Hence, we recorded more examinations involving interventional measures than patients. Merely second look endoscopies without further necessary interventions have not been calculated here.

Male/female	19/8	
Age	Median 72 years, range 40–88 years	
	Patients	Examinations
Upper GI bleeding	25	33
Lower GI bleeding	2	2
Bleeding source		
Ulcers	13	18
Tumor	2	4
Postinterventional	3	4
Diffuse bleeding	6	6
Reflux esophagitis	2	2
Others	1	1
Total examinations	27	35

TABLE 2: Bleeding sources as noted during emergency endoscopy, divided according to the kind of Hemospray application (primary treatment versus salvage therapy).

	Primary therapy	Salvage therapy
Bleeding source		
Ulcers	6	11
Tumor	2	2
Postinterventional	1	2
Diffuse bleeding	3	3
Variceal bleeding	1	1
Reflux esophagitis	0	2
Others	1	0
Total examinations	14	21

application of hemoclips was performed without effect until finally Hemospray was used.

Previous endoscopic therapy can be split into two categories. In seven patients, one procedure was conducted (ligature of esophageal varices and injection of fibrin glue in one patient each and injection of diluted suprarenin solution in five patients). Main indications of a sole injection therapy were diffuse larger bleeding sources without visible vessels. Here, the hemostatic powder was estimated as superior to mechanical or thermic alternatives.

In eight patients, two interventions were futile in achieving hemostasis. In all patients, diluted suprarenin was used, in combinations with through-the-scope (TTS) clips (four patients), over-the-scope clips (OTSC) (one patient), and the additional injection of fibrin glue (in three patients).

TABLE 3: Short-term success was defined as successful hemostasis during endoscopy persisting for at least 24 hours. Long-term success was defined as no further bleeding from the treated bleeding source within 30 days. One patient died during EE due to an aortoesophageal fistula. Three more patients died due to septic multiorganic failure during the hospital stay; one patient died due to liver failure following cirrhosis. These four fatalities were not linked to emergency endoscopy.

	Per examination	Per patient
Overall success		
Short-term	34/35 (97.1%)	**26/27 (96.3%)**
Long-term	23/35 (65.7%)	**17/27 (63.0%)**
Success upper GIB		
Examinations	33	**25**
Short-term success	32 (97,0%)	**24 (96%)**
Long-term success	21 (63,6%)	**15 (60%)**
Long-term success		
Primary therapy	9/14 (64,3%)	
Salvage therapy	14/21 (66,7%)	
Success lower GIB		
Endoscopy	2	2
Examinations	2 (100%)	2 (100%)
Short-term success	2 (100%)	2 (100%)
Long-term success	2 (100%)	2 (100%)
Unsuccessful treatment = recurrent bleeding	**11/33 (33.3%)**	**11/25 (44.0%)**
Ulcers	9	9
Carcinoma	2	2
Fatalities	**5/35 (14.2%)**	**5/27 (18.5%)**
Bleeding associated	1	1
Others	4	4
Further interventions	**10/35 (28,6%)**	**10/27 (37,0%)**
Emergency surgery	3	3
Reendoscopy	6	6
Radiologic coiling	1	1
Technical failure	1/35 (2.8%) Clotting of catheter	1/27 (3.7%)

In six patients, even a combination of diluted suprarenin solution and two further measures was insufficient in achieving hemostasis. In detail, the combination of TTS and argon-plasma-coagulation (APC) was used in two patients, the additional combination of fibrin glue and OTSC in one patient, and TTS and fibrin glue in three patients. The main problems of futile mechanical measures were mainly ulcers in the posterior wall of the duodenum, in which the bleeding area could not be grasped completely or oozing bleeding remained after previous therapy (Figures 1(a)–1(c)).

3.4. Hemospray as Primary Hemostasis Method. In the remaining 14 examinations (40%), Hemospray was used as singular approach (primary treatment) without previous

conventional treatment steps because of (at least) one of the following reasons:

1 of 27 patients (3.7%) required Hemospray application because of analgosedation failure with an extremely restless patient. Hemospray was applied to at least terminate the bleeding temporarily in order to improve sedation and vital parameters.

One fulminant arterial bleeding instance (3,7%) from the gastroduodenal artery required primary Hemospray to terminate bleeding temporarily and to gain some time for preparation of an emergency surgical procedure in stable conditions.

Further primary Hemospray applications were done in 4 patients (14,8%) presenting with diffuse gastric or duodenal bleeding in which the bleeding source could not be detected.

Finally, severely impaired coagulation due to liver cirrhosis or therapeutic anticoagulation stipulated Hemospray in 6 patients (22,2%).

3.5. Hemospray Application in Patients with Impaired Coagulation. Fifteen examinations (42,9%) were conducted with an impaired coagulation system. An impaired coagulation system was defined as thrombocytes < 50000/uL or an INR > 1,8 in an acute bleeding situation or the intake of NOAKs. In six patients, coagulation was altered medicamentously by Warfarin in two and Rivaroxaban in two patients. The coagulation was optimized in the patients on Warfarin with prothrombin concentrates before the examination. In these patients, endoscopic standard procedures were conducted and failed to achieve hemostasis. Hence Hemospray achieved hemostasis as salvage method. Both patients with Rivaroxaban showed diffuse bleeding. Here, Hemospray was successfully used as primary method.

Eight patients suffered from an impaired coagulation due to liver cirrhosis and one due to a liver transplant rejection. All of them received prothrombin concentrates, fresh frozen plasm, or thrombocyte concentrates, depending on the actual parameters. In five, first line interventions failed, while Hemospray was used as first treatment in four patients.

3.6. Analysis of Clinical Conditions with and without Hemospray Efficiency. Overall, Hemospray proved to obtain at least a short-term hemostasis in virtually all cases (34/35, 97.1%). Only in one patient (3.7%), in whom an esophageal carcinoma caused an aortoesophageal fistula with massive torrential bleeding, EE was performed during cardiopulmonal resuscitation. Here the application of Hemospray was ineffective because of the massive extent of bleeding. Hemospray application during resuscitation measures was further technically ineffective because of lacking space with air in the tubular esophagus flooded with blood from the aorta, causing repeated clotting of the application catheter.

In 16 of 27 patients (59.3%) in which Hemospray could be applied, a permanent success could be achieved without any rebleeding within 30 days from the same bleeding source. In the remaining 10 of 27 patients (37.0%) recurrent bleeding was encountered in patients either with extremely deep ulceration which had eroded an artery (mainly the gastroduodenal artery) or with malignant lesions.

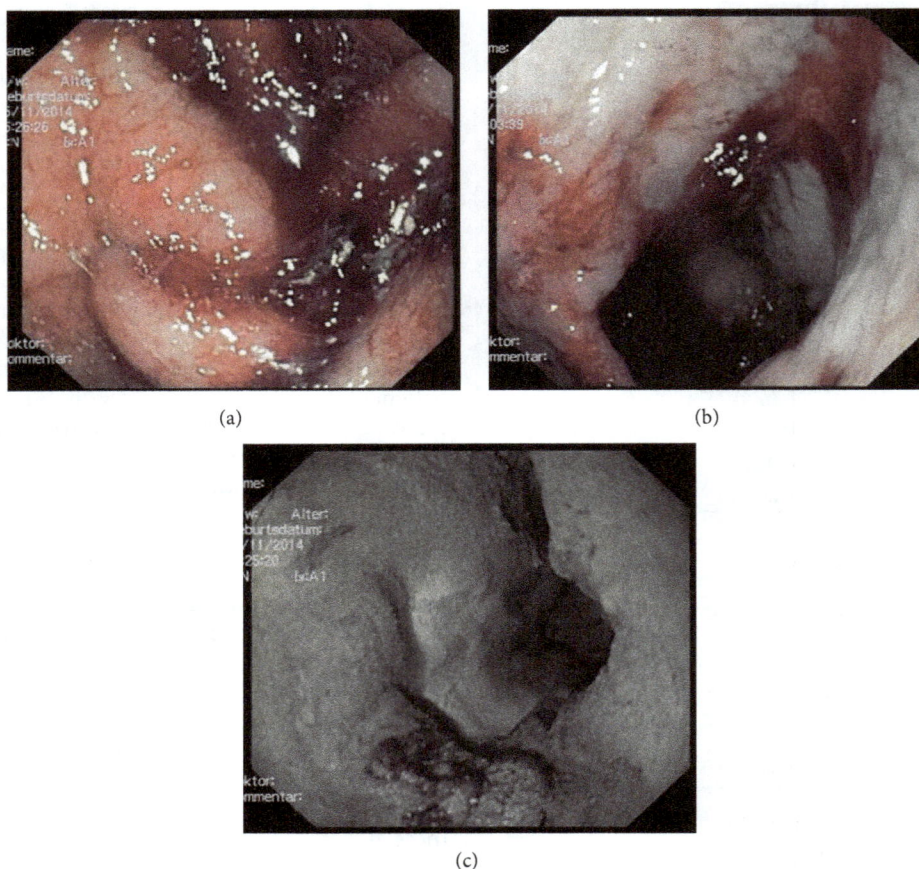

(a)   (b)

(c)

FIGURE 1: (a)–(c): acute antral bleeding (a), which cannot be terminated by injection of diluted epinephrine solution (200 mL in total) (b). After the application of Hemospray, hemostasis can finally be achieved (c).

At least, in these patients, the application of Hemospray stabilized the patients' conditions; hence further treatment (clip application in a second endoscopy, radiologic coiling of the corresponding artery, or a surgical procedure) could be conducted in a stable setting. Two of these patients suffered from gastric carcinoma causing diffuse bleeding. In these patients, rebleeding occurred, albeit all endoscopic measures were exhausted. In one patient, a gastrectomy was performed; in the second, coiling of the gastroduodenal artery was performed, terminating the GIB permanently.

In two patients suffering from esophageal varices, Hemospray was applied. In both, ligature was conducted as first line therapy. While in one, oozing bleeding was seen directly after the intervention, the second patient showed initially a sufficient hemostasis with recurring bleeding signs (fresh blood in the gastral probe) after 6 hours. As correlate, oozing bleeding next to one of the ligatures could be identified. In both, Hemospray application terminated the bleeding immediately and permanently. Hence further rescue interventions, for example, TIPS, could be spared.

3.7. Analysis of Mortality Cases from Gastrointestinal Bleeding (GIB). Of note, in this cohort with refractory or severe GIB 5 out of 27 patients (18.5%) died during the hospital stay. Three patients (11.1%) died due to septic multiorganic failure,

not related to EE. In these patients, death was not related to endoscopy or the GIB in any means.

In one patient, suffering from ethyl-toxic cirrhosis (3.7%), a duodenal ulcer caused an erosion of the gastroduodenal artery. In this patient, numerous endoscopies were performed in order to achieve hemostasis. Hemospray was only effective for achieving short-term hemostasis but could not induce long-term efficacy. Since this was not successful, the ulcer was even treated surgically twice. But no intervention was successful to cease the intermittent GIB including surgical measures. The patient developed several further complications, for example, renal failure and pneumonia; thus the medical treatment was then limited in due course.

In the fifth patient, an esophageal carcinoma caused an esophago-aorto fistula, requiring massive blood transfusions and mechanical life support. During EE the Hemospray proved to be ineffective in view of the massive bleeding and life resuscitation and, technically, the catheter could not be deployed appropriately due to clotting of the Hemospray within the catheters. Hence, no hemostasis could be reached and life support was terminated due to the infaust prognosis in this patient.

3.8. Major Adverse Events from Hemospray Application. In one patient (3.7%), EE was conducted due to melena following ischaemic colitis with complete colectomy and consecutive generalized peritonitis. The gastric anterior wall presented additionally with diffuse bleeding. Due to the compromised anticoagulation, Hemospray was administered. Immediately after the application, a new recess with white and fatty tissue appeared and could be documented. Hence laparotomy was performed rapidly after EE. Here an 8 cm perforation in this area was found and sewed. This major adverse event was closely related to Hemospray application. It seems possible that the forces which emerge during the release of the powder might have ruptured the tissue and caused the perforation of an apparently inflamed tissue.

4. Discussion

Hemospray is a new device for the treatment of GIB. Its efficient use in achieving hemostasis has been described as first line therapy previously [15, 16]. In our endoscopy department, Hemospray is normally only used as first line therapy in patients with a severely disturbed coagulation system. Otherwise, it is applied as salvage therapy, when other routine measures for the treatment of acute GIB fail (e.g., injection of epinephrine or fibrin, mechanical therapy by application of TTS or OTS clips, and thermal therapy). In various studies, a combination of these interventions has shown better short- and long-term effects in achieving hemostasis during EE [17, 18]. Hence a combination of two modalities is recommended in endoscopic guidelines [19]. In our patients, in which Hemospray was used as salvage therapy, a combination of at least two of the above listed traditional tools has normally been applied without achieving hemostasis. An exception presented patients with diffuse mucosal bleeding. After futile injection therapy, Hemospray was applied in several patients instead of mechanical or thermal alternatives.

When analyzing the cases where Hemospray was used as salvage therapy after unsuccessful conventional treatments, a subpopulation of 4.3% of all patients was identified among all EE with severe refractory GIB. Hence we represent real-life data of an unselected patient collective, since bleeding in most EE can be terminated by one or a combination of the mentioned methods. In these 4.3% of patients we found a substantial number of severe underlying diseases, such as liver cirrhosis and advanced stages of malignancies, complicating endoscopic hemostasis. If Hemospray would not have been available during these interventions, these patients would have very likely required emergency surgical or urgent radiological treatment. Thus, Hemospray represents a valuable emergency tool for approximately 5% of all patients with progredient GIB.

In our cohort, in total, Hemospray was found to be an efficient tool to achieve hemostasis during EE with a high short-term success rate of 97% and a moderate long-term success of 65,7%. Similar promising results have been described in literature [5, 9–11]. However, after the successful initial endoscopy, high rebleeding rates can be found, as we encountered in our population recurrent bleeding in 31% after all examinations. Thus, despite its rapid procoagulative and covering effects, Hemospray did not appear

to stimulate wound healing or tissue remodeling rapidly. Similar comparable rebleeding rates of 20–40% have been found in previous studies [9–14, 20]. In these studies, the rebleeding rate could be related to additional risk factors, such as antithrombotic therapy or malignancies [4, 12]. In our cohort, we can also confirm futile long-term hemostasis in advanced malignancies due to often accompanying necrotic tissue, exposed vessels, and increased contact-vulnerability of the tissue. Furthermore, we have encountered problems with, especially, long-term hemostasis, in ulcerations with an eroded artery in our collective.

For the long-term failure in arterial bleeding, covering the arterial vessel by Hemospray powder lasted very likely just not long enough to enable a sufficient fibrin clot formation or subsequent reendothelialization. Hence, when the Hemospray was washed off, rebleeding occurred. Similarly, in malignancies, progredient tissue destruction and necrosis contributed to several recurrences of GIB after Hemospray used in these areas. However, the application of Hemospray can be seen as partially successful in these patients, especially with regard to enabling the endoscopists to create an intermittent hemostasis for a restricted time in order to buy time to stabilize the cardiovascular situation of the patient, to administer blood transfusions and/or coagulation factors if necessary, and to organize further therapy (e.g., surgery). However, Hemospray does not represent a fire and forget device which guarantees a long-term hemostasis in all patients. Ten of 27 patients (37.0%) developed recurrent rebleeding within the observation period of 30 days.

During daily routine, we found the utilization of Hemospray beneficial in patients with markedly reduced anticoagulation (e.g., Warfarin or DOAC, or due to underlying diseases). In these situations, injection therapy or the application of clips can cause mucosal damage or may increase vessel lesions accidentally, resulting in further increasing the likelihood of severe or recurrent GIB. In several patients with reduced anticoagulation, especially with diffuse bleeding, Hemospray was used as first line therapy to create hemostasis and showed a high long-term success in all of these cases. Interestingly, in the case of DOAC bleeding the high rate of short-term success by Hemospray is of great value, because all DOAC have short half-lives of around 10–12 hours except in severe renal insufficiency or hepatic failure [4]. The intermittent hemostasis provided by Hemospray in nearly all cases helps to overcome their therapeutic anticoagulative effects. Thereafter, coagulation normalizes and the likelihood increases that vascular lesions may be closed by endogenous fibrin formation or after repeated endoscopic therapy. Thus, DOAC induced diffuse bleeding without significant obvious pathology represents a further valuable indication for Hemospray application.

As described above, previous studies applied Hemospray either as primary or as salvage therapy. In our cohort, the application was based on the choice of the endoscopists. Hence, we can compare the results of both indications in our cohort. On the one hand, the indications for primary (diffuse or malignant bleeding, especially with temporarily compromised coagulation parameters) and salvage therapy (bleeding ulcers, in which injection and mechanical therapy were insufficient, especially in hard to reach lesions) differed. On the other hand, we have found similar long-term results, with rebleeding in more than one third of the patients in every subgroup. In these patients, larger (arterial) vessels in inflamed ulcers or diffuse malignant lesions will not heal sufficiently for endoscopic hemostasis alone. Here, hemostasis can be reached for the moment, buying time to stabilize the patient and proceed to further treatments (surgical or radiological).

During the study period of 15 months, we encountered one possible complication caused by the application of Hemospray. In the above described setting, the pressure caused by the CO_2 release is deemed to be responsible for a perforation of the inflamed gastric wall. After Hemospray application an 8 cm large gastric perforation with view to the peritoneum appeared requiring surgery directly after gastroscopy. As reported from the literature this is a feared side effect of Hemospray application [14, 21], but this was the single one major complication resulting from 35 Hemospray applications in 27 patients (3,7%) in our population.

In our patient collective, we found a fairly high 30-day all-cause mortality rate of 18,5% with 5 deaths among 27 patients. However, only one death was directly caused by an untreatable massive GIB from a malignant aortoesophageal fistula, a condition where Hemospray was also ineffective due to technical reasons, bleeding extent and resuscitation. Bleeding related mortality was documented only in this patient (1/27; 3.7%). Thus, it is lower than reported from others in EE [3]. The other remaining fatalities resulted due to septic multiorganic failure in three (11,1%) and due to decompensated liver cirrhosis in one patient (3,7%), further demonstrating the number of challenges which are routinely encountered in this patient collective.

5. Conclusion

Hemospray enlarges the armament of emergency endoscopists. It is a safe and easy to use device which can be used in upper and lower endoscopy both as first line treatment and as salvage therapy with short-term effectiveness of 97%. However, it should not be assigned as a magic bullet, since long-term success was found to be only 60% after 30 days. We have encountered several rebleeding instances within 12–24 hours in up to 37% of patients, especially in malignancy or deep ulcerations of larger eroded arteries. These tend to rebleed after the elimination of Hemospray from the bleeding source. However, even these patients showed a benefit from the treatment, since intermittent bleeding cessation allows the stabilization of hemodynamic parameters and patients' clinical condition and gives time to plan onwards a definite treatment (e.g., surgery) in a controlled setting.

Appendix

Role of Hemospray and Its Indications in Emergency Endoscopy (EE)

Short-term hemostasis provided by Hemospray may give time

 (i) for cardiovascular stabilization,

 (ii) for substitution of blood products (erythrocyte concentrates) or coagulation factors,

 (iii) for spontaneous recovery of coagulation parameters in DOAC-treated patient,

 (iv) to organize further semielective radiological or surgical treatment,

 (v) to support the endoscopy team by experienced supervisors,

 (vi) to achieve rapid bleeding stop in restless patients, analog-sedation induced complications, or patients with high ASA scores (3-4).

Favourable Hemospray Indications

 (i) Diffuse bleeding (e.g., erosions, anticoagulated patients, or coagulopathy)

  (a) Superficial to deep ulcers without significant erosion of a large artery

  (b) Ulcerated lesions with venous bleeding

  (c) Quick hemostasis in restless patients (e.g., alcohol withdrawal and high comorbidity)

 (ii) Bleeding after endoscopic interventions (e.g., large polypectomy and papillectomy).

Unfavourable Hemospray Indications

 (i) Strong arterial bleeding and erosion of a submucosal or deeper located artery (e.g., gastroduodenalis)

  (a) Aortoesophageal fistula with great leakage.

Relative Contraindications

 (i) Ischaemic or severely inflamed gastrointestinal wall

  (a) Lesions with suspected covered perforation

  (b) Location near diverticula.

Abbreviations

DOAC: Direct oral anticoagulants
EE: Emergency endoscopy
GIB: Gastrointestinal bleeding
VKA: Vitamin K antagonists.

Competing Interests

The authors declare that they have no competing interests.

References

[1] J. D. Lewis, W. B. Bilker, C. Brensinger, J. T. Farrar, and B. L. Strom, "Hospitalization and mortality rates from peptic ulcer disease and GI bleeding in the 1990s: relationship to sales of nonsteroidal anti-inflammatory drugs and acid suppression medications," *American Journal of Gastroenterology*, vol. 97, no. 10, pp. 2540–2549, 2002.

[2] S. A. Hearnshaw, R. F. A. Logan, D. Lowe, S. P. L. Travis, M. F. Murphy, and K. R. Palmer, "Acute upper gastrointestinal bleeding in the UK: patient characteristics, diagnoses and outcomes in the 2007 UK audit," *Gut*, vol. 60, no. 10, pp. 1327–1335, 2011.

[3] B. S. Kim, B. T. Li, A. Engel et al., "Diagnosis of gastrointestinal bleeding: a practical guide for clinicians," *World Journal of Gastrointestinal Pathophysiology*, vol. 5, no. 4, pp. 467–478, 2014.

[4] I. L. Holster, V. E. Valkhoff, E. J. Kuipers, and E. T. T. L. Tjwa, "New oral anticoagulants increase risk for gastrointestinal bleeding: a systematic review and meta-analysis," *Gastroenterology*, vol. 145, no. 1, pp. 105.e15–112.e15, 2013.

[5] J. Jacques, R. Legros, S. Chaussade, and D. Sautereau, "Endoscopic haemostasis: an overview of procedures and clinical scenarios," *Digestive and Liver Disease*, vol. 46, no. 9, pp. 766–776, 2014.

[6] I. M. Gralnek, A. N. Barkun, and M. Bardou, "Management of acute bleeding from a peptic ulcer," *New England Journal of Medicine*, vol. 359, no. 9, pp. 928–937, 2008.

[7] D. J. Bjorkman, A. Zaman, M. B. Fennerty, D. Lieberman, J. A. DiSario, and G. Guest-Warnick, "Urgent vs. elective endoscopy for acute non-variceal upper-GI bleeding: an effectiveness study," *Gastrointestinal Endoscopy*, vol. 60, no. 1, pp. 1–8, 2004.

[8] N. I. Church and K. R. Palmer, "Diagnostic and therapeutic endoscopy," *Current Opinion in Gastroenterology*, vol. 15, no. 6, pp. 504–508, 1999.

[9] J. J. Y. Sung, D. Luo, J. C. Y. Wu et al., "Early clinical experience of the safety and effectiveness of Hemospray in achieving hemostasis in patients with acute peptic ulcer bleeding," *Endoscopy*, vol. 43, no. 4, pp. 291–295, 2011.

[10] M. Ibrahim, A. El-Mikkawy, I. Mostafa, and J. Devière, "Endoscopic treatment of acute variceal hemorrhage by using hemostatic powder TC-325: A Prospective Pilot Study," *Gastrointestinal Endoscopy*, vol. 78, no. 5, pp. 769–773, 2013.

[11] L. A. Smith, A. J. Stanley, J. J. Bergman et al., "Hemospray application in nonvariceal upper gastrointestinal bleeding: results of the survey to evaluate the application of hemospray in the luminal tract," *Journal of Clinical Gastroenterology*, vol. 48, no. 10, pp. e89–e92, 2014.

[12] I. L. Holster, E. J. Kuipers, and E. T. T. L. Tjwa, "Hemospray in the treatment of upper gastrointestinal hemorrhage in patients on antithrombotic therapy," *Endoscopy*, vol. 45, no. 1, pp. 63–66, 2013.

[13] M. C. Sulz, R. Frei, C. Meyenberger, P. Bauerfeind, G.-M. Semadeni, and C. Gubler, "Routine use of hemospray for gastrointestinal bleeding: prospective two-center experience in Switzerland," *Endoscopy*, vol. 46, no. 7, pp. 619–624, 2014.

[14] A. H. L. Yau, G. Ou, C. Galorport et al., "Safety and efficacy of Hemospray® in upper gastrointestinal bleeding," *Canadian Journal of Gastroenterology and Hepatology*, vol. 28, no. 2, Article ID 759436, pp. 72–76, 2014.

[15] E. Masci, M. Arena, E. Morandi, P. Viaggi, and B. Mangiavillano, "Upper gastrointestinal active bleeding ulcers: review of literature on the results of endoscopic techniques and our experience with Hemospray," *Scandinavian Journal of Gastroenterology*, vol. 49, no. 11, pp. 1290–1295, 2014.

[16] M. Bustamante-Balén and G. Plumé, "Role of hemostatic powders in the endoscopic management of gastrointestinal bleeding," *World Journal of Gastrointestinal Pathophysiology*, vol. 5, no. 3, pp. 284–292, 2014.

[17] M. Vergara, C. Bennett, X. Calvet, and J. P. Gisbert, "Epinephrine injection versus epinephrine injection and a second endoscopic method in high-risk bleeding ulcers," *The Cochrane Database of Systematic Reviews*, vol. 10, Article ID CD005584, 2014.

[18] R. Marmo, G. Rotondano, R. Piscopo, M. A. Bianco, R. D'Angella, and L. Cipolletta, "Dual therapy versus monotherapy in the endoscopic treatment of high-risk bleeding ulcers: a meta-analysis of controlled trials," *American Journal of Gastroenterology*, vol. 102, no. 2, pp. 279–289, 2007.

[19] J. H. Hwang, D. A. Fisher, T. Ben-Menachem et al., "The role of endoscopy in the management of acute non-variceal upper GI bleeding," *Gastrointestinal Endoscopy*, vol. 75, no. 6, pp. 1132–1138, 2012.

[20] I. L. Holster, E. Brullet, E. J. Kuipers, R. Campo, A. Fernández-Atutxa, and E. T. T. L. Tjwa, "Hemospray treatment is effective for lower gastrointestinal bleeding," *Endoscopy*, vol. 46, no. 1, pp. 75–78, 2014.

[21] L. A. Smith, A. J. Morris, and A. J. Stanley, "The use of hemospray in portal hypertensive bleeding; a case series," *Journal of Hepatology*, vol. 60, no. 2, pp. 457–460, 2014.

6

Replaceable Jejunal Feeding Tubes in Severely Ill Children

Tabea Pang, Sergio B. Sesia, Stefan Holland-Cunz, and Johannes Mayr

Department of Pediatric Surgery, University Children's Hospital Basel, Spitalstrasse 33, 4056 Basel, Switzerland

Correspondence should be addressed to Johannes Mayr; johannes.mayr@ukbb.ch

Academic Editor: Martin Hubner

Long-term enteral nutrition in chronically ill, malnourished children represents a clinical challenge if adequate feeding via nasogastric or gastrostomy tubes fails. We evaluated the usefulness and complications of a new type of surgical jejunostomy that allows for easier positioning and replacement of the jejunal feeding tube in children. We surgically inserted replaceable jejunal feeding tubes (RJFT) connected to a guide thread which exited through a separate tiny opening of the abdominal wall. In a retrospective case series, we assessed the effectiveness and complications of this technique in severely ill children suffering from malnutrition and complex disorders. Three surgical complications occurred, and these were addressed by reoperation. Four children died from their severe chronic disorders within the study period. The RJFT permitted continuous enteral feeding and facilitated easy replacement of the tube. After the postoperative period, jejunal feeding by RJFT resulted in adequate weight gain. This feeding access represents an option for children in whom sufficient enteral nutrition by nasogastric tubes or gastrostomy proved impossible. Further studies are required to investigate the safety and effectiveness of this surgical technique in a larger case series.

1. Introduction

Long-term enteral nutrition results in better bowel regeneration, a lower rate of infective complications, and fewer side effects when compared to long-term parenteral nutrition [1, 2]. In addition, enteral nutrition prevents parenteral nutrition-associated liver disease (PNALD) [3]. Moreover, extravasation of parenteral nutrition solution can result in soft tissue damage [4], and insertion of intravenous lines is painful for children and incurs stress to caregivers and hospital staff [5].

Gastrostomy feeding has gained widespread acceptance for long-term enteral nutrition in children unable to eat or drink sufficient quantities. It allows for bolus feeding and ensures safer administration of enteral nutrients when compared to other types of long-term enteral nutrition techniques. However, in children suffering from neurologic impairment, severe gastroesophageal reflux disease (GERD), or disorders of gastric or esophageal motility, feeding by gastrostomy is frequently accompanied by complications such as recurrent aspiration, regurgitation, aerophagia, recurrent vomiting, and weight loss [6, 7]. Although fundoplication has gained widespread acceptance among pediatric surgeons in the treatment of severe GERD, the high rate of GERD recurrence and more frequent postoperative complications in neurologically impaired, malnourished children have made jejunostomy feeding an accepted alternative to establish long-term enteral feeding access in these children [7–10]. Several techniques for insertion of jejunal feeding tubes have been proposed, such as JET-PEG [11–13], fine-needle catheter jejunostomy, endoscopically guided, laparoscopically controlled, percutaneously inserted jejunal feeding tubes or buttons [8, 12–14], or insertion of jejunal feeding tubes by laparotomy or laparoscopy [14].

In the past years, several problems associated with long-term use of jejunal feeding tubes have been reported, such as dislocation or blockage of the feeding tube and small bowel obstruction. Changing a jejunal feeding tube and correct placement of a new feeding tube may be hampered by several complications, including incorrect placement, kinking, or recurrent dislocation of the tube [15–17].

The introduction of a new insertion technique for jejunal feeding tubes permitting easier tube replacement together with a safer two-point fixation technique of the feeding tube addressed the problems formerly encountered with the use of jejunal feeding tubes in neurologically impaired, malnourished children [18].

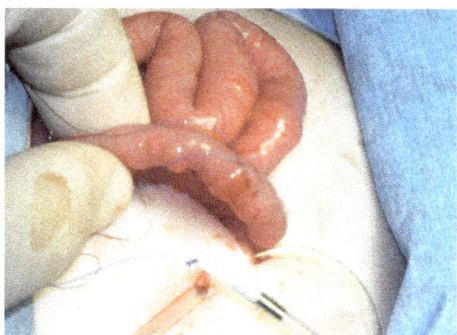

FIGURE 1: Placement of a purse string suture at antimesenteric aspect of the second jejunal loop. The feeding tube attached to a guide thread was introduced into the abdominal cavity (girl aged 2 months; patient 8).

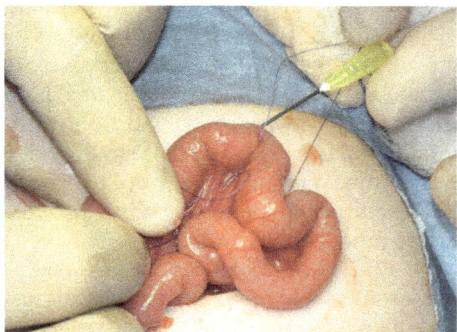

FIGURE 2: Insertion of the guide thread into the jejunal loop through the bore of a long injection needle (same patient as in Figure 1).

This single-center, retrospective case study aimed to describe the indications for jejunal feeding tube placement, postoperative complications, and weight gain observed in this group of critically ill children requiring mid-term or long-term enteral feeding access.

2. Patients and Methods

We conducted a retrospective, descriptive case study in patients who underwent jejunal feeding tube placement according to the surgical technique described by Schimpl et al. [18]. All children aged between 0 and 16 years who underwent jejunal tube placement between June 2005 and July 2011 were included in this investigation. We recorded patient demographics, main disorders of children, their medical and surgical histories, pre- and postoperative weight percentiles, type and number of postoperative complications, and nursing observations associated with jejunal tube feeding. The study protocol was approved by the ethical committee of Basel (protocol number: 2011/37).

3. Surgical Technique

After introduction of general anesthesia, children underwent surgical placement of an RJFT by a small transverse left upper abdominal incision (Figures 1, 2, 3, 4, 5, and 6). The

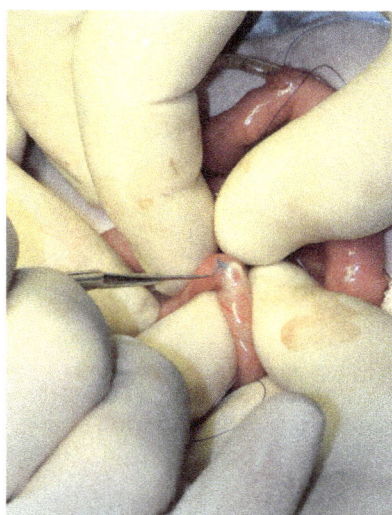

FIGURE 3: Because the small bowel in this very young patient (2 months) was too narrow to insert the needle over a distance of at least 8 cm without piercing the bowel wall inadvertently, we inserted the feeding tube equipped with a guide thread into the bowel lumen. An incision was made at the antimesenteric side of the jejunum loop at the planned exit site of the guide thread.

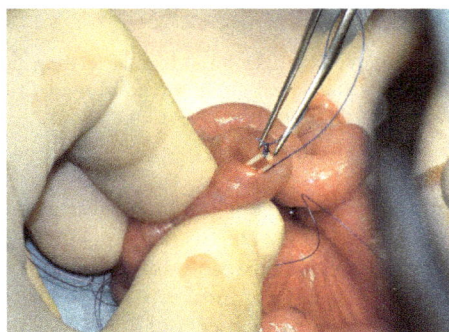

FIGURE 4: The guide thread was grasped and brought out through the abdominal wall using a needle.

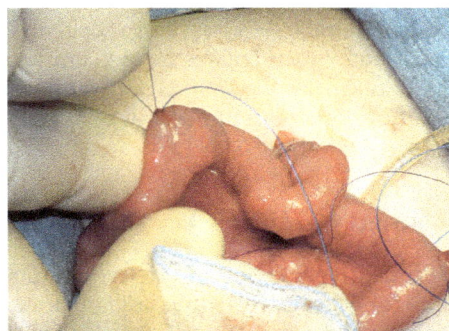

FIGURE 5: A suture was placed to close the opening of the bowel wall, and the suture was used to fix the bowel wall to the peritoneum of the abdominal wall.

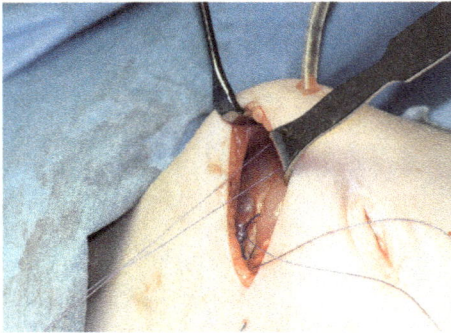

FIGURE 6: Both jejunal openings were sutured to the peritoneum of the abdominal wall. The guide thread exit site was placed to the right of the wound and the jejunostomy to the left.

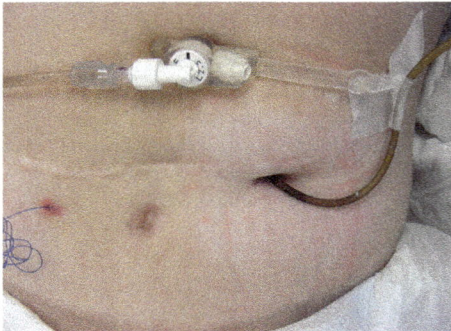

FIGURE 7: Photograph of a discolored jejunal feeding tube before tube exchange. Note the coiled guide thread to the left of the scar and gastrostomy button in the epigastrium.

chosen point of entry of the jejunal tube was at the second jejunal loop, approx. 15–20 cm from the ligament of Treitz. The exit point for the guide thread was 8–10 cm distally of the entry point. Both jejunal openings were secured with a purse string suture and fixed to the peritoneum of the abdominal wall using two absorbable stitches (Figure 6). The feeding tube (Freka® intestinal tube CH9 for PEG15; Fresenius Kabi, Schweiz AG, Stans, Switzerland) was attached to a 30 cm long 4-0 monofilament nonabsorbable thread for fixation and positioning of the tube tip within the jejunal loop. The guide thread was brought out through the abdominal wall and fixed to the abdominal wall at the epigastrium by applying adhesive tape. The laparotomy incision was closed, and jejunal tube feeding was initiated by slowly increasing the amount of nutrition solution infused continuously by a pump after a resting period of 6 h to 12 h [18].

4. Replacement of Jejunal Feeding Tube

We recommended replacement of the feeding tube at least every 6 months or when incrustations or discolorations of the feeding tube were observed (Figure 7). We applied anesthetic cream (Emla® Crème 5%, AstraZeneca, Zug, Switzerland) and an injectable anesthetic solution. A new monofilament nonabsorbable thread was sutured to the thread fixed to the

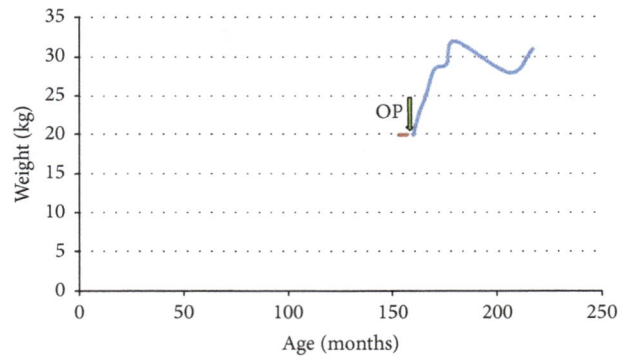

FIGURE 8: Weight development in patient 1 suffering from Wilkie syndrome [19].

tip of the feeding tube, and the feeding tube was withdrawn from the jejunostomy. A new feeding tube was sutured to the new thread, and the old thread and tube were discarded. The jejunal tube was reinserted into the jejunal loop, and the thread measuring 30 cm was coiled and fixed with adhesive tape to the abdominal skin surface close to the exit site of the thread. The new tube was fixed with one or two monofilament sutures and/or adhesive tape to the skin close to the point of entry of the tube. Parents and caregivers were instructed to replace the adhesive tapes at least once a week (or earlier if it became loose) and to apply gentle traction to the guide thread before fixing it to the skin surface. We advised parents and caregivers to apply continuous enteral feeds to prevent dumping syndrome.

5. Results

Eight children (6 girls, 2 boys) at a median age of 27 months (range: 2 months to 13 years) underwent laparotomy for surgical placement of an RJFT. All children suffered from severe malnutrition, defined by weight for age <3rd percentile and recurrent vomiting.

In the first patient, a girl aged 13 years suffering from congenital selenoprotein-defective myopathy, Wilkie syndrome [19], severe scoliosis, hypoxic brain disorder, pulmonary hypertension, and respiratory insufficiency necessitating continuous ventilation therapy for 2 months, insertion of the RJFT allowed for jejunal feeding and weight gain (Figure 8). The main clinical symptom encountered in the postoperative period was a recurrent chronic abdominal pain syndrome and recurrent Clostridium difficile enterocolitis.

In patient 2, a boy aged 4.5 years suffering from a complex congenital malformation syndrome with bilateral cleft palate, neurogenic scoliosis and dislocation of the hip, respiratory insufficiency with ventilator dependency for a period of 2 months, recurrent aspirations, cerebral palsy, and epilepsy, insertion of the RJFT resulted in weight gain (Figure 9) and less frequent pneumonia episodes.

Patient 3, a 4.5-year-old boy, suffered from VACTERL syndrome and Fanconi anemia and underwent allogenic stem cell transplantation [20]. Graft-versus-host disease (GvHD) of the gastrointestinal tract with recurrent blood-stained

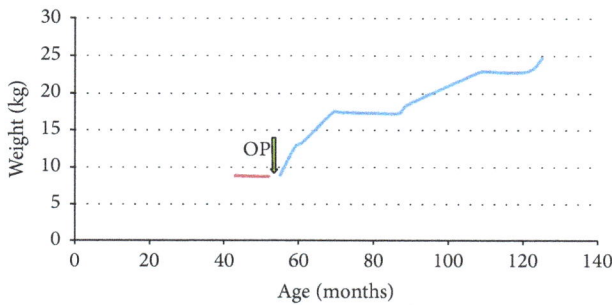

FIGURE 9: Weight development in patient 2 suffering from complex congenital malformation syndrome, respiratory insufficiency with ventilator dependency, recurrent aspirations, cerebral palsy, and epilepsy.

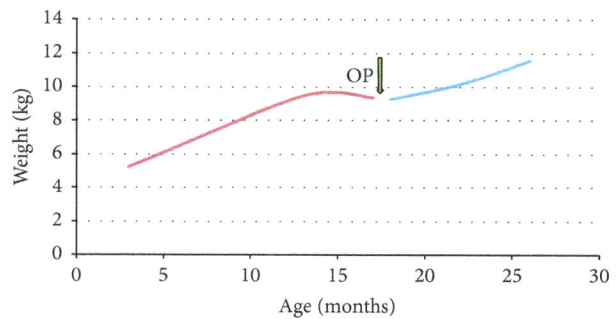

FIGURE 10: Weight development in patient 7 suffering from progressive encephalopathy caused by intractable epilepsy.

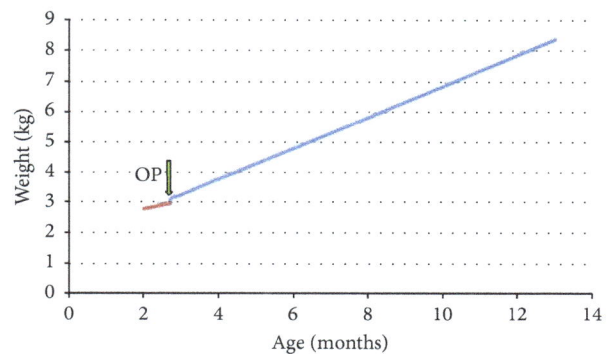

FIGURE 11: Weight development in patient 8 suffering from a microdeletion 22q11 syndromic disorder with cardiac malformation. After 3 months of RJFT use, the tube was removed, and the girl continued to grow well on oral feeding, with a weight for age at the 30th percentile.

vomiting occurred. Parenteral nutrition and immunosuppressive therapy were started, followed by insertion of an RJFT.

Patient 4, a 6-month-old girl, suffered from multiple congenital malformations, asplenia, psychomotoric retardation with generalized hypotonia, corpus callosum agenesis, and complex heart malformation complicated by an intracardial tumor. Impairment of laryngopharyngeal swallowing and inability to cough adequately resulted in recurrent aspiration episodes. Due to an absent sucking and swallowing reflex, neonatologists initiated tube feeding after birth. Within one year, the patient achieved a weight gain of 2.5 kg (from 10.0 kg to 12.5 kg).

In patient 5, a girl who underwent an operation for anaplastic ependymoma WHO grade III at the age of 5 months, occlusive hydrocephalus necessitated the placement of a ventriculoperitoneal shunt. We placed an RJFT to overcome the feeding problems associated with the neurological impairment characterized by dysphagia, swallowing dysfunction, hemiparesis, and facial nerve palsy. Because of a bacterial infection of the ventriculoperitoneal shunt device and influenza virus infection, we took down the jejunostomy 11 days after surgery and performed an external drainage of occlusive hydrocephalus. The patient died from tumor progression some days after removal of the RJFT.

Patient 6, a girl aged 3 years, suffered from progressive encephalopathy caused by intractable epilepsy, hypertrophic cardiomyopathy, pulmonary hypertension, central blindness, and neurogenic dislocation of the hip. Psychomotor retardation and recurrent aspirations complicated the clinical course, and treatment of epilepsy necessitated administration of a ketogenic diet. Because the girl was unable to swallow this diet, a nasogastric tube was placed, followed by percutaneous endoscopic gastrostomy placement (PEG). Feeding by PEG was poorly tolerated. Recurrent vomiting, massive tracheobronchial mucus secretion, recurrent aspiration episodes, and malnutrition complicated the clinical course. An RJFT was placed, which made adequate enteral nutrition and administration of the ketogenic diet possible. We enrolled the child in an outpatient enteral home-feeding program. The child died from progressive encephalopathy 6 months after the RJFT insertion.

Patient 7, the younger (15 months) sister of patient 6, suffered from the same disorders as her sister. Her main clinical problems comprised intractable epilepsy, recurrent vomiting episodes complicated by hematemesis, and insufficient weight gain (Figure 10).

Patient 8, a 2-month old girl, suffered from a microdeletion 22q11-syndromic disorder with cardiac malformation. Enteral nutrition by nasogastric tube was started due to pronounced swallowing dysfunction, absent sucking reflex, and aspiration episodes. After 4 weeks, the swallowing ability of the girl improved. Because an upper gastroesophageal contrast study revealed adequate swallowing with absent gastroesophageal reflux episodes, oral feeding was started and was well tolerated. After 3 months, the RJFT was removed and the girl continued to grow well with a weight for age at the 30th percentile (Figure 11).

6. Complications of RJFT Placement

Table 1 shows the complications after RJFT placement. In the first patient, the thread connected to the tip of the feeding tube used for correct placement of the tube within the jejunal loop became loose as the adhesive tape which held it in place detached itself from the skin. A long part of the thread

TABLE 1: Complications after RJFT placement.

Postoperative complications	n
Complications necessitating surgical intervention (volvulus, ventriculoperitoneal shunt infection, or small bowel obstruction)	3
Guide thread erroneously cut off*	1
Local skin infection at jejunostomy	5
Blockage of feeding tube due to incrustations	2
Dysfunction caused by kinking of feeding tube	2
Persistent jejunal fistula in an immunocompromised child suffering from Fanconi anemia and GvHD	1
Total	14

*In one child (patient 7), a nurse erroneously cut off the guide thread and the jejunal tube fell off. We inserted a new tube connected to a new guide thread by an endoscopically assisted procedure [26].

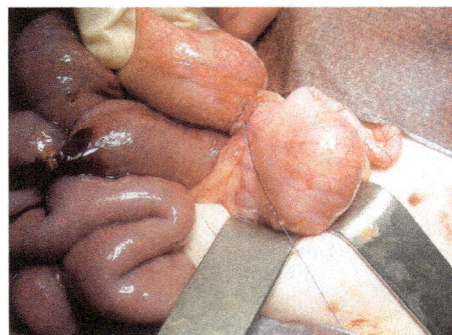

FIGURE 12: Acute small bowel obstruction in a girl aged 20 months. Bowel obstruction was caused by a loose guide thread and fibrous band crossing the terminal ileum. This complication occurred 18 months after RJFT insertion and was managed by resection of the fibrous band and guide thread (patient 7).

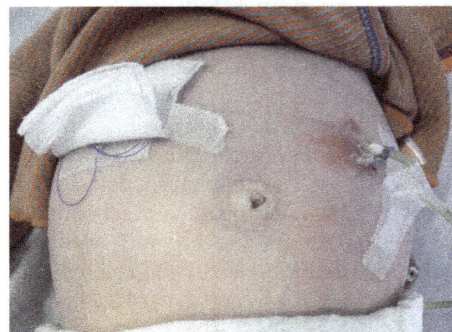

FIGURE 13: Local skin infection at the site of the jejunostomy. This infection was treated with antibiotic ointment and enterally administered antibiotics.

ran through the abdominal cavity and caused small bowel obstruction. At the revision surgery, we sutured the exit site of the thread at the antimesenteric boarder of the jejunum loop to the peritoneum of the abdominal wall. We applied this type of sutures in all further patients undergoing RJFT placement.

In patient 2, partial volvulus occurred 7 months after insertion of the RJFT when small bowel loops and colon became entrapped in a large congenital Morgagni hernia. Torsion occurred around the jejunostomy. We took down the jejunostomy by open surgery, reduced the volvulus, repaired the hernia, and placed a new RJFT.

In patient 3, who suffered from Fanconi anemia and GvHD after allogenic stem cell transplantation, enteral feeding was poorly tolerated due to bowel dysfunction related to Fanconi anemia and gastrointestinal GvHD. After several unsuccessful attempts to increase the volume of enteral feeding solution, we removed the feeding tube. However, the jejunostomy did not close spontaneously, and bacterial infection of the abdominal wall surrounding the jejunostomy occurred. The immunocompromised child died 3 weeks after the operation.

In patient 4, bacterial infection of the ventriculoperitoneal shunt occurred after insertion of the RJFT. The RJFT was removed after 11 days, and the ventriculoperitoneal shunt was exteriorized. Enteral feeding using a nasogastric tube was started again. Microbiological examination of the liquor revealed growth of *Enterobacter cloacae*. Due to incomplete resection of the brain tumor, the treatment situation was considered palliative, and the patient died from tumor progression.

In patient 6, the RJFT was used for 5 months. The feeding tube was replaced once because of massive incrustations from medications administered through the tube. The girl died from intractable epileptic seizures, hypertrophic cardiomyopathy, pulmonary hypertension, and pneumonia. An underlying autosomal recessive mitochondrial disorder was thought to be the cause of the condition of this girl and her sister (patient 7).

In patient 7, the younger sister of patient 6, the RJFT was used for 5.2 years. Eighteen months after surgical feeding

tube placement, acute small bowel obstruction occurred. Bowel obstruction was caused by entrapment of the ileocecal bowel segment in a loop of the guide thread. Small bowel obstruction was repaired surgically (Figure 12).

In this child, 3 episodes of skin infection occurred at the entrance site of the jejunal feeding tube within the regular follow-up period (Figure 13). These superficial skin infections were managed with antiseptic ointments and enteral antibiotics. Ten months after insertion of the feeding tube, the child developed pneumonia after aspiration of gastric contents. The RJFT was replaced uneventfully at intervals of 6 months.

In patient 8, RJFT use was monitored for a period of 3 months only. The tube underwent dislocation once, which was corrected by repositioning and fixation of the tube and thread using adhesive tape. An episode of local skin infection was managed with antibiotic ointments and systemic antibiotics.

7. Follow-Up of Patients

Long-term follow-up results beyond the study period are currently available for 4 patients. Patient 1 has been managed by enteral RJFT feeding for 11.8 years and patient 7 for 5.2 years. However, in patient 7 the RJFT was changed into a jejunal tube without guide thread during the surgical intervention for small bowel obstruction 18 months after insertion of the RJFT. Patient 2 died from his underlying disorders after 9.5 years of enteral RJFT feeding. Patient 8 has been eating normally since RJFT removal 6 years ago. None of these patients underwent any further surgical interventions. We observed further weight gain in all patients within the long-term follow-up period. Patients 3, 4, 5, and 6 died from their underlying disorders within the study period.

8. Discussion

Because of the retrospective nature of this single-center case series and the variable disorders of the children, the results must be interpreted with caution. All children suffered from disorders complicated by severe malnutrition and recurrent vomiting. In two children, a ketogenic diet was not tolerated when administered by the oral route or nasogastric tube, and insertion of an RJFT allowed for successful administration of the ketogenic diet.

When long-term feeding via gastrostomy is poorly tolerated because of recurrent aspiration, regurgitation, or gastroesophageal reflux disease jejunal application of enteral feedings is a promising option to facilitate enteral nutrition in children. Percutaneous gastrojejunostomy with transgastric jejunal insertion of a feeding tube using a neonatoscope and guidewire permits for a fast and safe insertion of a jejunal feeding tube with minimal exposure of the child to ionizing radiation. However, Michaud et al. reported that, in 27 patients followed up for a median period of 5.5 months, 31 tube dislodgements, 16 tube obstructions, 7 leakages around the tube, 6 internal ballon ruptures, and 1 intussusception occurred [17]. Additionally, 11 of 27 children required surgery, and the authors conclude that the high rate of complications and tube replacements limits the use of this jejunal feeding strategy [17]. Raval and Phillips reported that in a group of 20 children who did not tolerate gastrostomy feeding 14 children underwent image-guided jejunal feeding tube placement [20]. Half of these children ultimately underwent Roux-en-Y jejunostomy placements [20]. Image-guided jejunal feeding tube placement patients required 4.6 fluoroscopy-guided feeding tube revisions per year [20], which exposed them to a considerable amount of ionizing radiation.

Transgastric feeding tubes dislodge easily, and Kaplan et al. noted a rate of 84% jejunal feeding tube malfunctions, caused by tube dislodgements, tube obstructions, and leakages around the tube at a mean interval of 39 days after placement of the tube [21].

However, there are some reasons, why image-guided feeding tube placement represents a well-accepted first choice for jejunal feeding tube placement in children. These include a less invasive procedure, which can be performed in sedation in contrast to general anesthesia and easy discontinuation of the tube after treatment once the child no longer requires jejunal feeding [20].

In a 2-center study from Leeds and Manchester on the limitations and clinical usefulness of gastrojejunal feeding tubes in 18 children (12 of these suffered from neurological impairment) followed up for a median time interval of 10

months, the authors reported 65 tube related complications in 14 children [22]. Jejunal tube dislodgement was the most frequently observed complication, and 4 children suffered from recurrent aspiration, bilious vomiting, and diarrhea after onset of jejunal tube feeding [22]. In our study, 6 of 8 children suffered from neurological impairment. To the best of our knowledge, there exist no relevant systematic reviews or prospectively randomized controlled trials on gastrostomy or jejunostomy feeding in children with cerebral palsy [23].

Comparing our complication rate of surgical RJFT insertion to the complication rate of the "Omega"-jejunostomy tube technique, we noted a lower rate of complications for the second [24]. However, the small group of children we treated was younger (median age: 27 months) when compared to the patients treated by Schlager et al. with a "Omega" jejunostomy and button placement (median age at surgery: 11 years) [24]. Due to the low number of patients in both studies, further studies are required to confirm these results. We hypothesize that thread related complications observed in older children might be reduced by insertion of a small low profile button device into the jejunostomy after maturation of the jejunostomy, to avoid long-term use of the thread in older children. Further studies are required to evaluate this hypothesis.

Compared to esophagogastric disconnect, which is used when fundoplication failed and gastric feeding is no longer an option, the insertion of a RJFT is less technically demanding [24, 25].

Smith and Soucy followed up 57 pediatric patients in whom 64 surgical jejunostomies were placed [15]. They found a mean duration of jejunostomy use of 1.1 ± 2.4 years and an overall complication rate of 37.5% including 21.9% major complications, which is similar to our findings in neurologically impaired children. We agree with Smith and Soucy that the benefits of long-term usage of surgical jejunostomies outweigh the risks for most patients perhaps those who are neurologically impaired or suffer from intractable seizures [15].

The children we were able to follow up for a prolonged period of time underwent weight gain after surgical insertion of the RJFT. Caregivers also reported that the episodes of vomiting occurred less frequently and were less severe. Parents and caregivers were satisfied with the handling of the RJFT, although continuous administration of enteral nutrition solution was required. We discouraged parents and caregivers to apply bolus feeding due to the risk of dumping syndrome.

The RJFT was easily exchanged in the outpatient office, and application of lidocaine/prilocaine cream 5% (Emla cream® 5%, AstraZeneca, Zug, Switzerland) was considered helpful to avoid pain at the jejunostomy and exit site of the guide thread. However, in an older girl who was highly sensitive to pain, we exchanged the feeding tube under anesthesia or conscious sedation. We recommend to exchange the feeding tube at 6-month intervals and to rinse the tube with a small volume of water after every administration of enteral nutrition solution to avoid incrustation of the narrow tube. We discourage the routine administration of drugs using the jejunal tube to avoid blockage of the 9 CH tube lumen.

The immunocompromised child suffering from Fanconi anemia developed a jejunal fistula after removal of the feeding tube (Table 1). We noted that jejunal feeding was not adequately tolerated in this child and hypothesized that the impaired absorptive, digestive, and regenerative capacity of the bowel mucosa may be responsible for this phenomenon in children suffering from Fanconi anemia [27]. This situation may worsen when allogenic stem cell transplantation (STX) results in GvHD of the bowel mucosa [27]. We therefore do no longer recommend applying this feeding technique in children suffering from Fanconi anemia after allogenic STX.

9. Conclusions

The use of RJFT facilitated long-term jejunal feeding access in chronically ill children suffering from severe malnutrition, complex chronic disorders, and recurrent vomiting in whom feeding by nasogastric tube or PEG had failed. The most relevant surgical complication observed with RJFT placement was acute small bowel obstruction caused by the guide thread. Due to the limited number of children, the results of this retrospective study on the use of RJFT should be interpreted with caution. Further studies are required to investigate the effectiveness and safety of this feeding technique in children.

Competing Interests

The authors declare that there are no competing interests regarding the publication of this manuscript.

Authors' Contributions

Tabea Pang and Sergio B. Sesia contributed equally to this investigation. Tabea Pang, Sergio B. Sesia, and Johannes Mayr were responsible for designing the study and collecting the primary data. Stefan Holland-Cunz and Johannes Mayr were involved in the patient follow-up examinations. Sergio B. Sesia and Stefan Holland-Cunz approved the final version of the manuscript before submission.

References

[1] M. F. Goutail-Flaud, M. Sfez, A. Berg et al., "Central venous catheter-related complications in newborns and infants: a 587-case survey," *Journal of Pediatric Surgery*, vol. 26, no. 6, pp. 645–650, 1991.

[2] F. Yi, L. Ge, J. Zhao et al., "Meta-analysis: total parenteral nutrition versus total enteral nutrition in predicted severe acute pancreatitis," *Internal Medicine*, vol. 51, no. 6, pp. 523–530, 2012.

[3] S. J. Rangel, C. M. Calkins, R. A. Cowles et al., "Parenteral nutrition-associated cholestasis: an American pediatric surgical association outcomes and clinical trials committee systematic review," *Journal of Pediatric Surgery*, vol. 47, no. 1, pp. 225–240, 2012.

[4] A. M. Andrés, L. Burgos, J. C. López Gutiérrez et al., "Treatment protocol for extravasation lesions," *Cirugía pediátrica*, vol. 19, no. 3, pp. 136–139, 2006.

[5] P. Weber, "Das behinderte Kind," in *Pädiatrische Gastroenterologie, Hepatologie und Ernährung*, B. Rodeck and K. P. Zimmer, Eds., pp. 579–585, Springer, Heidelberg, Germany, 2008.

[6] C. Pedrón Giner, C. Martínez-Costa, V. M. Navas-López et al., "Consensus on paediatric enteral nutrition access," *Nutrición Hospitalaria*, vol. 26, no. 1, pp. 1–15, 2011.

[7] C. Egnell, S. Eksborg, and L. Grahnquist, "Jejunostomy enteral feeding in children: outcome and safety," *Journal of Parenteral and Enteral Nutrition*, vol. 38, no. 5, pp. 631–636, 2014.

[8] C. T. Albanese, R. B. Towbin, I. Ulman, J. Lewis, and S. D. Smith, "Percutaneous gastrojejunostomy versus Nissen fundoplication for enteral feeding of the neurologically impaired child with gastroesophageal reflux," *The Journal of Pediatrics*, vol. 123, no. 3, pp. 371–375, 1993.

[9] C. Esposito, F. Alicchio, M. Escolino, G. Ascione, and A. Settimi, "Laparoscopy-assisted jejunostomy in neurological patients with chronic malnutrition and GERD. Technical considerations and analysis of the results," *La Pediatria Medica e Chirurgica*, vol. 35, no. 3, pp. 125–129, 2013.

[10] M. A. Gilger, C. Yeh, J. Chiang, C. Dietrich, M. L. Brandt, and H. B. El-Serag, "Outcomes of surgical fundoplication in children," *Clinical Gastroenterology and Hepatology*, vol. 2, no. 11, pp. 978–984, 2004.

[11] M. Classen and A. T. R. Axon, *Gastroenterologische Endoskopie*, 2004.

[12] J. Stein, *Praxishandbuch Klinische Ernährung und Infusionstherapie*, 2003.

[13] C. Löser and M. Keymling, *Praxis der Enteralen Ernährung: Indikationen—Technik—Nachsorge*, 2001.

[14] D. Belsha, M. Thomson, D. R. Dass, R. Lindley, and S. Marven, "Assessment of the safety and efficacy of percutaneous laparoscopic endoscopic jejunostomy (PLEJ)," *Journal of Pediatric Surgery*, vol. 51, no. 3, pp. 513–518, 2016.

[15] D. Smith and P. Soucy, "Complications of long-term jejunostomy in children," *Journal of Pediatric Surgery*, vol. 31, no. 6, pp. 787–790, 1996.

[16] D. Al-Zubeidi, H. Demir, W. P. Bishop, and R. M. Rahhal, "Gastrojejunal feeding tube use by gastroenterologists in a pediatric academic center," *Journal of Pediatric Gastroenterology and Nutrition*, vol. 56, no. 5, pp. 523–527, 2013.

[17] L. Michaud, S. Coopman, D. Guimber, R. Sfeir, D. Turck, and F. Gottrand, "Percutaneous gastrojejunostomy in children: efficacy and safety," *Archives of Disease in Childhood*, vol. 97, no. 8, pp. 733–734, 2012.

[18] G. Schimpl, J. Mayr, and M. W. L. Gauderer, "Jejunostomy with replaceable feeding tube: a new technique," *Journal of the American College of Surgeons*, vol. 184, no. 6, pp. 652–654, 1997.

[19] S. Fiorini, M. M. S. Tejeira, C. Tennina, S. Tomezzoli, and N. Requejo, "Superior mesenteric artery syndrome (Wilkie syndrome). Case report," *Archivos Argentinos de Pediatría*, vol. 106, no. 6, pp. 546–548, 2008.

[20] M. V. Raval and J. D. Phillips, "Optimal enteral feeding in children with gastric dysfunction: surgical jejunostomy vs image-guided gastrojejunal tube placement," *Journal of Pediatric Surgery*, vol. 41, no. 10, pp. 1679–1682, 2006.

[21] D. S. Kaplan, U. K. Murthy, and W. G. Linscheer, "Percutaneous endoscopic jejunostomy: long-term follow-up of 23 patients," *Gastrointestinal Endoscopy*, vol. 35, no. 5, pp. 403–406, 1989.

[22] P. Godbole, G. Margabanthu, D. C. Crabbe et al., "Limitations and uses of gastrojejunal feeding tubes," *Archives of Disease in Childhood*, vol. 86, no. 2, pp. 134–137, 2002.

[23] G. Sleigh and P. Brocklehurst, "Gastrostomy feeding in cerebral palsy: a systematic review," *Archives of Disease in Childhood*, vol. 89, no. 6, pp. 534–539, 2004.

[24] A. Schlager, K. Arps, R. Siddharthan, P. Rajdev, and K. F. Heiss, "The 'omega' jejunostomy tube: a preferred alternative for postpyloric feeding access," *Journal of Pediatric Surgery*, vol. 51, no. 2, pp. 260–263, 2016.

[25] P. D. Danielson and R. W. Emmens, "Esophagogastric disconnection for gastroesophageal reflux in children with severe neurological impairment," *Journal of Pediatric Surgery*, vol. 34, no. 1, pp. 84–87, 1999.

[26] G. De Bernardis and J. Mayr, "Replacement of a string jejunostomy if the suture is lost: first time a technique with no need to cut," *Surgical Laparoscopy, Endoscopy and Percutaneous Techniques*, vol. 23, no. 3, pp. 360–361, 2013.

[27] R. Peffault de Latour, R. Porcher, J.-H. Dalle et al., "Allogeneic hematopoietic stem cell transplantation in Fanconi anemia: the European Group for Blood and Marrow Transplantation experience," *Blood*, vol. 122, no. 26, pp. 4279–4286, 2013.

7

Involvement of Reduced Microbial Diversity in Inflammatory Bowel Disease

Dawei Gong,[1] **Xiaojie Gong,**[2] **Lili Wang,**[1] **Xinjuan Yu,**[1] **and Quanjiang Dong**[1]

[1]*Department of Central Laboratories and Gastroenterology, Qingdao Municipal Hospital, School of Medicine, Qingdao University, Qingdao 266071, China*
[2]*Department of Emergency Surgery, The Fifth People's Hospital of Ji'nan, Ji'nan 250022, China*

Correspondence should be addressed to Quanjiang Dong; jiangacer@126.com

Academic Editor: Tamar Ringel-Kulka

A considerable number of studies have been conducted to study the microbial profiles in inflammatory conditions. A common phenomenon in inflammatory bowel disease (IBD) is the reduction of the diversity of microbiota, which demonstrates that microbial diversity negatively correlates with disease severity in IBD. Increased microbial diversity is known to occur in disease remission. Species diversity plays an important role in maintaining the stability of the intestinal ecosystem as well as normal ecological function. A reduction in microbial diversity corresponds to a decrease in the stability of the ecosystem and can impair ecological function. Fecal microbiota transplantation (FMT), probiotics, and prebiotics, which aim to modulate the microbiota and restore its normal diversity, have been shown to be clinically efficacious. In this study, we hypothesized that a reduction in microbial diversity could play a role in the development of IBD.

1. Introduction

Inflammatory bowel disease (IBD) is a chronic disease, and the two main forms of IBD are ulcerative colitis (UC) and Crohn's disease (CD). IBD has been shown to be associated with increased morbidity in developed countries and developing countries that are gradually adopting a more modern lifestyle. IBD has been reported to be caused by a multitude of factors such as genetics, environment, immune system, and gut microbiota. Although its exact pathogenesis remains unclear, dysbiosis of the microbiota in the intestinal tract is widely accepted to initiate or promote intestinal inflammation [1–3].

An increasing number of studies have used noncultured *16S* rRNA sequencing technology to reveal intestinal microbial profiles in IBD and healthy controls. Some meaningful features were found. The gastrointestinal tract contains several hundred microbial species [4–7], most of which belong to the Firmicutes, Bacteroidetes, Proteobacteria, and Actinobacteria phyla [8, 9]. A balanced microbial population in the human gut could benefit the human body by providing nutrients, maintaining immune homeostasis, and granting niche protection. However, recent studies have demonstrated a dysbiosis in IBD patients. CD patients had significantly higher populations of *Streptococcus* and *Enterococcus* and lower populations of *Coprococcus*, *Roseburia*, *Faecalibacterium*, and *Ruminococcus* compared with healthy controls [10]. Furthermore, the abundance of *Bacteroides*, *Enterococcus*, *Blautia*, and *Escherichia-Shigella* genera was significantly increased in patients with UC, and the abundance of *Coprococcus* decreased compared with healthy controls [10]. Andoh et al. found that the abundance of *Clostridium* was decreased in patients with active UC and inactive/active CD patients, whereas the abundance of *Bacteroides* significantly increased in the patients with CD [11]. Although the altered microbial profiles did not show any consistent results across many studies, a common feature, that is, reduced microbiota diversity, emerged in all patients with IBD [7, 12–16].

The diversity of microbiota is closely associated with disease conditions. In a study on microbiota signatures in eczema, Nylund et al. found that the severity of eczema was inversely correlated with the microbial diversity ($r = -0.54$; $P = 0.005$), indicating that the lower the microbial diversity, the higher the severity of eczema [17]. Additionally, the microbial diversity increased with improvement of symptoms in eczema [17]. A similar relationship was found between the microbial diversity and disease severity in human IBD [18]. Russell et al. treated neonatal mice with vancomycin and reported that this resulted in a reduction in microbial diversity accompanied by an increase in the severity of asthma [19]. The level of diversity is also related to the response to therapy in patients. For example, children with UC who responded to corticosteroid medication were reported to have a higher diversity than nonresponders [20].

Little attention has been paid to the role of reduced microbial diversity in the function of the intestinal ecosystem. This review intends to reveal the relationship between a reduction in diversity and IBD from a biological perspective.

2. Reduced Microbial Diversity in IBD

A previous study compared the intestinal microbial flora between patients with active CD and healthy controls using *16S* rRNA gene sequencing. The mean Shannon diversity was lower in CD patients than in the healthy controls [21]. Similar to these findings, in a multicenter study, fecal samples collected from 161 patients with CD and 121 healthy individuals found that the active/inactive CD patients had a significantly lower Shannon diversity than the healthy controls [22]. Sha et al. analyzed the diversity of fecal microbiota in IBD patients compared with healthy controls using denaturing gradient gel electrophoresis. The participants included patients with UC, patients with CD, and healthy controls. The microbial diversity was remarkably lower in IBD patients than in the healthy control group, and the reduced microbial diversity was more obvious in the active UC and active CD groups [13]. Additionally, studies of microbial profiles from UC patients revealed that these patients have lower fecal microbial diversity and lower abundance of major anaerobic bacteria (*Bacteroides* and *Clostridium* subcluster XIVa) compared with healthy controls [23]. In another study, microarray hybridization was used to study the characteristics of the microbiota from healthy controls and children hospitalized with severe UC. The richness, evenness, and biodiversity of the gut microbiota were all significantly reduced in children with UC compared with healthy controls; furthermore, a reduction in the abundance of *Clostridium* and an increase in the class Gammaproteobacteria were found [20].

The precise causal relationship between the inflammatory state and a reduction in bacterial diversity remains unknown. To determine whether defects in the mucosal barrier and bacterial dysbiosis are inherently abrogated in the terminal ileum (TI) of patients with UC (where inflammation is absent), the TI was biopsied from patients with CD and UC and from healthy controls without IBD [24]. Despite the absence of ileitis, UC patients displayed ileal barrier depletion and a reduction in the α-diversity compared with pediatric patients without IBD [24]. In a study on mice, when antibiotics were used to deplete the gut microbiota, a reduction in diversity and mild gut inflammation occurred [25]. In another study, microbial profiles of patients with CD, their healthy siblings, and unrelated healthy individuals were sequenced and analyzed. Healthy siblings who were at a higher risk of developing CD had lower core microbial diversity than low-risk healthy controls (although the microbial diversity in the siblings was higher than that in the CD patients), suggesting that the loss of core microbial diversity may be a fundamental step in the pathogenesis of CD [26]. Interestingly, the hygiene hypothesis suggests that improved hygiene conditions may lead to a reduction in the intestinal microbial diversity and that it may in turn be responsible for the development of IBD [27].

3. Attempt to Restore Normal Diversity to Alleviate IBD

FMT involves the transfer of fecal suspension from a healthy donor to the intestinal tract of a recipient, modulating imbalanced gut microbiota and restoring normal diversity and bacterial composition of the intestine. FMT therapy is currently used in treatment of intestinal inflammation [28].

FMT has received extended attention in the treatment of IBD [29–31]. Many studies have revealed that FMT can induce the remission of some IBD patients. Moayyedi et al. conducted FMT in patients with active UC in a randomized controlled trial. In their study, patients with UC were examined using flexible sigmoidoscopy at the start of the study and were randomly assigned to groups that received an enema of either 50 mL of FMT (from healthy anonymous donors, $n = 38$) or 50 mL of placebo (water, $n = 37$) once per week for six weeks. The primary outcome was remission of UC, defined as a Mayo score ≤ 2 with an endoscopic Mayo score of 0 at week 7 of treatment. In their study, nine of the patients who received FMT (24%) and 2 who received placebo (5%) achieved remission ($P = 0.03$) [32]. Additionally, the fecal samples of patients receiving FMT had greater microbial diversity compared with baseline [33]. A systematic review and meta-analysis from a large multigroup sample after FMT therapy found that remission after FMT could reach 36.2% [34]. A subgroup analysis revealed that the clinical remission of the UC group and the remission rate of the CD group reached 22% and 60.5%, respectively [34]. FMT has also been reported to have the best efficacy in treating patients when first diagnosed [32].

Clostridium difficile infection (CDI) is caused by toxin-producing *C. difficile* and features a range of symptoms from mild diarrhea to potentially lethal conditions such as pseudomembranous colitis. Low et al. found that the microbial diversity was lower in patients with CDI than in healthy controls, and alterations in the composition included a reduction in the abundance of Firmicutes and Bacteroidetes as well as an increased abundance of Proteobacteria [35]. Notably, a study on CDI reported that the reduction in microbial diversity occurs prior to the occurrence of CDI, emphasizing the promoting effect of reduced diversity on intestinal inflammation [36]. Antibiotic therapy for CDI cannot achieve the desired effect and can induce recurrent *Clostridium difficile* infection (rCDI) [37]. In other studies, increased microbiota diversity could be achieved in recipients who achieved remission after FMT [35, 38, 39]. Accordingly, when FMT was used to treat CDI, a significant curative effect could be achieved [28, 40]. van Nood et al. studied the efficacy of FMT in rCDI compared with vancomycin to treat recurrent infection. They found a significantly higher rate in the resolution of *C. difficile*-associated diarrhea in the FMT group with the resolution of symptoms in nearly all patients in the FMT group [40]. After the FMT procedure, the recipients showed increased microbial diversity at levels similar to the microbial features of the healthy donor [40]. To investigate the eradication of *C. difficile* and changes in the microbiome following FMT in children with and without IBD, 8 children (5 with IBD and 3 without IBD) with a history of recurrent CDI (≥3 recurrences) received FMT via colonoscopy. All 8 children showed the resolution of CDI symptoms and eradication of *C. difficile* at 10–20 weeks and 6 months after the administration of FMT [41]. There was also an increase in the intestinal microbial diversity after FMT therapy [41]. Three systematic reviews and a meta-analysis on CDI treated with FMT showed an average curative rate of approximately 90% [42–44]. Furthermore, a controlled trial revealed that the curative rate of rCDI treated with FMT could reach 81% [40]. FMT therapy is associated with fewer adverse reactions [45, 46]. The most successful application of FMT was reported in the treatment of CDI [47]. Although the pathogenesis of CDI is significantly different from that of IBD, the microbiota of patients with both conditions have been found to be similar, and both conditions have shown successful outcomes following FMT treatment, especially in CDI, indicating that the normal intestinal microbiota plays an indispensable role in human homeostasis and that reduced diversity of the microbiota could cause intestinal inflammation.

4. Potential Factors Contributing to a Reduction in Microbial Diversity

The gastrointestinal tract environment may be considered as an ecosystem. It includes the mucosal epithelium, mucus layer, bacteria, viruses, funguses, parasites, and archaea [4]. The health of the gastrointestinal ecosystem is primarily represented by its microbial diversity. A balanced ecosystem represents normal ecological function and gut health. However, the ecological environment is disturbed in IBD, resulting in reduced microbial diversity. Therefore, the question arises: what are the factors that induce a reduction in microbial diversity? Knowing the exact mechanism could help reduce the risks associated with reduced diversity and provide therapeutic strategies to treat it.

4.1. Role of Antibiotics, Diet, and Environments. Antibiotics are widely used and can lead to significant changes in the composition of the intestinal microbial flora [48–51]. Jakobsson et al. studied the effects of metronidazole and clarithromycin on intestinal microbiota and found that the drugs caused a significant diversity reduction [52]. The antibiotics disrupted the microbiota and caused antibiotic-associated diarrhea [53, 54]. Diet is also responsible for altering the composition of the intestinal microbiota [55]. In a recent study, Sonnenburg et al. reported that a diet low in dietary fiber could decrease the diversity of intestinal microbiota in mice and that a diet that is persistently low in dietary fiber resulted in a progressive loss of microbial diversity in subsequent generations of mice. Conversely, a diet rich in dietary

fiber helped maintain high intestinal microbiota diversity in mice of all generations [56]. This phenomenon may explain the higher morbidity of IBD in Western countries, which tend to have high-fat low-fiber diets. Recently, a systematic review focusing on the impact of diet on gut microbiota also indicated that a fiber-rich diet could elevate microbial diversity [57]. Environmental factors can also significantly impact the microbial profile [58]; the microbial profiles in Malawian and Venezuelan populations are more diverse than those of adults and children residing in the US [59].

4.2. Role of Genetics, Immune System, and Mucus. To study the potential role of the chromatin remodeler CHD1 in shaping the gut microbiome of *Drosophila melanogaster*, Sebald et al. performed deep *16S* rRNA gene sequencing of gut microbiota from $Chd1^{-/-}$ and control $Chd1^{WT/WT}$ flies, which carried a wild-type *Chd1* rescue transgene in a Chd1-deficient genetic background. Interestingly, principal coordinate analysis revealed clear distinctions between the microbiota of mutant and wild-type flies. The $Chd1^{-/-}$ flies had a significantly lower microbial diversity than the $Chd1^{WT/WT}$ controls [60]. This implies the genetic function in shaping the structure and composition of microbiota. Lim et al. investigated the effect of heritability and host genetics on gut microbiota and metabolic syndrome and reported that the patients with metabolic syndrome had lower microbial diversity than healthy individuals. The microbial profiles were significantly associated with the special host genotype [61, 62]. The role of adaptive immunity on the gut microbiota was investigated in a mouse model to determine the role of immunity in the regulation of gut microflora. The microbiota of immunodeficient $Rag1^{-/-}$ mice and wild-type mice housed in the same conditions were analyzed using *16S* rRNA sequencing [63]. The results demonstrated that $Rag1^{-/-}$ mice had distinct microbiota and had a higher increase in microbial diversity with increasing age compared to wild-type mice [63]. To a certain extent, this study may imply that immune enhancement could suppress microbial diversity. Furthermore, the human intestinal tract surface is covered with a mucus layer that prevents intimate interaction between the intestinal epithelium and bacteria [64, 65]. The colon mucus layer in humans consists of an inner layer and an outer layer. The viscosity of the outer layer is low, making it easy to penetrate by bacteria. However, the inner layer of the mucus is viscous and sterile [66]. The mucus plays an indispensable role in maintaining homeostasis in the human intestinal tract. During inflammation, the mucus layer is impaired and infiltrated by microbes [64]. *MUC2*, which is primarily produced by goblet cells, is a major component of the colonic mucus layer [66, 67]. In a *MUC2*-deficient mouse model, mice lacking *MUC2* were found to develop spontaneous colitis [68, 69]. Mucin is an energy source for intestinal microbiota and could regulate the composition of intestinal microflora [70]. Bel et al. studied $TMF^{-/-}$ mice lacking TMF/ARA160 and found that these mice produce thick and uniform colonic mucus. The microbial features of $TMF^{-/-}$ knockout mice and wild-type mice were analyzed and the Shannon diversity index was higher in the former than in the latter group [71]. When dextran sulfate sodium (DSS) was used to induce colitis in two mice groups, the results showed that the knockout mice (with higher diversity) exhibited an attenuated response to DSS compared to their wild-type counterparts. Both groups of mice were cohoused for 4 weeks, and the diversity of microbiota was higher in the cohoused wild-type mice than in the wild-type mice housed alone; additionally, the cohoused wild-type mice had diminished susceptibility to induced colitis [71].

Many studies have already reported the association between these factors and IBD. Interestingly, these factors, which contribute a reduction in microbial diversity, are also risk factors for developing IBD [72–76].

5. Mechanism of Reduction in Diversity

Biodiversity plays an important role in maintaining a balanced ecosystem by contributing to the stability of an ecosystem as well as ecological functioning [77–79]. A high diversity provides the ecosystem with strong stability, which is defined as the ability to resist disturbance and to maintain normal ecological function [80]. When diversity is lost, the stability of an ecosystem decreases, which means that it is more susceptible to even minor assaults. This may explain why the lower gut microbial diversity observed in Western populations is associated with a higher morbidity rate of IBD. Consequently, IBD patients who achieve remission but still have lower microbial diversity are more likely to experience relapse.

Biodiversity is positively correlated with ecological function, and ecological function can maintain a balanced state when the biodiversity is at a certain level for functional redundancy [81, 82]. When the balance is disrupted, the biodiversity reduces and the normal function of the ecosystem is transformed to another state, which is undesirable [83]. To determine the precise dysfunction in the intestinal ecosystem of patients with IBD, Morgan et al. studied microbial metabolism in IBD patients and healthy subjects using shotgun metagenomes. They identified major shifts in metabolic pathways, including an increase in the occurrence of oxidative stress pathways and a decrease in basic metabolism and short-chain fatty acid (SCFA) production [84]. The microbiome of patients with ileal CD is known to exhibit heightened virulence and secretion pathways [84]. One study compared the metagenome of the microbiota between children with active CD with a reduced diversity and altered stool microbial composition and healthy controls. Modules that were more abundant in the CD group included ubiquinone and lipopolysaccharide (LPS) biosynthesis, as well as the twin-arginine translocation system; sulfur reduction was also noted, whereas key processes such as fatty acid biosynthesis were overrepresented in the controls [21]. LPS can activate the toll-like receptor 4 (TLR-4) signaling pathway to induce inflammation [85]. Duboc et al. compared stool samples from IBD patients and healthy subjects to study the impact of dysbiosis in IBD on metabolism to bile acids and inflammation of the epithelium. The microbiota of IBD patients exhibited impaired deconjugation, transformation, and desulfation to bile acids, demonstrating an increase in the conjugated bile

acid rates and fecal 3-OH-sulfated bile acids as well as a decrease in the secondary bile acids. The results also showed that secondary bile acids could lead to anti-inflammation activities [86].

The reduction in diversity, accompanied by alterations in the microbial structure, could induce a disturbance in normal intestinal ecological function, which is harmful to the host [84]. These phenomena suggest that a reduction in microbial diversity has a far-reaching impact on the gut ecosystem, deteriorating the gut environment and inducing intestinal inflammation. Future research should further investigate the relationship between microbial diversity and intestinal health to promote the clinical remission of intestinal inflammation via biotherapy.

6. Conclusion

The diversity of microbiota contributes to the stability of the intestinal ecosystem and its ecological function. A loss of diversity could initiate an inflammatory reaction and promote the development of inflammatory disease. Bacterial therapy, including FMT, probiotics, and prebiotics, has obtained curative efficacy accompanied by an improvement in diversity [87–92]. The restoration of normal microbiota diversity represents a promising prospect in curing corresponding inflammatory disease.

Abbreviations

IBD: Inflammatory bowel disease
FMT: Fecal microbiota transplantation
UC: Ulcerative colitis
CD: Crohn's disease
TI: Terminal ileum
CDI: *Clostridium difficile* infection
rCDI: Recurrent *Clostridium difficile* infection
SCFA: Short-chain fatty acid
LPS: Lipopolysaccharide
TLR-4: Toll-like receptor 4.

Competing Interests

The authors declare that they have no competing interests.

References

[1] B. Chassaing and A. T. Gewirtz, "Gut microbiota, low-grade inflammation, and metabolic syndrome," *Toxicologic Pathology*, vol. 42, no. 1, pp. 49–53, 2014.

[2] S. Brugman, K.-Y. Liu, D. Lindenbergh-Kortleve et al., "Oxazolone-induced enterocolitis in zebrafish depends on the composition of the intestinal microbiota," *Gastroenterology*, vol. 137, no. 5, pp. 1757e1–1767e1, 2009.

[3] P. M. Munyaka, N. Eissa, C. N. Bernstein, E. Khafipour, and J. E. Ghia, "Antepartum antibiotic treatment increases offspring susceptibility to experimental colitis: a role of the gut microbiota," *PLoS ONE*, vol. 10, no. 11, Article ID e0142536, 2015.

[4] F. Sommer and F. Bäckhed, "The gut microbiota-masters of host development and physiology," *Nature Reviews Microbiology*, vol. 11, no. 4, pp. 227–238, 2013.

[5] Human Microbiome Project C, "Structure, function and diversity of the healthy human microbiome," *Nature*, vol. 486, pp. 207–214, 2012.

[6] J. J. Faith, J. L. Guruge, M. Charbonneau et al., "The long-term stability of the human gut microbiota," *Science*, vol. 341, no. 6141, Article ID 1237439, 2013.

[7] J. Qin, R. Li, J. Raes et al., "A human gut microbial gene catalogue established by metagenomic sequencing," *Nature*, vol. 464, no. 7285, pp. 59–65, 2010.

[8] L. Rigottier-Gois, "Dysbiosis in inflammatory bowel diseases: the oxygen hypothesis," *ISME Journal*, vol. 7, no. 7, pp. 1256–1261, 2013.

[9] P. De Cruz, S. Kang, J. Wagner et al., "Association between specific mucosa-associated microbiota in Crohn's disease at the time of resection and subsequent disease recurrence: a pilot study," *Journal of Gastroenterology and Hepatology*, vol. 30, no. 2, pp. 268–278, 2015.

[10] L. Chen, W. Wang, R. Zhou et al., "Characteristics of fecal and mucosa-associated microbiota in Chinese patients with inflammatory bowel disease," *Medicine*, vol. 93, no. 8, article e51, 2014.

[11] A. Andoh, H. Imaeda, T. Aomatsu et al., "Comparison of the fecal microbiota profiles between ulcerative colitis and Crohn's disease using terminal restriction fragment length polymorphism analysis," *Journal of Gastroenterology*, vol. 46, no. 4, pp. 479–486, 2011.

[12] K. Ray, "IBD: Gut microbiota in IBD goes viral," *Nature Reviews Gastroenterology and Hepatology*, vol. 12, article no. 122, 2015.

[13] S. Sha, B. Xu, X. Wang et al., "The biodiversity and composition of the dominant fecal microbiota in patients with inflammatory bowel disease," *Diagnostic Microbiology and Infectious Disease*, vol. 75, no. 3, pp. 245–251, 2013.

[14] J. Dicksved, J. Halfvarson, M. Rosenquist et al., "Molecular analysis of the gut microbiota of identical twins with Crohn's disease," *ISME Journal*, vol. 2, no. 7, pp. 716–727, 2008.

[15] C. Manichanh, L. Rigottier-Gois, E. Bonnaud et al., "Reduced diversity of faecal microbiota in Crohn's disease revealed by a metagenomic approach," *Gut*, vol. 55, no. 2, pp. 205–211, 2006.

[16] S. J. Ott, M. Musfeldt, D. F. Wenderoth et al., "Reduction in diversity of the colonic mucosa associated bacterial microflora in patients with active inflammatory bowel disease," *Gut*, vol. 53, no. 5, pp. 685–693, 2004.

[17] L. Nylund, M. Nermes, E. Isolauri, S. Salminen, W. M. de Vos, and R. Satokari, "Severity of atopic disease inversely correlates with intestinal microbiota diversity and butyrate-producing bacteria," *Allergy*, vol. 70, no. 2, pp. 241–244, 2015.

[18] E. Papa, M. Docktor, C. Smillie et al., "Non-invasive mapping of the gastrointestinal microbiota identifies children with inflammatory bowel disease," *PLoS ONE*, vol. 7, no. 6, Article ID e39242, 2012.

[19] S. L. Russell, M. J. Gold, M. Hartmann et al., "Early life antibiotic-driven changes in microbiota enhance susceptibility to allergic asthma," *EMBO Reports*, vol. 13, no. 5, pp. 440–447, 2012.

[20] S. Michail, M. Durbin, D. Turner et al., "Alterations in the gut microbiome of children with severe ulcerative colitis," *Inflammatory Bowel Diseases*, vol. 18, no. 10, pp. 1799–1808, 2012.

[21] C. Quince, U. Z. Ijaz, N. Loman et al., "Extensive modulation of the fecal metagenome in children with Crohn's disease during exclusive enteral nutrition," *American Journal of Gastroenterology*, vol. 110, no. 12, pp. 1718–1729, 2015.

[22] A. Andoh, H. Kuzuoka, T. Tsujikawa et al., "Multicenter analysis of fecal microbiota profiles in Japanese patients with Crohn's disease," *Journal of Gastroenterology*, vol. 47, no. 12, pp. 1298–1307, 2012.

[23] H. Nemoto, K. Kataoka, H. Ishikawa et al., "Reduced diversity and imbalance of fecal microbiota in patients with ulcerative colitis," *Digestive Diseases and Sciences*, vol. 57, no. 11, pp. 2955–2964, 2012.

[24] M. Alipour, D. Zaidi, R. Valcheva et al., "Mucosal barrier depletion and loss of bacterial diversity are primary abnormalities in paediatric ulcerative colitis," *Journal of Crohn's and Colitis*, vol. 10, no. 4, pp. 462–471, 2016.

[25] L. Grasa, L. Abecia, R. Forcén et al., "Antibiotic-induced depletion of murine microbiota induces mild inflammation and changes in toll-like receptor patterns and intestinal motility," *Microbial Ecology*, vol. 70, no. 3, pp. 835–848, 2015.

[26] C. Hedin, C. J. van der Gast, G. B. Rogers et al., "Siblings of patients with Crohn's disease exhibit a biologically relevant dysbiosis in mucosal microbial metacommunities," *Gut*, vol. 65, no. 6, pp. 944–953, 2016.

[27] G. A. W. Rook, "99th Dahlem conference on infection, inflammation and chronic inflammatory disorders: darwinian medicine and the 'hygiene' or 'old friends' hypothesis," *Clinical and Experimental Immunology*, vol. 160, no. 1, pp. 70–79, 2010.

[28] T. J. Borody and J. Campbell, "Fecal microbiota transplantation. Techniques, applications, and issues," *Gastroenterology Clinics of North America*, vol. 41, no. 4, pp. 781–803, 2012.

[29] S. Kunde, A. Pham, S. Bonczyk et al., "Safety, tolerability, and clinical response after fecal transplantation in children and young adults with ulcerative colitis," *Journal of Pediatric Gastroenterology and Nutrition*, vol. 56, no. 6, pp. 597–601, 2013.

[30] T. J. Borody, E. F. Warren, S. Leis, R. Surace, and O. Ashman, "Treatment of ulcerative colitis using fecal bacteriotherapy," *Journal of Clinical Gastroenterology*, vol. 37, no. 1, pp. 42–47, 2003.

[31] L. P. Smits, K. E. C. Bouter, W. M. De Vos, T. J. Borody, and M. Nieuwdorp, "Therapeutic potential of fecal microbiota transplantation," *Gastroenterology*, vol. 145, no. 5, pp. 946–953, 2013.

[32] P. Moayyedi, M. G. Surette, P. T. Kim et al., "Fecal microbiota transplantation induces remission in patients with active ulcerative colitis in a randomized controlled trial," *Gastroenterology*, vol. 149, no. 1, Article ID 59708, pp. 102–109, 2015.

[33] Y. Shi, Y. Dong, W. Huang et al., "Fecal microbiota transplantation for ulcerative colitis: a systematic review and meta-analysis," *PLOS ONE*, vol. 11, no. 6, Article ID e0157259, 2016.

[34] R. J. Colman and D. T. Rubin, "Fecal microbiota transplantation as therapy for inflammatory bowel disease: a systematic review and meta-analysis," *Journal of Crohn's and Colitis*, vol. 8, no. 12, pp. 1569–1581, 2014.

[35] D. E. Low, D. Shahinas, M. Silverman et al., "Toward an understanding of changes in diversity associated with fecal microbiome transplantation based on 16s rRNA gene deep sequencing," *mBio*, vol. 3, no. 5, Article ID e00338-12, 2012.

[36] C. Vincent, D. A. Stephens, V. G. Loo et al., "Reductions in intestinal Clostridiales precede the development of nosocomial *Clostridium difficile* infection," *Microbiome*, vol. 1, no. 1, article 18, 2013.

[37] L. V. McFarland, "Alternative treatments for *Clostridium difficile* disease: what really works?" *Journal of Medical Microbiology*, vol. 54, no. 2, pp. 101–111, 2005.

[38] R. A. Britton and V. B. Young, "Role of the intestinal microbiota in resistance to colonization by *Clostridium difficile*," *Gastroenterology*, vol. 146, no. 6, pp. 1547–1553, 2014.

[39] M. Rupnik, M. H. Wilcox, and D. N. Gerding, "Clostridium difficile infection: new developments in epidemiology and pathogenesis," *Nature Reviews Microbiology*, vol. 7, no. 7, pp. 526–536, 2009.

[40] E. van Nood, A. Vrieze, M. Nieuwdorp et al., "Duodenal infusion of donor feces for recurrent *Clostridium difficile*," *The New England Journal of Medicine*, vol. 368, no. 5, pp. 407–415, 2013.

[41] S. K. Hourigan, L. A. Chen, Z. Grigoryan et al., "Microbiome changes associated with sustained eradication of *Clostridium difficile* after single faecal microbiota transplantation in children with and without inflammatory bowel disease," *Alimentary Pharmacology and Therapeutics*, vol. 42, no. 6, pp. 741–752, 2015.

[42] Z. Kassam, C. H. Lee, Y. Yuan, and R. H. Hunt, "Fecal microbiota transplantation for clostridium difficile infection: systematic review and meta-analysis," *American Journal of Gastroenterology*, vol. 108, no. 4, pp. 500–508, 2013.

[43] N. G. Rossen, J. K. MacDonald, E. M. de Vries et al., "Fecal microbiota transplantation as novel therapy in gastroenterology: a systematic review," *World Journal of Gastroenterology*, vol. 21, no. 17, pp. 5359–5371, 2015.

[44] Y.-T. Li, H.-F. Cai, Z.-H. Wang, J. Xu, and J.-Y. Fang, "Systematic review with meta-analysis: long-term outcomes of faecal microbiota transplantation for Clostridium difficile infection," *Alimentary Pharmacology and Therapeutics*, vol. 43, no. 4, pp. 445–457, 2016.

[45] J. Landy, H. O. Al-Hassi, S. D. McLaughlin et al., "Review article: faecal transplantation therapy for gastrointestinal disease," *Alimentary Pharmacology and Therapeutics*, vol. 34, no. 4, pp. 409–415, 2011.

[46] T. Spector and R. Knight, "Authors' reply to Mawer and Wilcox and Mullish and Williams," *British Medical Journal*, vol. 351, Article ID h6132, 2015.

[47] T. J. Borody and A. Khoruts, "Fecal microbiota transplantation and emerging applications," *Nature Reviews Gastroenterology and Hepatology*, vol. 9, no. 2, pp. 88–96, 2012.

[48] C. G. Buffie, I. Jarchum, M. Equinda et al., "Profound alterations of intestinal microbiota following a single dose of clindamycin results in sustained susceptibility to Clostridium difficile-induced colitis," *Infection and Immunity*, vol. 80, no. 1, pp. 62–73, 2012.

[49] J. Yin, X.-X. Zhang, B. Wu, and Q. Xian, "Metagenomic insights into tetracycline effects on microbial community and antibiotic resistance of mouse gut," *Ecotoxicology*, vol. 24, no. 10, pp. 2125–2132, 2015.

[50] G. Dubourg, J. C. Lagier, C. Robert et al., "Culturomics and pyrosequencing evidence of the reduction in gut microbiota diversity in patients with broad-spectrum antibiotics," *International Journal of Antimicrobial Agents*, vol. 44, no. 2, pp. 117–124, 2014.

[51] L. Dethlefsen, S. Huse, M. L. Sogin, and D. A. Relman, "The pervasive effects of an antibiotic on the human gut microbiota, as revealed by deep 16s rRNA sequencing," *PLoS Biology*, vol. 6, no. 11, article no. e280, pp. 2383–2400, 2008.

[52] H. E. Jakobsson, C. Jernberg, A. F. Andersson, M. Sjölund-Karlsson, J. K. Jansson, and L. Engstrand, "Short-term antibiotic treatment has differing long-term impacts on the human throat and gut microbiome," *PLoS ONE*, vol. 5, no. 3, Article ID e9836, 2010.

[53] P. A. Johanesen, K. E. Mackin, M. L. Hutton et al., "Disruption of the gut microbiome: clostridium difficile infection and the threat of antibiotic resistance," *Genes*, vol. 6, no. 4, pp. 1347–1360, 2015.

[54] J. Momper, Y. Mulugeta, and G. Burckart, "Failed pediatric drug development trials," *Clinical Pharmacology & Therapeutics*, vol. 98, no. 3, pp. 245–251, 2015.

[55] E. P. Halmos, C. T. Christophersen, A. R. Bird, S. J. Shepherd, P. R. Gibson, and J. G. Muir, "Diets that differ in their FODMAP content alter the colonic luminal microenvironment," *Gut*, vol. 64, no. 1, pp. 93–100, 2015.

[56] E. D. Sonnenburg, S. A. Smits, M. Tikhonov, S. K. Higginbottom, N. S. Wingreen, and J. L. Sonnenburg, "Diet-induced extinctions in the gut microbiota compound over generations," *Nature*, vol. 529, no. 7585, pp. 212–215, 2016.

[57] H. L. Simpson and B. J. Campbell, "Review article: dietary fibre-microbiota interactions," *Alimentary Pharmacology and Therapeutics*, vol. 42, no. 2, pp. 158–179, 2015.

[58] P. J. Turnbaugh, M. Hamady, T. Yatsunenko et al., "A core gut microbiome in obese and lean twins," *Nature*, vol. 457, no. 7228, pp. 480–484, 2009.

[59] T. Yatsunenko, F. E. Rey, M. J. Manary et al., "Human gut microbiome viewed across age and geography," *Nature*, vol. 486, no. 7402, pp. 222–227, 2012.

[60] J. Sebald, M. Willi, I. Schoberleitner et al., "Impact of the chromatin remodeling factor CHD1 on gut microbiome composition of *Drosophila melanogaster*," *PLoS ONE*, vol. 11, no. 4, Article ID e0153476, 2016.

[61] M. Y. Lim, H. J. You, H. S. Yoon et al., "The effect of heritability and host genetics on the gut microbiota and metabolic syndrome," *Gut*, 2016.

[62] D. N. Frank, C. E. Robertson, C. M. Hamm et al., "Disease phenotype and genotype are associated with shifts in intestinal-associated microbiota in inflammatory bowel diseases," *Inflammatory Bowel Diseases*, vol. 17, no. 1, pp. 179–184, 2011.

[63] H. Zhang, J. B. Sparks, S. V. Karyala, R. Settlage, and X. M. Luo, "Host adaptive immunity alters gut microbiota," *ISME Journal*, vol. 9, no. 3, pp. 770–781, 2015.

[64] M. E. V. Johansson, J. K. Gustafsson, J. Holmen-Larsson et al., "Bacteria penetrate the normally impenetrable inner colon mucus layer in both murine colitis models and patients with ulcerative colitis," *Gut*, vol. 63, no. 2, pp. 281–291, 2014.

[65] L. A. Van Der Waaij, H. J. M. Harmsen, M. Madjipour et al., "Bacterial population analysis of human colon and terminal ileum biopsies with 16S rRNA-based fluorescent probes: commensal bacteria live in suspension and have no direct contact with epithelial cells," *Inflammatory Bowel Diseases*, vol. 11, no. 10, pp. 865–871, 2005.

[66] M. E. V. Johansson, M. Phillipson, J. Petersson, A. Velcich, L. Holm, and G. C. Hansson, "The inner of the two Muc2 mucin-dependent mucus layers in colon is devoid of bacteria," *Proceedings of the National Academy of Sciences of the United States of America*, vol. 105, no. 39, pp. 15064–15069, 2008.

[67] M. E. V. Johansson, J. M. H. Larsson, and G. C. Hansson, "The two mucus layers of colon are organized by the MUC2 mucin, whereas the outer layer is a legislator of host-microbial interactions," *Proceedings of the National Academy of Sciences of the United States of America*, vol. 108, supplement 1, pp. 4659–4665, 2011.

[68] C. K. Heazlewood, M. C. Cook, R. Eri et al., "Aberrant mucin assembly in mice causes endoplasmic reticulum stress and spontaneous inflammation resembling ulcerative colitis," *PLoS Medicine*, vol. 5, no. 3, article no. e54, 2008.

[69] M. Van der Sluis, B. A. E. De Koning, A. C. J. M. De Bruijn et al., "Muc2-deficient mice spontaneously develop colitis, indicating

that MUC2 is critical for colonic protection," *Gastroenterology*, vol. 131, no. 1, pp. 117–129, 2006.

[70] S. Etzold and N. Juge, "Structural insights into bacterial recognition of intestinal mucins," *Current Opinion in Structural Biology*, vol. 28, no. 1, pp. 23–31, 2014.

[71] S. Bel, Y. Elkis, H. Elifantz et al., "Reprogrammed and transmissible intestinal microbiota confer diminished susceptibility to induced colitis in TMF$^{-/-}$ mice," *Proceedings of the National Academy of Sciences of the United States of America*, vol. 111, no. 13, pp. 4964–4969, 2014.

[72] A. N. Ananthakrishnan, H. Khalili, G. G. Konijeti et al., "A prospective study of long-term intake of dietary fiber and risk of Crohn's disease and ulcerative colitis," *Gastroenterology*, vol. 145, no. 5, pp. 970–977, 2013.

[73] X. Li, J. Sundquist, K. Hemminki, and K. Sundquist, "Risk of inflammatory bowel disease in first- and second-generation immigrants in Sweden: a nationwide follow-up study," *Inflammatory Bowel Diseases*, vol. 17, no. 8, pp. 1784–1791, 2011.

[74] S. Y. Shaw, J. F. Blanchard, and C. N. Bernstein, "Association between the use of antibiotics in the first year of life and pediatric inflammatory bowel disease," *The American Journal of Gastroenterology*, vol. 105, no. 12, pp. 2687–2692, 2010.

[75] D. K. Amre, S. D'Souza, K. Morgan et al., "Imbalances in dietary consumption of fatty acids, vegetables, and fruits are associated with risk for crohn's disease in children," *American Journal of Gastroenterology*, vol. 102, no. 9, pp. 2016–2025, 2007.

[76] C. S. J. Probert, V. Jayanthi, D. Pinder, A. C. Wicks, and J. F. Mayberry, "Epidemiological study of ulcerative proctocolitis in Indian migrants and the indigenous population of Leicestershire," *Gut*, vol. 33, no. 5, pp. 687–693, 1992.

[77] Y. Feng, "Species diversity and managed ecosystem stability," *Chinese Journal of Applied Ecology*, vol. 14, no. 6, pp. 853–857, 2003.

[78] A. S. Mori, T. Furukawa, and T. Sasaki, "Response diversity determines the resilience of ecosystems to environmental change," *Biological Reviews*, vol. 88, no. 2, pp. 349–364, 2013.

[79] T. H. Oliver, M. S. Heard, N. J. Isaac et al., "Biodiversity and resilience of ecosystem functions," *Trends in Ecology & Evolution*, vol. 30, no. 11, pp. 673–684, 2015.

[80] F. Isbell, D. Craven, J. Connolly et al., "Biodiversity increases the resistance of ecosystem productivity to climate extremes," *Nature*, vol. 526, no. 7574, pp. 574–577, 2015.

[81] M. Loreau, "Biodiversity and ecosystem functioning: the mystery of the deep sea," *Current Biology*, vol. 18, no. 3, pp. R126–R128, 2008.

[82] P. Balvanera, A. B. Pfisterer, N. Buchmann et al., "Quantifying the evidence for biodiversity effects on ecosystem functioning and services," *Ecology Letters*, vol. 9, no. 10, pp. 1146–1156, 2006.

[83] M. Scheffer, S. Carpenter, J. A. Foley, C. Folke, and B. Walker, "Catastrophic shifts in ecosystems," *Nature*, vol. 413, no. 6856, pp. 591–596, 2001.

[84] X. C. Morgan, T. L. Tickle, H. Sokol et al., "Dysfunction of the intestinal microbiome in inflammatory bowel disease and treatment," *Genome Biology*, vol. 13, article no. R79, 2012.

[85] A. Poltorak, X. He, I. Smirnova et al., "Defective LPS signaling in C3H/HeJ and C57BL/10ScCr mice: mutations in *Tlr4* gene," *Science*, vol. 282, no. 5396, pp. 2085–2088, 1998.

[86] H. Duboc, S. Rajca, D. Rainteau et al., "Connecting dysbiosis, bile-acid dysmetabolism and gut inflammation in inflammatory bowel diseases," *Gut*, vol. 62, no. 4, pp. 531–539, 2013.

[87] S. Oliva, G. Di Nardo, F. Ferrari et al., "Randomised clinical trial: the effectiveness of *Lactobacillus reuteri* ATCC 55730 rectal enema in children with active distal ulcerative colitis," *Alimentary Pharmacology and Therapeutics*, vol. 35, no. 3, pp. 327–334, 2012.

[88] W. Kruis, E. Schütz, P. Fric, B. Fixa, G. Judmaier, and M. Stolte, "Double-blind comparison of an oral *Escherichia coli* preparation and mesalazine in maintaining remission of ulcerative colitis," *Alimentary Pharmacology and Therapeutics*, vol. 11, no. 5, pp. 853–858, 1997.

[89] B. J. Rembacken, A. M. Snelling, P. M. Hawkey, D. M. Chalmers, and A. T. R. Axon, "Non-pathogenic *Escherichia coli* versus mesalazine for the treatment of ulcerative colitis: a randomised trial," *The Lancet*, vol. 354, no. 9179, pp. 635–639, 1999.

[90] W. Kruis, P. Frič, J. Pokrotnieks et al., "Maintaining remission of ulcerative colitis with the probiotic *Escherichia coli* Nissle 1917 is as effective as with standard mesalazine," *Gut*, vol. 53, no. 11, pp. 1617–1623, 2004.

[91] D. Jonkers, J. Penders, A. Masclee, and M. Pierik, "Probiotics in the management of inflammatory bowel disease: a systematic review of intervention studies in adult patients," *Drugs*, vol. 72, no. 6, pp. 803–823, 2012.

[92] J. Shen, Z.-X. Zuo, and A.-P. Mao, "Effect of probiotics on inducing remission and maintaining therapy in ulcerative colitis, Crohn's disease, and pouchitis: meta-analysis of randomized controlled trials," *Inflammatory Bowel Diseases*, vol. 20, no. 1, pp. 21–35, 2014.

8

Novel Implications in Molecular Diagnosis of Lynch Syndrome

Raffaella Liccardo,[1] **Marina De Rosa,**[1] **Paola Izzo,**[1,2] **and Francesca Duraturo**[1]

[1]Department of Molecular Medicine and Medical Biotechnology, University of Naples "Federico II", 80131 Naples, Italy
[2]CEINGE Biotecnologie Avanzate, University of Naples "Federico II", 80131 Naples, Italy

Correspondence should be addressed to Francesca Duraturo; duraturo@dbbm.unina.it

Academic Editor: Haruhiko Sugimura

About 10% of total colorectal cancers are associated with known Mendelian inheritance, as Familial Adenomatous Polyposis (FAP) and Lynch syndrome (LS). In these cancer types the clinical manifestations of disease are due to mutations in high-risk alleles, with a penetrance at least of 70%. The LS is associated with germline mutations in the DNA mismatch repair (MMR) genes. However, the mutation detection analysis of these genes does not always provide informative results for genetic counseling of LS patients. Very often, the molecular analysis reveals the presence of variants of unknown significance (VUSs) whose interpretation is not easy and requires the combination of different analytical strategies to get a proper assessment of their pathogenicity. In some cases, these VUSs may make a more substantial overall contribution to cancer risk than the well-assessed severe Mendelian variants. Moreover, it could also be possible that the simultaneous presence of these genetic variants in several MMR genes that behave as low risk alleles might contribute in a cooperative manner to increase the risk of hereditary cancer. In this paper, through a review of the recent literature, we have speculated a novel inheritance model in the Lynch syndrome; this could pave the way toward new diagnostic perspectives.

1. Introduction

Colorectal cancer (CRC) is a multifactorial disease in which genetic and environmental factors are involved. Familial CRC, in which one or more first-degree and/or second-degree relatives of the index case manifest CRC, constitutes approximately 20% of the total CRC burden [1]. High penetrance mutations confer a predisposition to CRC in the so-called hereditary syndromes, responsible for about 2–6% of the total CRC. Low penetrance mutations are found in the remaining part of CRC (about 96%), representing a risk factor in both sporadic and familial cases [2, 3]. CRC syndromes are defined on the basis of clinical, pathological, and, more recently, genetic findings [3] (Table 1).

Accordingly, the identification of predisposing genes allows for accurate risk assessment and more precise screening approaches. Lynch syndrome (LS) is the most common hereditary form of CRC with an incidence of 3–5% of all CRCs whereas its primary genetic counterpart, namely, Familial Adenomatous Polyposis (FAP), accounts for less than 1% of the total CRC burden [4].

LS and FAP are diseases with autosomal dominant inheritance, caused by germline mutations in the DNA mismatch repair genes (MMR) or in the Adenomatous Polyposis Coli tumor suppressor gene (APC), respectively. These syndromes may also occur in more attenuated forms. In FAP syndrome, attenuated forms (AFAP) are caused by low penetrance mutations (missense mutations) in the main APC gene or by biallelic loss of the MYH gene (MAP, MUTYH-associated polyposis with autosomal recessive inheritance), encoding a protein of the Base Excision Repair complex (BER) [5]. Variant clinic forms of LS are characterized by the presence of additional tumors of still unclear etiology in extracolonic locations. Recent studies suggest that an interaction between main genes (MMR) and modifier genes and/or environmental factors may beat the basis of these tumors. These variant syndromes include Muir-Torre syndrome (autosomal dominant) due to MSH2 and MLH1 genes mutations and characterized by the presence of cutaneous manifestations (multiple sebaceous adenomas, epithelioma, and keratoacanthoma) associated with colorectal and endometrial cancers and Turcot syndrome (autosomal dominant) associated with

APC, PMS2, and MLH1 genes mutations and characterized by brain cancers (glioblastoma and cerebellar medulloblastoma) are associated with colorectal cancer [6, 7].

In the process of colorectal carcinogenesis many other genes are involved such as oncogenes and tumor suppressor genes that play a key role in the control of cell cycle. Mutations in these genes are at the basis of rarer inherited CRC syndromes. These are mainly "hamartomatous polyposis syndromes" characterized by the presence of benign adenomas arising from epithelial and/or stromal intestinal tissue, which increase the risk of developing CRC. These syndromes, whose characteristics are summarized in Table 1, include Peutz-Jeghers syndrome, juvenile polyposis, Cowden syndrome, and Bannayan-Riley-Ruvalcaba syndrome [8–11].

In this review we intend to highlight new insights into the molecular features of Lynch syndrome in favor of a novel inheritance model in contrast with the classical monogenic transmission; this could suggest new genetic and clinical surveillance approaches.

2. Lynch Syndrome (LS)

2.1. Genetics Features. LS is an autosomal dominant disease with recessive phenotype caused by a defect in one of the mismatch repair (MMR) genes. The main clinical-pathological features of the Lynch syndrome are as follows [1–11, 13]:

> Autosomal dominant inheritance
>
> Penetrance for colorectal cancer (CRC) of 85–90%
>
> Earlier age of onset of CRC (~45 years) with respect to general population (69 years)
>
> Preferential tumor localization in the right-sided colon
>
> Presence of multiple synchronous and metachronous colorectal cancers
>
> Better prognosis than CRCs
>
> Increased risk for extracolonic cancers
>
> Accelerated carcinogenesis
>
> Poorly differentiated tumors, with a marked lymphocytic peritumoral inflammation recalling features of the so-called "Crohn's reaction"
>
> Microsatellite instability

The mismatch repair system was first studied in bacteria in which three proteins, MutS, MutL, and MutH, were identified. In humans, at least seven mismatch repair genes are involved in mismatch repair and their names derive from their structural homology to the bacterial proteins: the MutS homologues (MSH), MSH2 on chromosome 2p16, MSH3 on chromosome 5q11, and MSH6 on chromosome 2p16; the MutL homologues (MLH), MLH1 on chromosome 3p21 and MLH3 on chromosome 2p16; the postmeiotic segregation homologues (PMS), PMS1 and PMS2 on chromosome 7p22. No MutH homologues have been identified in humans [14]. MSH2 and MSH6 bind together to form a heteroduplex (MutSa) that predominantly identifies base pairs mismatched, while MSH2 and MSH3 (MutSβ) combine to identify short insertions or deletions. MSH2 is essential for both complexes to function, while a functional overlap exists between MSH3 and MSH6. MLH1 and PMS2 (MutLα) or MLH3 (Mutlγ) also bind together to form a heteroduplex that interacts with MutSα or MutSβ complex, stimulating excision and resynthesis of the abnormal DNA. Similarly to MSH2, also MLH1 is essential for both complexes to repair mismatches. Altogether, this group of four proteins recruits exonuclease-1 (EXO1), the proliferating cell nuclear antigen (PCNA), DNA polymerase (Polδ or Polε), two replication factor (RPA and RFC), and a ligase, to repair DNA on the daughter strand at the mismatch point. If any of the four major proteins (MSH2, MLH1, MSH6, or PMS2) is functionally inactive, mismatches are not repaired [15, 16].

2.2. Microsatellite Instability. Consequently, a defective DNA MMR system increases the mutation rate and makes the cell vulnerable to mutations in genes controlling cell growth (tumor suppressor genes and oncogenes), resulting in an increased cancer risk.

In case of a defective MMR system, mutations occur frequently in small (usually mononucleotide or dinucleotide) repetitive DNA sequences, known as microsatellites. In MMR-deficient tumor cells the number of microsatellite repeat units can deviate from the corresponding normal DNA; the number of repeats is usually decreased even though it is occasionally found to be increased [17].

Length or size microsatellite variation is known as MSI (microsatellite instability). MSI (formerly referred to as MIN or, RER, replication error) is the molecular hallmark of LS since approximately 95% of all LS-associated cancers show MSI [13]. Although most microsatellite sequences are located in noncoding sequences (telomeres and centromeres), many genes contain repetitive sequences in their coding regions and some of these genes play key roles in the regulation of cell growth. Identification of an even growing number of guide genes and target genes of the mutator phenotype can lead to discover new complex molecular mechanisms that underlie the process of colorectal tumorigenesis [18].

MSI thereby serves as a reliable phenotypic marker of MMR deficiency in order to preselect patients eligible for germline mutation analysis in the MMR genes [19].

However, despite the fact that MSI is a reliable marker for MMR deficiency, however until 15% of sporadic CRCs showed an MSI phenotype. This is mainly caused by somatic hypermethylation of the MLH1-gene promoter. Methylation of the MSH2 promoter has also been reported but it is to be considered as a heritable somatic methylation because it is caused by a deletion of the last exon of EPCAM that is adjacent to MSH2 on chromosome 2 [18].

Hypermethylation of CpG islands in the MLH1 promoter (CIMP phenotype) causes severe inhibition of gene transcription thereby mimicking an inactivating gene mutation. If both copies of the gene are inactivated (biallelic hypermethylation), the MLH1 function is lost. This leads to microsatellite unstable cancers, especially in older patients. Therefore, in MLH1-deficient microsatellite unstable (MSI-H) tumors the MLH1 hypermethylation can be assessed to

TABLE 1: Hereditary colon cancer syndromes: clinical and genetic features. (AD, autosomal dominant; AR, autosomal recessive).

Disease (OMIM)	Gene	Incidence	Inheritance	Mutation identified (%)	Penetrance	Clinical features
Hereditary nonpolyposis colorectal cancer (HNPCC) (114500)	MLH1, MSH2, MSH6, PMS2, MLH3, EPCAM	1 in 400	AD	Point mutation, large rearrangements (60–80%)	90%	Proximal CRC, endometrial carcinoma, ovarian tumors, small bowel carcinoma, urinary tract carcinoma
Classical familial adenomatous polyposis (FAP) (175100)	APC	1 in 8000	AD	Point mutation, large rearrangements (80–90%)	<100%	100 to >500 adenomatous polyps of large bowel, duodenum, stomach
Attenuated FAP (AFAP) (175100)	APC	<1 in 8000	AD	Point mutation, large rearrangements (20–30%)	<100%	10 to 100 adenomatous polyps of large bowel, duodenum, stomach
MUTYH-associated polyposis (MAP) (608456)	MUTYH	<1 in 10000	AR	Point mutation, large rearrangements (15–20%)	<100%	20 to 100 adenomatous polyps of large bowel, duodenum, stomach
Muir Torre syndrome (HNPCC) (158320)	MLH1, MSH2	<1 in 400	AD	Point mutation, large rearrangements (60–80%)	90%	CRC, endometrial carcinoma multiple sebaceous adenomas, epithelioma, keratoacanthoma
Turcot syndrome (HNPCC) (276300)	APC, PMS2, MLH1	<1 in 400	AD	Point mutation, large rearrangements (60–80%)	90%	CRC, glioblastoma, cerebellar medulloblastoma
Peutz-Jeghers syndrome (PJS) (175200)	STK11 (LKB1)	1 in 200000	AD	Point mutation, large rearrangements (90%)	95–100%	<20 juvenile polyps (PJ) of large bowel, duodenum, stomach, mucocuta-neous/perioral hyperpigmentation, ovarian tumors, breast cancer
Juvenile polyposis syndrome (JPS) (174900)	SMAD4, BMPR1A	1 in 100000	AD	Point mutation, large rearrangements (60%)	90–100%	5 to 100 JP of large bowel, duodenum, stomach, gastric cancer
Cowden syndrome (CS) (158350)	PTEN	1 in 200000	AD	Point mutation, large rearrangements (80%)	90–95%	Multiple JP/lipomas of large bowel, duodenum, stomach, mucocutaneous tumors, breast cancer, endometrial carcinoma, thyroid cancer
Bannayan-Ruvalcaba-Riley syndrome (BRRS) (153480)	PTEN	1 in 200000	AD	Point mutation, large rearrangements (60%)	90–95%	Multiple JP/lipomas of large bowel, duodenum, stomach, microcephaly, developmental delay, hemangiomatosis

distinguish sporadic CRCs from LS-related cancers. Moreover, recent findings have also identified the BRAF gene as a marker to distinguish LS from sporadic cases of colon cancer [20, 21]. Indeed, an oncogenic BRAF mutation has been described only in one case among several LS tumors [22]. Specific activating mutations in the BRAF oncogene, usually the V600E missense mutation, can be detected in 40–87% of all sporadic microsatellite unstable tumors [13]. In this case, the survival in the subjects with MSI-H tumors and BRAF mutation is higher than sporadic tumors with BRAF mutation and MSI stable; therefore, the good prognosis of MSI-H tumors is not affected by the BRAF genotype [23]. Also in another study, the MSI-H/BRAF mutation group had a good prognosis [24]. This emphasizes even more the need to evaluate both BRAF mutation and MSI status in patients with CRC for an accurate prognosis [23]. These results indicate that in cases of MSI, BRAF mutations closely correlate with MLH1 promoter methylation in sporadic MSI CRCs, in contrast to LS characterized by germline mutations in the MMR genes.

In 1997 the National Cancer Institute recommended a panel, known as the "panel of Bethesda," comprising five microsatellites: two mononucleotide repeats (BAT25, BAT26) and three dinucleotide repeats (D2S123, D17S250, D5S346) [25]. Tumors showing instability at two or more of these repeats (40% of markers) are defined at high instability (MSI-H); those with instability between 20–40% are classified as low instability (MSI-L) [26]; tumors without alteration (20% or less) are classified as stable (MSS). Subsequently, in order to improve the sensitivity rate and the predictive specificity, Bethesda guidelines were revised and other loci were enclosed in the panel test: BAT-25 and BAT-26 besides three other quasimonomorphic mononucleotide repeats, namely, NR21, NR22, and NR24 [27–29].

MSI testing is also very important because several pieces of evidence suggested that MSI-H tumors (stage II) are associated with a favorable prognosis when patients are not treated with 5-fluorouracil compared to MSI-L and MSS CRC [30, 31]. These different features are probably related to the lymphocytic infiltrate characteristic of MMR-deficient tumors that determines an antitumor immune response which may be abrogated by the immunosuppressive effects of the chemotherapy [17].

Besides MSI testing, analysis of MMR protein expression by immunohistochemistry (IHC) is routinely performed to identify patients with suspected Lynch syndrome. IHC testing is a specific (100%) and sensitive (92,3%) screening tool to identify MSI-H tumors [13, 32]. A more detailed discussion on MMR IHC is available in a recent review article [33].

2.3. Clinical Features. LS is characterized by a high lifetime risk for tumor development, especially in the case of CRC (20–70%), endometrial cancer (15–70%), and other extracolonic tumors (15%). These extracolonic malignancies include carcinomas of small intestine, stomach, pancreas and biliary tract, ovarium, brain, upper urinary tract, and skin. More recently, gastric cancers have been included in the tumor spectrum of LS [34]. The molecular and

clinical-pathological profiles of gastric cancers in LS mutation carriers have been evaluated and compared with the profiles of sporadic gastric cancers, and several differences have been identified, while there are similarities with canonical HNPCC spectrum malignancies. Stomach can thus be considered as a target tissue in which somatic inactivation ("second hit") of MMR genes may occur in carriers of a germline mutation ("first hit") [34, 35].

2.4. Clinical Diagnosis of Lynch Syndrome. Identification of MMR gene mutation carriers is critical for improving cancer surveillance and effectiveness of prevention. Before MMR genes and their causal role in hereditary CRC cancer were identified, the International Collaborative Group on hereditary nonpolyposis colorectal cancer had established the Amsterdam criteria I in 1990. These criteria were used to identify families eligible for molecular analysis. Subsequently modified guidelines (Amsterdam criteria II) were designed to include extracolonic LS-related cancers [1]. Nevertheless, Amsterdam criteria resulted to be very restrictive and failed to identify a large portion of MMR gene mutation carriers. To overcome this issue, Bethesda guidelines, which were less restrictive and had a sensitivity greater than 90% even with a lower specificity (25%), were later defined [25].

3. New Insights into the Molecular Features of Lynch Syndrome

A long time, literature data report that in addition to the postreplicative repair, MMR proteins have developed various other functions that may have relevant roles in carcinogenesis [16]. These new roles include the following:

(1) DNA damage signalling caused by exogenous carcinogens (heterocyclic amines, oxidative agents, and UV radiation) that is achieved through a synergistic action between the p53-homologous proteins (p53, p63 and p73) and the MutSα-MutLα complex; furthermore, in response to an exogenous damage, MLH1 interacts with the protein MRE11, a component of the "BRCA1 associated surveillance complex" (BASC), and regulates the cell cycle and the apoptotic pathway [36, 37]

(2) Prevention of reparative recombination (gene conversion) between nonidentical sequences [38]

(3) Promotion of meiotic crossover; several studies in *S. Cerevisiae* and knockout mice have shown that homologous chromosome recombination during meiosis is controlled by MMR proteins, in order to avoid mutational events due to deletions, insertions, or mismatched bases. Among the MMR proteins, MLH1, PMS2, and MLH3 are involved in this process. In fact, experimental murine deficiency of one of these three proteins is associated with male infertility (defective spermatogenesis) [38, 39]

(4) Immunoglobulin diversification based on the "somatic hypermutation" (SHM) process, which is regulated by the MutSα-MutLα complex, in combination

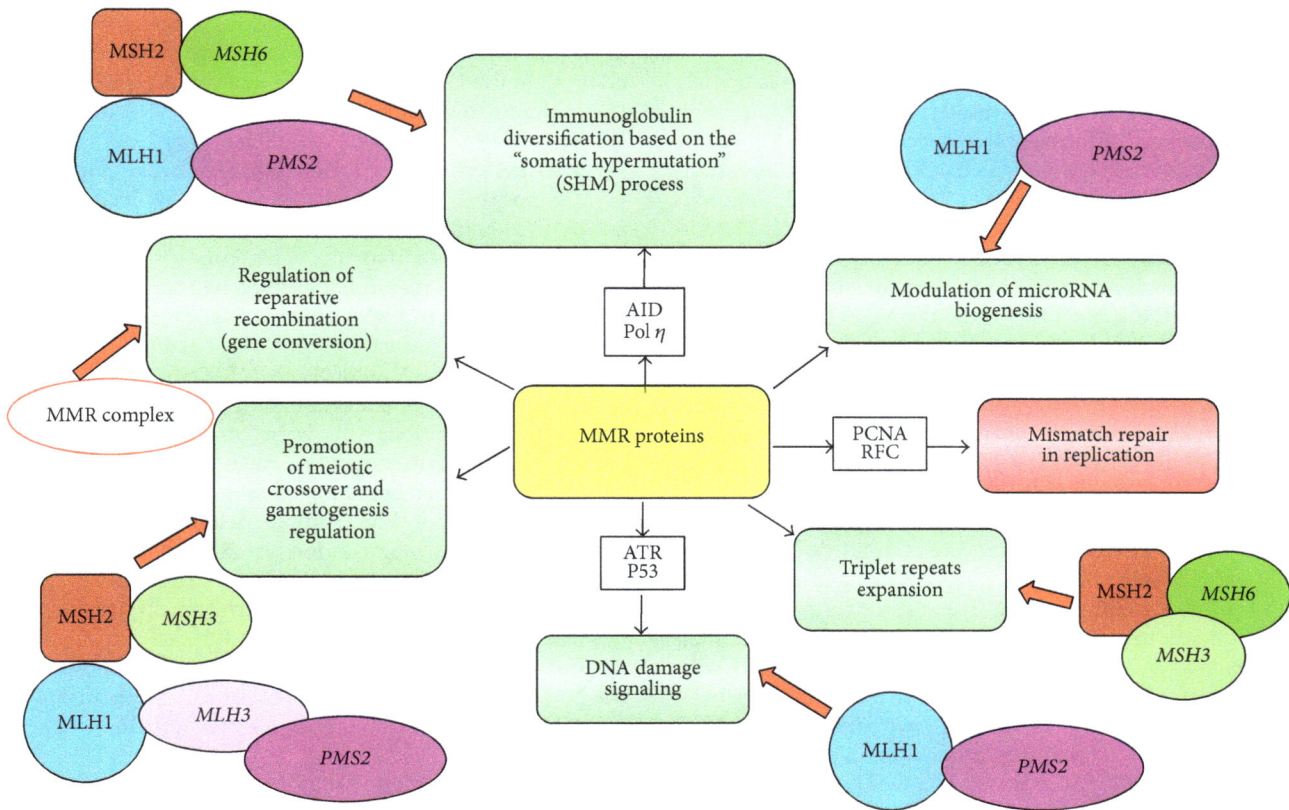

FIGURE 1: New role for MMR proteins.

with two other proteins, AID (activation-induced cytidine deaminase) and Polμ (DNA Polymerase "error-prone") [40]; in particular, MutSα deficiency is associated with neoplastic transformation of T lymphocytes [41]

(5) Expansion of repeated triplets (CTG, CGG) that underlie the pathogenesis of various neurodegenerative diseases such as Huntington's Disease, Myotonic Dystrophy, and Fragile X Syndrome. This mechanism is still unknown; however experimental evidence indicates that, although MutSβ binds these expansions, the repair is prevented by looping conformations of these regions [42]. Since the triplet expansion is at the basis of the anticipation of the disease in the family, loss of function of MutSβ may have a protective role against the intergenerational instability [43, 44]

(6) Modulation of microRNA biogenesis by interaction of MMR proteins with the microprocessor complex; in particular, MutLα specifically binds pri-miRNAs and the complex Drosha/DGCR8 in order to stimulate the processing of pri-miRNAs to pre-miRNAs in a manner dependent on MutLα ATPase activity [45]

These new features indicate that MMR deficiency strongly affects cellular resistance to reparative and/or apoptotic response to DNA damage because impairment of postreplicative MMR complexes associated with impairment of components of other cell systems (Figure 1).

4. Genotype-Phenotype Associations in Lynch Syndrome

4.1. Canonical Features. Germline mutations are distributed unevenly along each MMR gene, denoting the absence of mutational hot spots. Even the nature of the germline alterations is varied.

Absence of redundant functions for MSH2 and MLH1 proteins stresses the importance of these two genes; therefore, mutations in these genes are associated with aggressive forms of HNPCC, characterized by early age of onset, typically around 45 years of age, high penetrance, and high degree of microsatellite instability (MSI-H) [46]. The CRC incidence is similar in subjects with mutations in MLH1 and MSH2 (84% and 71% resp.); however, individuals with alterations in the MSH2 gene show a higher incidence (48–61%) of extracolonic malignancy (endometrial, gastric, ovarian, and kidney cancer) than those carrying mutations in the MLH1 gene (11–42%) [47].

The clinical phenotype is different when minor genes are involved. Mutations in MSH6, for example, seem to cause a form of "attenuated" HNPCC, characterized by lower penetrance, later age of onset, usually around 60 years of age, and MSI-L [48].

Defects in the PMS2 gene are instead associated with early tumor development and microsatellite instability, although some features are different with respect to cancers caused by the MLH1 and MSH2 mutations. PMS2 mutations are associated with combined presence of multiple colorectal adenomas and glioblastomas (Turcot syndrome). The specificity of brain tumor is probably linked to the accumulation of mutations in target genes (oncogenes, tumor suppressor) more specifically expressed in the brain [49]. Recently, MLH3 variants were associated with brain cancer predisposition [50].

In the MSH3 gene, missense, silent, and intronic variations have been mainly identified; these mutations are associated with a severe phenotype in the case they are inherited in combination with each other or associated with variants in the MSH2 gene [51]. In fact, MSH3 knockout mice showed a low susceptibility to cancer development that caused late-onset colorectal cancer, whereas double mutant MSH3-MSH6 mice showed a very similar phenotype to that found in mice lacking MSH2. These results are justified by the redundant function of the MSH3 and MSH6 genes [52]. Moreover, MSH3 inactivation is primarily associated with instability of tetranucleotide repeats (EMAST) that has been frequently observed in moderately or poorly differentiated adenocarcinomas as well as in other cancers including lung, kidney, ovarian, and bladder cancer [14, 53].

In recent years, numerous studies have found an association between the development of hematopoietic and intestinal tumors in infant age and the presence of homozygous mutations in the MLH1, MSH2, MSH6, and PMS2 genes [54, 55]. This phenotype was also associated with heterozygous mutations in two or more MMR genes, suggesting a mechanism of compound heterozygosity [56–58].

In a subset of LS patients, a germline mutation at the $3'$ end of the EPCAM (TACSTD1) gene has been identified resulting in allelic-specific methylation and transcription silencing of MSH2, which is located upstream of the EPCAM gene. The EPCAM gene encodes for the Epithelial Cell Adhesion Molecule protein that is involved in cell signalling, migration, proliferation, and differentiation. Accordingly, this mutation may contribute to the development of extra-colonic cancers [59].

4.2. Noncanonical Features. Recently a group of Lynch-like syndrome patients was described [60]. This group may account for as much as 70% of suspected Lynch syndrome subjects. Unlike sporadic MSI cancer, Lynch-like patients are nearly impossible to differentiate from Lynch patients; they are MSI-positive and cancer tissues express abnormal MMR protein, not only for MLH1 as in sporadic MSI cancers but also for the other MMR proteins, such as MSH2, MSH6, and PMS2, as in Lynch syndrome cancers. Lynch-like patients show a mean age of onset comparable to LS. The only differentiating features between these two syndromes are the lower incidence for CRC and other LS-associated cancers and the absence of MMR genes germline mutation in Lynch-like syndrome. There are likely three potential reasons for cancer onset in Lynch-like patients: (a) a genetic process within the tumors other than germline mutations coupled with second allele inactivation, (b) unknown germline mutations in other genes than the DNA MMR genes that can drive MSI, and/or (c) unidentified germline mutations in the DNA MMR genes [12, 61].

Mensenkamp et al. [62] noted that a considerable number of MSI-positive tumors lack any known molecular mechanism for their development. Patients were screened for somatic mutations and for loss of heterozygosity in MLH1 and MSH2 genes. This research identified two somatic mutations in 13 of 25 tumors, 8 of which were MLH1-deficient and 5 were MSH2-deficient, indicating that such acquired mutations underlie more than 50% of the MMR-deficient tumors that have not been found associated with germline mutations or promoter methylation. This is in contrast with LS that is associated with germline mutations in the MMR genes.

Moreover, other hereditary factors might play a role in tumor development. For example, deletions affecting genes that regulate MSH2 degradation were shown to lead to MMR deficiency and undetectable levels of MSH2 protein. Moreover, cells lacking SETD2 (H3K36 trimethyltransferase SET domain containing protein 2) display MSI due to the loss of an epigenetic histone mark that is essential for the recruitment of the MSH2-MSH6 complex. Whether these mechanisms lead to MSH2-deficient colorectal cancer remains to be clarified [63].

In these cases high-throughput sequencing procedures play an important role to identify new constitutive and somatic mutations in putative genes associated with hereditary predisposition to cancer [64].

It is also noteworthy that, in addition to canonical inactivation via gene mutation, MMR activity can also be modulated by changes in MMR gene expression. This type of alteration may be the result of mutations occurring in regions that are not always routinely analyzed such as the promoter and the $5'$ and $3'$-untraslated regions.

Previous studies have defined and characterized the core promoter regions of hMSH2 (from −300 to −17 upstream of the start codon) [65] and hMLH1 (from −220 to −39 upstream of the start codon) [66]; subsequent studies have been carried out to demonstrate that germline mutations in these regions are involved in LS [67, 68].

Regarding mutations in the $3'$UTR of MMR genes, a 3-nucleotide (TTC) deletion in the MLH1 $3'$UTR was found in leukemia patients [69]. This alteration was shown to destroy a binding site for miR-422a and there is a downregulation suggesting a possible role for the miRNA in regulation of MLH1expression [69].

Therefore, cell levels of MMR are likely to be under a tight regulation in order to prevent the overproduced protein which may sequester other factors involved in controlling the mutation rate. Potentially adverse consequences of overproduced MLH1 and MSH2 are highlighted by a report showing that apoptosis is induced in a human cell line when these two genes were expressed under the control of the cytomegalovirus (CMV) promoter [70]. The dangerous excess of MMR protein can also be the effect of homodimerization complex as shown by a study in yeast cells of Shcherbakova et al. [71] showing that the MLH1-MLH1 homodimer replaced the MLH1-PMS1/PMS2/MLH3 heterodimer, inactivating also the MutSα and MutSβ functions, thus resulting in nonfunctional MMR complex.

This concept is also partially extended to other minor MMR genes; overexpression of the MSH3 gene in cultured mammalian cells selectively inactivates MutSα because MSH2 is sequestered into a MSH2-MSH3 (MutSβ) complex, resulting in reduced MutSα-dependent repair of base-base mismatches and a strong base substitution mutator phenotype [72].

Finally, several MSI tumors with unknown cause of MMR inactivation could display a miRNA down- or upexpression genotype that specifically modulate MMR genes [73, 74]. miRNA expression is in turn regulated by DNA damage [75]. miRNAs able to regulate the mismatch repair function are miR-155 and miR-21 that significantly downregulate the core MMR proteins, MSH2, MSH6, and MLH1, and have been associated with a mutator phenotype, in particular with MSI inflammatory bowel diseases (IBD) CRCs [76, 77].

5. Characterization of the "Variants of Uncertain Significance" (VUS) in the MMR Genes

Several mutations identified in the MMR genes are missense, silent, or intronic variants. The influence of these variants on the development of cancer is often a controversial topic; therefore they are classified as "VUS," Variant of Uncertain Significance [78, 79].

Several criteria can be applied to assess the possible pathogenicity of a VUS, [57, 80]; these criteria are as follows: (1) de novo appearance; (2) segregation with the disease; (3) absence in normal individuals; (4) change of amino acid polarity or size; (5) occurrence of the amino acid change in a domain that is evolutionary conserved between species and/or shared between proteins belonging to the same protein family (in silico analysis); (6) effects on splicing or on protein function; (7) loss of the nonmutated allele due to a large deletion in the tumor DNA (loss of heterozygosity (LOH)); (8) loss of protein expression in the tumor; (9) evaluation of MSI in tumor tissues. All studies conducted to date show that none of the above criteria, including functional assays, is an indicator of pathogenicity, if taken alone; it is necessary that a combination of strategies be used in order to lead to a correct assessment of the pathogenicity of uncertain variants [81]. According to these observations, a classification of MMR sequence variants identified by genetic testing has been proposed based on a 5-class system, using a multifactorial likelihood model (Table 2).

Variant-Class 5 includes coding sequence variation resulting in a stop codon (nonsense or frameshift), splicing aberration variants by mRNA assay, large genomic deletions or duplications, abrogated mRNA/protein function variants based either on laboratory assays, on evidence for cosegregation with disease, and on MSI tumor, and/or loss of MMR protein expression.

Variant-Class 4 includes IVS+-1 or IVS+-2 mutations resulting in splicing aberrations, variants abrogating mRNA/protein function based on laboratory assays, evidence of cosegregation with disease or MSI tumor, and/or loss of MMR protein expression.

Variant-Class 3 includes large genomic duplications, missense alterations, small in-frame insertions/deletions, silent variants, intronic variants, and promoter and regulatory region variants for which insufficient molecular evidence is available and with intermediate clinical effects or low penetrance alleles.

Variant-Class 2 includes synonymous substitutions and intronic variants with no associated mRNA aberration, with a proficient protein expression/function, and lack of cosegregation and/or MSS tumor.

Variant-Class 1 includes variants reported in control reference groups and excluded as founder pathogenic sequence variant.

According to this classification, most of the VUS tested for the MMR genes are likely to be pathogenetic and thus they can be associated with the HNPCC phenotype.

For the MLH1 gene, 52 out of 73 VUS resulted to be pathogenetic (70%), similar pathogenicity has been demonstrated for 25 out of 35 VUS identified in the MSH2 gene, (71%) (https://www.insight-group.org).

For minor MMR genes, the percentage of pathogenic VUSs is reduced due to the milder mutational contribution of these genes to the development of the disease. For the MSH6 gene, only 1 out of 8 variants studied (13%) was found to have aberrant effects on protein function; for the PMS2 gene, 4 variants were analyzed and all (100%) seem to have a causative role in Lynch syndrome; for the MLH3 gene, however, functional assays have not identified any variant with certain pathogenetic significance; finally, for the MSH3 gene relevant functional studies have not yet been reported (https://www.insight-group.org).

6. Probability of a "Synergistic Effect" between Low Risk Allelic Variants in the MMR Genes

With the advent of high-throughput technologies it is becoming even more possible to analyze a great number of polymorphic variants in large cohorts of cases and controls of specific cancers, such as breast, prostate, and colorectal cancer, thus providing new insights into common mechanisms of carcinogenesis. In some cases, VUSs make a more substantial overall contribution to cancer risk than the well-assessed severe Mendelian variants. It is also possible that the simultaneous presence of some polymorphisms and VUSs in cancer predisposition genes that behave as low risk alleles might contribute in a cooperative manner to increase the risk of hereditary cancer [12, 64]. Therefore, current literature data suggest a significant proportion of the inherited susceptibility to relatively common human diseases may be due to the addition of the effects of a series of low frequency variants of different genes, probably acting in a dominant and independent manner, with each of them conferring a moderate but even detectable increase in the relative cancer risk [50, 51, 75, 81–83]. Therefore, several functional studies based on GWAS data related to cancer susceptibility have

TABLE 2: Proposed classification system for MMR variant interpretation *(Colon Cancer Family Registry 2009, InSiGHT Variant Interpretation Committee 2011)*.

Class	Description	Probability of being pathogenic
5	Definitely pathogenic	>0.99
4	Likely pathogenic	0.95–0.99
3	Uncertain	0.05–0.949
2	Likely not pathogenic or of little clinical significance	0.001–0.049
1	Not pathogenic or of no clinical significance	<0.001

been performed in an attempt to demonstrate the effective association and to test the hypothesis of synergistic effects between low risk allelic variants [80, 81].

In a recent study on yeast genome, it has been shown that the minor alleles of the MMR complex cause a weak mutator phenotype; however, their interaction causes a more severe mutator phenotype [82]. In this study, 11 polymorphisms and 14 missense variants of uncertain significance previously identified in the MSH2, MLH1, MSH6, and PMS2 genes were studied by complementation tests. The mutator effect of these variants was tested singly and in combination with each other.

In 2011, Kumar et al. showed that some variants occurring in domain I of the MSH2 gene in yeast strains (msh2Δ1) behave as weak alleles in the presence of a functional protein MSH6, as they do not alter the stability of the MutSα complex. However, by combining these variants with weak alleles falling in the N-terminal region (NTR) (DNA binding domain) of the MSH6 gene, a strong mutator phenotype was found. Moreover, the mutator synergistic effect is also found between different systems of DNA damage response. A recent population study by Smith et al. [83] has shown that the simultaneous presence of mutations in the TP53 gene and single nucleotide polymorphisms (SNPs) in genes belonging to different repair systems as BER, NER, MMR, and DSBR (Double-Strand Break Repair) complex is associated with an earlier age of onset of breast cancer (<50 years). Therefore, in this case, the authors suggest an additive or multiplicative effect.

The additive effect of low penetrance genes could also be the cause of atypical Lynch syndromes such as familial CRC type X [84]. With respect to LS, the familial CRC type X is more often located in the distal colon; extracolonic cancers are less frequent than in LS, and the age of onset is delayed. The sine qua non condition for this diagnosis is the absence of molecular genetic evidence of LS (MSI, IHC, or MMR mutations).

7. Scientific Hypothesis and Our Results

Molecular characterization of patients with a clinical diagnosis of Lynch syndrome currently relies on the identification of point mutations and large rearrangements [85, 86] by DHPLC and MLPA, respectively, in the major MMR genes, MLH1 and MSH2.

This strategy does not always provide informative results for genetic counseling. Indeed, many families selected according to international diagnostic criteria (Amsterdam Criteria and Bethesda Guidelines) do not have a molecular diagnosis of Lynch syndrome. In our experience, we have identified several patients carrying genetic VUS (missense, intronic, and silent variants) not only in main genes, MLH1 and MSH2 [80], but also in other MMR genes. According to international recommendations (Colon cancer Family Registry 2009, InSiGHT Variant Interpretation Committee 2011) we used a multifactorial likelihood model in an attempt to define a pathogenetic role for numerous VUS identified in MMR genes [50, 51, 64, 85]. The segregation analysis, population studies (to exclude the polymorphic nature of the variant), assessment of MSI in tumor tissues, detection of loss of protein expression in tumor tissues by immunohistochemical analysis (IHC), in silico analysis by a variety of bioinformatics tools, and gene expression studies are strategies that have to be used to assess an exhaustive evaluation of the pathogenicity of uncertain variants [85].

In light of literature data indicated that "minor" MMR proteins have other functions besides the postreplicative repair that could be highly relevant in carcinogenesis; in our laboratories, we have also analyzed the minor MMR genes, MSH6, PMS2, MLH3, and MSH3 for germline variants detected in patients negative for germline mutations in the major MMR genes. Many of the subjects analyzed in our series [50, 51, 64, 85] showed coinheritance of different genetic alterations in the minor MMR genes (Table 3) we speculate a likely additive role of low penetrance alleles in the disease development, in favor of a putative polygenic inheritance for Lynch syndrome, according to recent literature data [87–89].

8. Conclusion

The recent literature data describe the MMR proteins increasingly new roles. It is now known that MMR proteins not only have an exclusive role in the repair of DNA mismatch but are also involved in many other processes relevant in carcinogenesis. Therefore, some genetic variants may not affect the repair function but may be responsible for the loss of other important functions related to MMR proteins. In the light of these new roles of the MMR proteins it is essential to widen the mutations detection in all genes that are part of MMR complex. This will lead to the identification of numerous VUS in these genes. However, the study of VUS identified in MMR genes provides important information

TABLE 3: Patients carrying variants in several MMR genes: MSH6, PMS2, MSH3, and MLH3; *patient 504 showing also the UV in MSH2 gene (c.984 C>T) [64].

Patients	MSH6	PMS2	MLH3	MSH3	Phenotype
9525	ex4 c.2633 T>C (Val>Ala)	ex14 c.2324 A>G (Asn>Ser)	ex1 c.2530 C>T (Pro>Ser) c.2533 T>C (Ser>Pro)	IVS7 -9 T>C	Amsterdam +
013		ex6 c.665G>C (Ser>Thr) IVS6 +16A>G	ex1 c.2533 T>C (Ser>Pro)		No Amsterdam MSI-H
103	ex5 c.3261_62insC (Phe>stop)		ex1 c.2533 T>C (Ser>Pro)	ex12 c.1860G>A (Asp>Asn)	No Amsterdam later onset MSI-H
423		IVS12-4G>A	ex1 c.2530 C>T (Pro>Ser) c.2533 T>C (Ser>Pro)		Amsterdam + later onset MSI-L
015	ex5 c.3295_97delTT (Ile>stop)		ex1 c.666 G>A (Lys) c.2191 G>T (Val>Phe) c.2533A>G (Ser>Gly)		Amsterdam + MSI-H
210	ex4 c.2941 A>G (Ile>Val)	IVS6+16A>G ex13 c.2324 T>C (Phe)	ex1 c.2530 C>T (Pro>Ser)	IVS6-64 C>T	Amsterdam + MSI not detected
211	ex4 c.2941 A>G (Ile>Val)	IVS12-4 G>A		IVS6-64 C>T	Amsterdam + MSI not detected
416		ex11 c.1714C>A (Thr>Lys)	ex 1 c.2027G>A (Arg>Lys)	IVS6-64 C>T	Amsterdam + MSI-H
504*				ex4 c.693G>A (Pro) ex20 c.2732 T>G (Leu>Trp)	Amsterdam + MSI-H

on the pathogenicity of the many genetic variants that are identifying in patients with suspected diagnosis of Lynch syndrome. Very often these variants are causing the disease, perhaps with a different degree of pathogenicity. Sometimes the simultaneous presence of molecular alterations in several MMR genes could be causing the onset of tumor. All these reassess the classical model of monogenic transmission in favor of a polygenic inheritance of Lynch syndrome.

Therefore, these recent findings allow clarifying better the genotype-phenotype correlations in Lynch syndrome, demonstrating the importance of molecular analysis to improve the genetic counseling and, consequently, the clinical surveillance.

Competing Interests

The authors declare that they have no competing interests regarding the manuscript.

Acknowledgments

This paper is supported by agreement 2010–2012 between CEINGE and Campania Regional Authority and POR Campania FSE 2007–2013.

References

[1] H. T. Lynch, K. Drescher, J. Knezetic, and S. Lanspa, "Genetics, biomarkers, hereditary cancer syndrome diagnosis, heterogeneity and treatment: a review," *Current Treatment Options in Oncology*, vol. 15, no. 3, pp. 429–442, 2014.

[2] C. C. Chung and S. J. Chanock, "Current status of genome-wide association studies in cancer," *Human Genetics*, vol. 130, no. 1, pp. 59–78, 2011.

[3] L. Valle, "Genetic predisposition to colorectal cancer: where we stand and future perspectives," *World Journal of Gastroenterology*, vol. 20, no. 29, pp. 9828–9849, 2014.

[4] M. De Rosa, R. J. Dourisboure, G. Morelli et al., "First genotype characterization of Argentinean FAP patients: identification of 14 novel APC mutations," *Human Mutation*, vol. 23, no. 5, pp. 523–524, 2004.

[5] M. De Rosa, M. Galatola, S. Borriello, F. Duraturo, S. Masone, and P. Izzo, "Implication of adenomatous polyposis coli and MUTYH mutations in familial colorectal polyposis," *Diseases of the Colon and Rectum*, vol. 52, no. 2, pp. 268–274, 2009.

[6] N. J. Samadder, K. Jasperson, and R. W. Burt, "Hereditary and common familial colorectal cancer: evidence for colorectal screening," *Digestive Diseases and Sciences*, vol. 60, no. 3, pp. 734–747, 2015.

[7] M. De Rosa, U. Pace, D. Rega et al., "Genetics, diagnosis and management of colorectal cancer (Review)," *Oncology Reports*, vol. 34, no. 3, pp. 1087–1096, 2015.

[8] N. Carlomagno, F. Duraturo, M. Candida et al., "Multiple splenic hamartomas and familial adenomatous polyposis: a case report and review of the literature," *Journal of Medical Case Reports*, vol. 9, no. 1, article no. 154, 2015.

[9] M. Galatola, L. Paparo, F. Duraturo et al., "Beta catenin and cytokine pathway dysregulation in patients with manifestations of the "PTEN hamartoma tumor syndrome"," *BMC Medical Genetics*, vol. 13, article no. 28, 2012.

[10] L. Paparo, G. B. Rossi, P. Delrio et al., "Differential expression of PTEN gene correlates with phenotypic heterogeneity in three cases of patients showing clinical manifestations of PTEN hamartoma tumour syndrome," *Hereditary Cancer in Clinical Practice*, vol. 11, article 8, 2013.

[11] M. Galatola, E. Miele, C. Strisciuglio et al., "Synergistic effect of interleukin-10-receptor variants in a case of early-onset ulcerative colitis," *World Journal of Gastroenterology*, vol. 19, no. 46, pp. 8659–8670, 2013.

[12] J. M. Carethers, "Differentiating lynch-like from lynch syndrome," *Gastroenterology*, vol. 146, no. 3, pp. 602–604, 2014.

[13] M. G. F. van Lier, A. Wagner, M. E. van Leerdam et al., "A review on the molecular diagnostics of Lynch syndrome: a central role for the pathology laboratory," *Journal of Cellular and Molecular Medicine*, vol. 14, no. 1-2, pp. 181–197, 2010.

[14] D. C. Hegan, L. Narayanan, F. R. Jirik, W. Edelmann, R. M. Liskay, and P. M. Glazer, "Differing patterns of genetic instability in mice deficient in the mismatch repair genes Pms2, Mlh1, Msh2, Msh3 and Msh6," *Carcinogenesis*, vol. 27, no. 12, pp. 2402–2408, 2006.

[15] S.-H. Jun, T. G. Kim, and C. Ban, "DNA mismatch repair system: classical and fresh roles," *FEBS Journal*, vol. 273, no. 8, pp. 1609–1619, 2006.

[16] J. Jiricny, "The multifaceted mismatch-repair system," *Nature Reviews Molecular Cell Biology*, vol. 7, no. 5, pp. 335–346, 2006.

[17] F. A. Sinicrope and D. J. Sargent, "Molecular pathways: microsatellite instability in colorectal cancer: prognostic, predictive, and therapeutic implications," *Clinical Cancer Research*, vol. 18, no. 6, pp. 1506–1512, 2012.

[18] P. Alhopuro, H. Sammalkorpi, I. Niittymäki et al., "Candidate driver genes in microsatellite-unstable colorectal cancer," *International Journal of Cancer*, vol. 130, no. 7, pp. 1558–1566, 2012.

[19] A. Zaanan, K. Meunier, F. Sangar, J.-F. Fléjou, and F. Praz, "Microsatellite instability in colorectal cancer: from molecular oncogenic mechanisms to clinical implications," *Cellular Oncology*, vol. 34, no. 3, pp. 155–176, 2011.

[20] K. Imai and H. Yamamoto, "Carcinogenesis and microsatellite instability: the interrelationship between genetics and epigenetics," *Carcinogenesis*, vol. 29, no. 4, pp. 673–680, 2008.

[21] S. G. Sharma and M. L. Gulley, "BRAF mutation testing in colorectal cancer," *Archives of Pathology and Laboratory Medicine*, vol. 134, no. 8, pp. 1225–1228, 2010.

[22] L. Wang, J. M. Cunningham, J. L. Winters et al., "BRAF mutations in colon cancer are not likely attributable to defective DNA mismatch repair," *Cancer Research*, vol. 63, no. 17, pp. 5209–5212, 2003.

[23] Y. Nakaji, E. Oki, R. Nakanishi et al., "Prognostic value of BRAF V600E mutation and microsatellite instability in Japanese patients with sporadic colorectal cancer," *Journal of Cancer Research and Clinical Oncology*, vol. 143, no. 1, pp. 151–160, 2017.

[24] P. Lochhead, A. Kuchiba, Y. Imamura et al., "Microsatellite instability and BRAF mutation testing in colorectal cancer prognostication," *Journal of the National Cancer Institute*, vol. 105, no. 15, pp. 1151–1156, 2013.

[25] C. R. Boland, S. N. Thibodeau, S. R. Hamilton et al., "A National Cancer Institute workshop on microsatellite instability for cancer detection and familial predisposition: development of international criteria for the determination of microsatellite instability in colorectal cancer," *Cancer Research*, vol. 58, no. 22, pp. 5248–5257, 1998.

[26] E. Vilar, M. E. Mork, A. Cuddy et al., "Role of microsatellite instability-low as a diagnostic biomarker of Lynch syndrome in colorectal cancer," *Cancer Genetics*, vol. 207, no. 10-12, pp. 495–502, 2014.

[27] R. M. Xicola, X. Llor, E. Pons et al., "Performance of different microsatellite marker panels for detection of mismatch repair-deficient colorectal tumors," *Journal of the National Cancer Institute*, vol. 99, no. 3, pp. 244–252, 2007.

[28] A. Umar, C. R. Boland, J. P. Terdiman et al., "Revised Bethesda Guidelines for hereditary nonpolyposis colorectal cancer (Lynch syndrome) and microsatellite instability," *Journal of the National Cancer Institute*, vol. 96, no. 4, pp. 261–268, 2004.

[29] N. Suraweera, A. Duval, M. Reperant et al., "Evaluation of tumor microsatellite instability using five quasimonomorphic mononucleotide repeats and pentaplex PCR," *Gastroenterology*, vol. 123, no. 6, pp. 1804–1811, 2002.

[30] D. J. Sargent, S. Marsoni, G. Monges et al., "Defective mismatch repair as a predictive marker for lack of efficacy of fluorouracil-based adjuvant therapy in colon cancer," *Journal of Clinical Oncology*, vol. 28, no. 20, pp. 3219–3226, 2010.

[31] J. H. Kim and G. H. Kang, "Molecular and prognostic heterogeneity of microsatellite-unstable colorectal cancer," *World Journal of Gastroenterology*, vol. 20, no. 15, pp. 4230–4243, 2014.

[32] H. T. Lynch, P. M. Lynch, S. J. Lanspa, C. L. Snyder, J. F. Lynch, and C. R. Boland, "Review of the Lynch syndrome: history, molecular genetics, screening, differential diagnosis, and medicolegal ramifications," *Clinical Genetics*, vol. 76, no. 1, pp. 1–18, 2009.

[33] J. Shia, S. Holck, G. Depetris, J. K. Greenson, and D. S. Klimstra, "Lynch syndrome-associated neoplasms: a discussion on histopathology and immunohistochemistry," *Familial Cancer*, vol. 12, no. 2, pp. 241–260, 2013.

[34] G. Corso, D. Marrelli, and F. Roviello, "Familial gastric cancer: update for practice management," *Familial Cancer*, vol. 10, no. 2, pp. 391–396, 2011.

[35] A. Gylling, W. M. Abdel-Rahman, M. Juhola et al., "Is gastric cancer part of the tumour spectrum of hereditary nonpolyposis colorectal cancer? A Molecular Genetic Study," *Gut*, vol. 56, no. 7, pp. 926–933, 2007.

[36] V. O'Brien and R. Brown, "Signalling cell cycle arrest and cell death through the MMR System," *Carcinogenesis*, vol. 27, no. 4, pp. 682–692, 2006.

[37] K. Yamane, J. E. Schupp, and T. J. Kinsella, "BRCA1 activates a G2-M cell cycle checkpoint following 6-thioguanine-induced DNA mismatch damage," *Cancer Research*, vol. 67, no. 13, pp. 6286–6292, 2007.

[38] A. Nicholson, M. Hendrix, S. Jinks-Robertson, and G. F. Crouse, "Regulation of mitotic homeologous recombination in yeast: functions of mismatch repair and nucleotide excision repair genes," *Genetics*, vol. 154, no. 1, pp. 133–146, 2000.

[39] G. Ji, Y. Long, Y. Zhou, C. Huang, A. Gu, and X. Wang, "Common variants in mismatch repair genes associated with increased risk of sperm DNA damage and male infertility," *BMC Medicine*, vol. 10, article 49, 2012.

[40] S. Roa, Z. Li, J. U. Peled, C. Zhao, W. Edelmann, and M. D. Scharff, "MSH2/MSH6 complex promotes error-free repair of AID-Induced dU:G mispairs as well as error-prone hypermutation of A:T Sites," *PLoS ONE*, vol. 5, no. 6, Article ID e11182, 2010.

[41] C. Jiang, M.-L. Zhao, K. M. Waters, and M. Diaz, "Activation-induced deaminase contributes to the antibody-independent role of B cells in the development of autoimmunity," *Autoimmunity*, vol. 45, no. 6, pp. 440–448, 2012.

[42] S. Tomé, I. Holt, W. Edelmann et al., "ATPase domain mutation affects CTG*CAG repeat instability in transgenic mice," *PLoS Genetics*, vol. 5, no. 5, Article ID e1000482, 2009.

[43] E. Dragileva, A. Hendricks, A. Teed et al., "Intergenerational and striatal CAG repeat instability in Huntington's disease knock-in mice involve different DNA repair genes," *Neurobiology of Disease*, vol. 33, no. 1, pp. 37–47, 2009.

[44] A. Seriola, C. Spits, J. P. Simard et al., "Huntington's and myotonic dystrophy hESCs: down-regulated trinucleotide repeat instability and mismatch repair machinery expression upon differentiation," *Human Molecular Genetics*, vol. 20, no. 1, pp. 176–185, 2011.

[45] G. Mao, X. Pan, and L. Gu, "Evidence that a mutation in the MLH1 3′-untranslated region confers a mutator phenotype and mismatch repair deficiency in patients with relapsed leukemia," *Journal of Biological Chemistry*, vol. 283, no. 6, pp. 3211–3216, 2008.

[46] P. Hsieh and K. Yamane, "DNA mismatch repair: molecular mechanism, cancer, and ageing," *Mechanisms of Ageing and Development*, vol. 129, no. 7-8, pp. 391–407, 2008.

[47] J. J. Koornstra, M. J. Mourits, R. H. Sijmons, A. M. Leliveld, H. Hollema, and J. H. Kleibeuker, "Management of extracolonic tumours in patients with Lynch syndrome," *The Lancet Oncology*, vol. 10, no. 4, pp. 400–408, 2009.

[48] E. Lucci-Cordisco, V. Rovella, S. Carrara et al., "Mutations of the 'minor' mismatch repair gene MSH6 in typical and atypical hereditary nonpolyposis colorectal cancer," *Familial Cancer*, vol. 1, no. 2, pp. 93–99, 2001.

[49] E. C. Chao and S. M. Lipkin, "Molecular models for the tissue specificity of DNA mismatch repair-deficient carcinogenesis," *Nucleic Acids Research*, vol. 34, no. 3, pp. 840–852, 2006.

[50] F. Duraturo, R. Liccardo, and P. Izzo, "Coexistence of MLH3 germline variants in colon cancer patients belonging to families with Lynch syndrome-associated brain tumors," *Journal of Neuro-Oncology*, vol. 129, no. 3, pp. 577–578, 2016.

[51] F. Duraturo, R. Liccardo, A. Cavallo, M. D. Rosa, M. Grosso, and P. Izzo, "Association of low-risk MSH3 and MSH2 variant alleles with Lynch syndrome: probability of synergistic effects," *International Journal of Cancer*, vol. 129, no. 7, pp. 1643–1650, 2011.

[52] J. Huang, S. A. Kuismanen, T. Liu et al., "MSH6 and MSH3 are rarely involved in genetic predisposition to nonpolypotic colon cancer," *Cancer Research*, vol. 61, no. 4, pp. 1619–1623, 2001.

[53] S.-Y. Lee, H. Chung, B. Devaraj et al., "Microsatellite alterations at selected tetranucleotide repeats are associated with morphologies of colorectal Neoplasias," *Gastroenterology*, vol. 139, no. 5, pp. 1519–1525, 2010.

[54] P. Bandipalliam, "Syndrome of early onset colon cancers, hematologic malignancies & features of neurofibromatosis in HNPCC families with homozygous mismatch repair gene mutations," *Familial Cancer*, vol. 4, no. 4, pp. 323–333, 2005.

[55] J. C. Herkert, R. C. Niessen, M. J. W. Olderode-Berends et al., "Paediatric intestinal cancer and polyposis due to bi-allelic PMS2 mutations: case series, review and follow-up guidelines," *European Journal of Cancer*, vol. 47, no. 7, pp. 965–982, 2011.

[56] J.-W. Poley, A. Wagner, M. M. C. P. Hoogmans et al., "Biallelic germline mutations of mismatch-repair genes: a possible cause for multiple pediatric malignancies," *Cancer*, vol. 109, no. 11, pp. 2349–2356, 2007.

[57] S. E. Plon, D. M. Eccles, D. Easton et al., "Sequence variant classification and reporting: recommendations for improving the interpretation of cancer susceptibility genetic test results," *Human Mutation*, vol. 29, no. 11, pp. 1282–1291, 2008.

[58] A. Peters, H. Born, R. Ettinger, P. Levonian, and K. B. Jedele, "Compound heterozygosity for MSH6 mutations in a pediatric lymphoma patient," *Journal of Pediatric Hematology/Oncology*, vol. 31, no. 2, pp. 113–115, 2009.

[59] S. Y. Kang, C. K. Park, D. K. Chang et al., "Lynch-like syndrome: characterization and comparison with EPCAM deletion carriers," *International Journal of Cancer*, vol. 136, no. 7, pp. 1568–1578, 2015.

[60] D. D. Buchanan, C. Rosty, M. Clendenning, A. B. Spurdle, and A. K. Win, "Clinical problems of colorectal cancer and endometrial cancer cases with unknown cause of tumor mismatch repair deficiency (suspected Lynch syndrome)," *Application of Clinical Genetics*, vol. 7, pp. 183–193, 2014.

[61] C. R. Boland, "The mystery of mismatch repair deficiency: lynch or lynch-like?" *Gastroenterology*, vol. 144, no. 5, pp. 868–870, 2013.

[62] A. R. Mensenkamp, I. P. Vogelaar, W. A. G. Van Zelst-Stams et al., "Somatic mutations in *MLH1* and *MSH2* are a frequent cause of mismatch-repair deficiency in lynch syndrome-like tumors," *Gastroenterology*, vol. 146, no. 3, pp. 643.e8–646.e8, 2014.

[63] F. Li, G. Mao, D. Tong et al., "The histone mark H3K36me3 regulates human DNA mismatch repair through its interaction with MutSα," *Cell*, vol. 153, no. 3, pp. 590–600, 2013.

[64] F. Duraturo, R. Liccardo, A. Cavallo, M. De Rosa, and P. Izzo, *Synergistic Effects of Low-Risk Variant Alleles in Cancer Predisposition*, Carcinogenesis, edited by Kathryn Tonissen, InTech, Rijeka, Croatia, 2013.

[65] Y. Iwahashi, E. Ito, Y. Yanagisawa et al., "Promoter analysis of the human mismatch repair gene hMSH2," *Gene*, vol. 213, no. 1-2, pp. 141–147, 1998.

[66] E. Ito, Y. Yanagisawa, Y. Iwahashi et al., "A core promoter and a frequent single-nucleotide polymorphism of the mismatch repair gene hMLH1," *Biochemical and Biophysical Research Communications*, vol. 256, no. 3, pp. 488–494, 1999.

[67] M. Mrkonjic, S. Raptis, R. C. Green et al., "MSH2 −118T>C and MSH6 −159C>T promoter polymorphisms and the risk of colorectal cancer," *Carcinogenesis*, vol. 28, no. 12, pp. 2575–2580, 2007.

[68] S. Raptis, M. Mrkonjic, R. C. Green et al., "MLH1 −93G>A promoter polymorphism and the risk of microsatellite-unstable colorectal cancer," *Journal of the National Cancer Institute*, vol. 99, no. 6, pp. 463–474, 2007.

[69] G. Mao, S. Lee, J. Ortega, L. Gu, and G.-M. Li, "Modulation of microRNA processing by mismatch repair protein MutLα," *Cell Research*, vol. 22, no. 6, pp. 973–985, 2012.

[70] G. Zhang, E. Gibbs, Z. Kelman, M. O'Donnell, and J. Hurwitz, "Studies on the interactions between human replication factor C and human proliferating cell nuclear antigen," *Proceedings of the National Academy of Sciences of the United States of America*, vol. 96, no. 5, pp. 1869–1874, 1999.

[71] P. V. Shcherbakova, M. C. Hall, M. S. Lewis et al., "Inactivation of DNA mismatch repair by increased expression of yeast MLH1," *Molecular and Cellular Biology*, vol. 21, no. 3, pp. 940–951, 2001.

[72] G. Marra, I. Iaccarino, T. Lettieri, G. Roscilli, P. Delmastro, and J. Jiricny, "Mismatch repair deficiency associated with overexpression of the MSH3 gene," *Proceedings of the National Academy of Sciences of the United States of America*, vol. 95, no. 15, pp. 8568–8573, 1998.

[73] D.-A. Landau and F. J. Slack, "MicroRNAs in mutagenesis, genomic instability, and DNA repair," *Seminars in Oncology*, vol. 38, no. 6, pp. 743–751, 2011.

[74] Y. Dong, J. Yu, and S. S. M. Ng, "MicroRNA dysregulation as a prognostic biomarker in colorectal cancer," *Cancer Management and Research*, vol. 6, pp. 405–422, 2014.

[75] Y. Wang and T. Taniguchi, "MicroRNAs and DNA damage response: implications for cancer therapy," *Cell Cycle*, vol. 12, no. 1, pp. 32–42, 2013.

[76] N. Valeri, P. Gasparini, C. Braconi et al., "MicroRNA-21 induces resistance to 5-fluorouracil by down-regulating human DNA MutS homolog 2 (hMSH2)," *Proceedings of the National Academy of Sciences of the United States of America*, vol. 107, no. 49, pp. 21098–21103, 2010.

[77] M. Svrcek, N. El-Murr, K. Wanherdrick et al., "Overexpression of microRNAs-155 and 21 targeting mismatch repair proteins in inflammatory bowel diseases," *Carcinogenesis*, vol. 34, no. 4, pp. 828–834, 2013.

[78] F. J. Couch, L. J. Rasmussen, R. Hofstra, A. N. A. Monteiro, M. S. Greenblatt, and N. de Wind, "Assessment of functional effects of unclassified genetic variants," *Human Mutation*, vol. 29, no. 11, pp. 1314–1326, 2008.

[79] S. Syngal, E. A. Fox, C. Li et al., "Interpretation of genetic test results for hereditary nonpolyposis colorectal cancer: implications for clinical predisposition testing," *JAMA*, vol. 282, no. 3, pp. 247–253, 1999.

[80] A. P. Shaik, A. S. Shaik, and Y. A. Al-Sheikh, "Colorectal cancer: a review of the genome-wide association studies in the kingdom of Saudi Arabia," *Saudi Journal of Gastroenterology*, vol. 21, no. 3, pp. 123–128, 2015.

[81] L. Le Marchand, "Genome-wide association studies and colorectal cancer," *Surgical Oncology Clinics of North America*, vol. 18, no. 4, pp. 663–668, 2009.

[82] D. E. Goldgar, D. F. Easton, G. B. Byrnes, A. B. Spurdle, E. S. Iversen, and M. S. Greenblatt, "Genetic evidence and integration of various data sources for classifying uncertain variants into a single model," *Human Mutation*, vol. 29, no. 11, pp. 1265–1272, 2008.

[83] T. R. Smith, W. Liu-Mares, B. O. Van Emburgh et al., "Genetic polymorphisms of multiple DNA repair pathways impact age at diagnosis and TP53 mutations in breast cancer," *Carcinogenesis*, vol. 32, no. 9, pp. 1354–1360, 2011.

[84] N. M. Lindor, K. Rabe, G. M. Petersen et al., "Lower cancer incidence in Amsterdam-I criteria families without mismatch repair deficiency: familial colorectal cancer type X," *JAMA*, vol. 293, no. 16, pp. 1979–1985, 2005.

[85] F. Duraturo, R. Liccardo, A. Cavallo, M. De Rosa, G. B. Rossi, and P. Izzo, "Multivariate analysis as a method for evaluating the pathogenicity of novel genetic MLH1 variants in patients with colorectal cancer and microsatellite instability," *International Journal of Molecular Medicine*, vol. 36, no. 2, pp. 511–517, 2015.

[86] F. Duraturo, A. Cavallo, R. Liccardo et al., "Contribution of large genomic rearrangements in Italian Lynch syndrome patients: characterization of a novel alu-mediated deletion," *BioMed Research International*, vol. 2013, Article ID 219897, 7 pages, 2013.

[87] T. A. Muranen, N. Mavaddat, S. Khan et al., "Polygenic risk score is associated with increased disease risk in 52 Finnish breast cancer families," *Breast Cancer Research and Treatment*, vol. 158, no. 3, pp. 463–469, 2016.

[88] J. Yuan, Y. Li, T. Tian et al., "Risk prediction for early-onset gastric carcinoma: a case-control study of polygenic gastric cancer in Han Chinese with hereditary background," *Oncotarget*, vol. 7, no. 23, pp. 33608–33615, 2016.

[89] B. A. Talseth-Palmer, D. C. Bauer, W. Sjursen et al., "Targeted next-generation sequencing of 22 mismatch repair genes identifies Lynch syndrome families," *Cancer Medicine*, vol. 5, no. 5, pp. 929–941, 2016.

9

Chemotherapy Plus Cetuximab versus Chemotherapy Alone for Patients with KRAS Wild Type Unresectable Liver-Confined Metastases Colorectal Cancer: An Updated Meta-Analysis of RCTs

W. Lv,[1] G. Q. Zhang,[1,2] A. Jiao,[1] B. C. Zhao,[1] Y. Shi,[1] B. M. Chen,[1] and J. L. Zhang[1]

[1]*Department of Hepatobiliary and Transplantation Surgery, The First Hospital of China Medical University, Shenyang, Liaoning Province, China*
[2]*Department of Clinical Medicine, First Affiliated Hospital of Zhengzhou University, Zhengzhou, Henan Province, China*

Correspondence should be addressed to J. L. Zhang; jlz2000@yeah.net

Academic Editor: Nicola Silvestris

Purpose. Our study analyses clinical trials and evaluates the efficacy of adding cetuximab in systematic chemotherapy for unresectable colorectal cancer liver-confined metastases patients. *Materials and Methods.* Search EMBASE, PubMed, and the Cochrane Central Register of Controlled Trials for RCTs comparing chemotherapy plus cetuximab with chemotherapy alone for KRAS wild type patients with colorectal cancer liver metastases (CRLMs). We calculated the relative risks (RRs) with 95% confidence interval and performed meta-analysis of hazard ratios (HRs) for the R0 resection rate, the overall response rate (ORR), the progression-free survival (PFS) and overall survival (OS). *Results.* 1173 articles were retrieved and 4 RCTs were available for our study. The four studies involved 504 KRAS wild type patients with CRLMs. The addition of cetuximab significantly improved all the 4 outcomes: the R0 resection rate (RR 2.03, $p = 0.004$), the ORR (RR 1.76, $p < 0.00001$), PFS (HR 0.63, $p < 0.0001$), and also OS (HR 0.74, $p = 0.04$); the last outcome is quite different from the conclusion published before. *Conclusions.* Although the number of patients analysed was limited, we found that the addition of cetuximab significantly improves the outcomes in KRAS wild type patients with unresectable colorectal cancer liver-confined metastases. Cetuximab combined with systematic chemotherapy perhaps suggests a promising choice for KRAS wild type patients with unresectable liver metastases.

1. Introduction

Liver is well known as the most common site of colorectal cancer metastasis. Liver metastases have already been found in about 25% patients when establishing the diagnosis of colorectal cancer [1]. Colorectal cancer liver metastasis now has already become a focused point for the researchers recently. Surgery is an effective measure to improve survival rate for patients with resectable metastases. Unfortunately, only about 10% patients with colorectal cancer liver metastases (CRLMs) are accessible to get a surgery treatment at the time of diagnosis [2], and at least two-thirds of the rest of 90% patients died for the reason of unresectable CRLMs (5-year survival rate is almost zero) [3].

During the past decade, the median survival of patients with CRLMs increased quite significantly by systematic chemotherapy [4]. In addition, the median survival has also been improved from 6–8 months to over 20 months by the use of targeted therapy [5]. Recently, the epidermal growth factor receptor (EGFR) has become a promising target for it is activated in colorectal tumors [6]. Inhibition of the active target seems to be a potential choice for patients with CRLMs. For this reason, cetuximab, a strong EGFR inhibitor, has already been focused on the treatment of CRLMs. KRAS is an effector gene in the downstream of EGFR, a paper reported that patients with KRAS mutant type could not benefit from adjuvant chemotherapy and were not sensitive to

EGFR inhibitor, and cetuximab is also not effective to KRAS mutant type patients with CRLMs [7, 8].

However, a lot of papers revealed the efficacy of anti-EGFR plus chemotherapy treatment for patients with CRLMs, and four RCT studies have already been published before 2011 [9–12], and even a meta-analysis has been published in 2012 [13] showing a higher level of evidence-based medical evidence on the benefit and disadvantages using anti-EGFR agents in combination with chemotherapy treatment for patients with colorectal cancer, but there are still some controversial issues such as whether cetuximab increases overall survival (OS) or not. According to a new meta-analysis published in 2016, cetuximab does increase the OS of patients with unresectable metastases colorectal cancer [14]. But this study failed to mention the results of patients with colorectal cancer liver-limited metastases. In addition, a randomized controlled trial published in 2013 gave the conclusion that cetuximab benefits the OS of patients with colorectal cancer liver-limited metastases [15], and both the conclusions imply that the conclusion of the meta-analysis studied on the patients only with colorectal cancer liver-limited metastases published in 2012 may be a little unreasonable.

Therefore in this article we perform a meta-analysis of RCTs comparing cetuximab plus chemotherapy with chemotherapy alone with the aim of identifying whether cetuximab plus chemotherapy improves the outcomes of R0 resection rate, overall response rate, progression-free survival, and overall survival of KRAS wild type patients only with colorectal cancer liver-limited metastases or not at a higher level of evidence-based medical evidence.

2. Materials and Methods

2.1. Search Strategy. A search of PubMed, EMBASE, and Cochrane Library databases (all databases from January 2004 to July 2016) was performed to extract the relevant literature that reports R0 section rate, overall response rate, and outcome on progression-free survival and overall survival of patients with liver-limited metastases which originated from KRAS wild type colorectal cancer and are treated by chemotherapy with or without cetuximab in a randomized controlled trial (RCT). Search terms were as follows: "colorectal cancer metastases" (or "carcinoma" or "malignant tumor") and "cetuximab". The latest search was executed on July 13, 2016 and had no limit for language. We start the search from January 2004 because the cetuximab for the treatment of patients with advanced colon cancer was approved by FDA in 2004 [16]. Meanwhile, we included the conference literature as well.

2.1.1. Types of Studies. Only randomized controlled trials (RCTs) provided the outcomes of KRAS wild type colorectal cancer liver-confined metastases patients that were included in the meta-analysis for ensuring the study level. Other nonrandomized trials were all excluded.

2.1.2. Characteristics of Patients Included. The inclusion criteria of patients were as follows:

(1) Patients should have been given a confirmed diagnosis of metastatic and liver-limited colorectal cancer (extrahepatic resection must be excluded) and have not received any primary treatments of the metastases till the trial began.

(2) Patients included must be KRAS wild type.

(3) The liver-limited metastases must be unresectable (according to the definition of single participant).

(4) All the patients who did not meet the above criteria should be excluded.

2.1.3. Types of Intervention. Patients who met the criteria (1)–(3) were randomly assigned to chemotherapy alone group or chemotherapy plus cetuximab group in each included study.

2.1.4. The Measurement of Outcomes. The radical resection (R0 resection) rate of liver-confined metastases was the first outcome we measure, and overall response rate (ORR), progression-free survival (PFS), and overall survival (OS) would also be measured in turn.

2.2. Data Selection, Extraction, and Analysis

2.2.1. Selection of Studies. This job was executed by two authors (W. Lv and G. Q. Zhang) independently abiding by the above inclusion criteria. Studies would be chosen if they contained the following items:

(1) Total population of KRAS wild type patients with liver-limited metastases colorectal cancer

(2) The number of R0 resection in the group

(3) Either the number of responses or relative risk (RR) (if available)

(4) Either PFS months or hazard ratio (HR) (if available)

(5) Either OS months or HR (if available)

Once a study contained the 1st and 2nd items, it also contained any of the items of the 3rd to 5th items, and the study would be included. Any discrepancies between the authors were resolved through discussion, rechecking the article content until the authors reached a consensus.

2.2.2. Data Extraction. The data were extracted as follows: the first author, publication year, region, number of patients in each arm, treatments, R0 resection rate (and RR), response rate (and RR), PFS time (and HR), and OS time (and HR).

Three authors (W. Lv, G. Q. Zhang, and A. Jiao) extracted the data independently by the items described above. HRs and their 95% confidence interval (CI) for PFS and OS (if available) were obtained from each primary study. The events of total R0 resections and responses were directly extracted from the studies included or obtained by calculating through the percentages provided by each study included. The proportion of patients with the R0 resection and response outcomes and 95% CIs has been calculated and presented as well as RRs.

2.2.3. Quality Assessment. Two authors (W. Lv and G. Q. Zhang) assessed the quality of the included trials using the quality checklist recommended by the Cochrane Handbook [17]. The following domains on the risk of bias were assessed: randomization, patients blinding, concealed allocation, intention-to-treat analysis, and completeness to follow-up. We resolved all disagreements by discussion and referral to a third author (A. Jiao) for adjudication.

2.2.4. Statistical Analysis. HRs and RRs were both performed in our meta-analysis, and we used Cochran's Q test to evaluate the statistical heterogeneity among the studies which had been included in our meta-analysis, and I^2 statistic and p value were both used to evaluate the statistical heterogeneity. It is considered that I^2 statistic > 50% and $p < 0.1$ represented significant statistical heterogeneity [18]. In our study, there was no statistical heterogeneity presented in our study, so we cited the fixed effect model in our study. At last, we assessed potential publication biases and two tailed $p < 0.05$ would be identified as significant statistical difference [17].

We evaluated the publication bias existing in our meta-analysis or not according to Begg's test and Egger's test, calculated by software Stata/SE 12.0.

Finally, the results of our meta-analysis were reported as forest plots. Statistical analyses were performed with Stata/SE 12.0 and Review Manager 5.3 (Review Manager (RevMan) [Computer program], Version 5.3, Copenhagen: The Nordic Cochrane Centre, The Cochrane Collaboration, 2014).

3. Results

3.1. Overview of Studies. A total of 1173 articles have been retrieved by the search strategy described in Materials and Methods. Most of the studies were excluded only by screening the title for various reasons (Figure 1). There were 139 RCTs left after screening. Furthermore, 135 papers were excluded with the reasons given in Figure 1. Finally, 4 papers (data extracted from 2 published articles and 1 conference abstract that pooled the analysis of another 2 published trials) were considered eligible for inclusion [10–12, 15, 19]. These 4 papers were all RCTs. All trials included chemotherapy plus C arms and chemotherapy alone arms. Characteristics of these studies and the summary of the outcomes had been represented in Table 1, and 504 patients (250 in experimental arms and 254 in control arms) were enrolled in the 4 RCTs. Unresectability criteria were according to the definition of single participant because they were not clearly described.

3.2. Quality Assessment. We evaluated the quality of each trial according to five domains: randomization, patients blinding, concealed allocation, intention-to-treat analysis, and completeness to follow-up (Table 2). All included articles described their study design as prospective randomized controlled trials. No studies reported that patient blinding and concealed allocation clearly and all the studies included used intention-to-treat analysis. All the follow-up of the studies has been finished, and all studies had greatly adequate follow-up durations.

3.3. Effect of Interventions

3.3.1. R0 Resection Rate. Data on R0 resection rates in KRAS wild type colorectal cancer patients with liver-confined metastases were available in all RCTs [10–12, 15] (504 patients). A fixed effect model has been chosen because the heterogeneity was 28% ($p = 0.25$). The results of our meta-analysis showed that the rate of radical resection of liver metastases was significantly increased from 8.7% to 17.6% by the use of cetuximab (RR 2.03, 95% CI 1.25–3.29; $p = 0.004$; Figure 2).

3.3.2. Response Rate. Data on response rates in KRAS wild type colorectal cancer patients with liver-confined metastases were available in 3 RCTs [10, 12, 15] (326 patients). A fixed effect model has been chosen because the heterogeneity was 0% ($p = 0.68$). The results of our meta-analysis showed that the likelihood of response of the liver metastases was significantly increased from 37.4% to 65.6% by the use of cetuximab (RR 1.76, 95% CI 1.40–2.21; $p < 0.00001$; Figure 3).

3.3.3. Progression-Free Survival. Data on progression-free survival in KRAS wild type colorectal cancer patients with liver-confined metastases were available in all RCTs [10–12, 15] (504 patients). A fixed effect model has been chosen because the heterogeneity was 0% ($p = 0.94$). The results of our meta-analysis showed that the risk of progression was significantly reduced by the use of cetuximab (HR 0.63, 95% CI 0.50–0.79; $p < 0.0001$; Figure 4).

3.3.4. Overall Survival. Data on the HRs for death in KRAS wild type colorectal cancer patients with liver-confined metastases were available in 3 RCTs [10, 12, 15] (326 patients). A fixed effect model has been chosen because the heterogeneity was 16% ($p = 0.31$). The results of our meta-analysis showed that the risk of death was significantly reduced by the use of cetuximab (HR 0.74, 95% CI 0.55–0.98; $p = 0.04$; Figure 5), while this outcome is quite different from the conclusion given by the previous studies.

3.4. Risk of Bias in the 4 RCTs. According to Begg's test ($p = 0.734$) and Egger's test ($p = 0.680$), we could give the conclusion that publication bias did not exist in our meta-analysis.

4. Discussion

The liver is the most common metastatic site of colorectal cancer, and the resection of liver metastases usually has a significant impact on the prognosis [20]. Systematic chemotherapy had already been regarded as an effective way to shrink the size of liver metastases for resection. Some studies reported that systematic chemotherapy does have credible ability to reduce the tumor size and has made a few patients with unresectable liver metastases undergo hepatic resection after chemotherapy treatment (12.5%, 3.3%) [2, 21]. But the rate is still not high enough.

In order to identify the effect of the addition of cetuximab more systematically we performed our meta-analysis for a

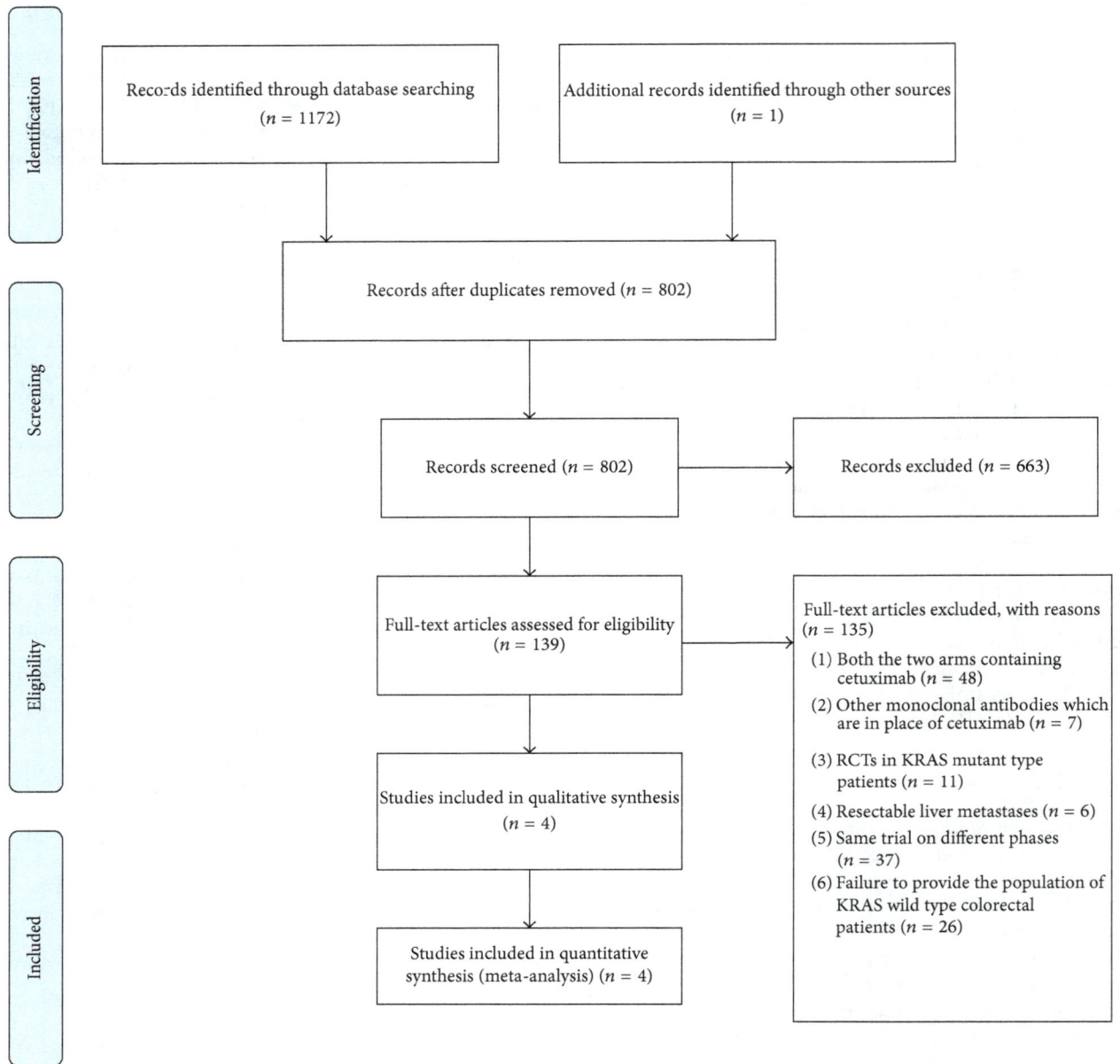

FIGURE 1: Flowchart of the included studies.

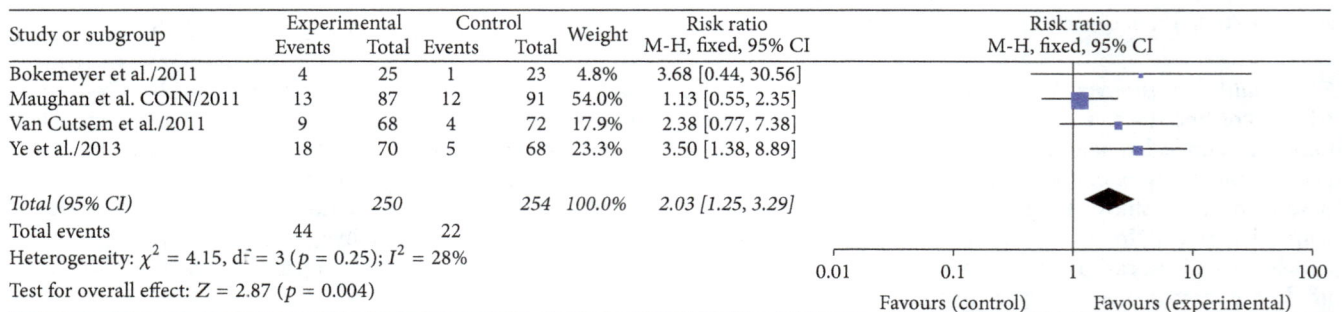

| Study or subgroup | Experimental | | Control | | Weight | Risk ratio M-H, fixed, 95% CI | Risk ratio M-H, fixed, 95% CI |
	Events	Total	Events	Total			
Bokemeyer et al./2011	4	25	1	23	4.8%	3.68 [0.44, 30.56]	
Maughan et al. COIN/2011	13	87	12	91	54.0%	1.13 [0.55, 2.35]	
Van Cutsem et al./2011	9	68	4	72	17.9%	2.38 [0.77, 7.38]	
Ye et al./2013	18	70	5	68	23.3%	3.50 [1.38, 8.89]	
Total (95% CI)		250		254	100.0%	2.03 [1.25, 3.29]	
Total events	44		22				

Heterogeneity: $\chi^2 = 4.15$, df = 3 ($p = 0.25$); $I^2 = 28\%$

Test for overall effect: $Z = 2.87$ ($p = 0.004$)

FIGURE 2: Meta-analysis R0 resection comparing chemotherapy ± cetuximab in patients with liver-limited metastases.

TABLE 1: Characteristics of the RCT studies included in our meta-analysis.

Author year	Number of LCM wt pts (exp/ctr)	Treatments (exp/ctr) arms	R0 resection% (exp/ctr) RR (p)	Response rate% (exp/ctr) RR (p)	PFS months exp versus ctr/HR (p)	OS months exp versus ctr/HR (p)
Bokemeyer et al./2011 (OPUS)	48 (25/23)	FOLFOX + C versus FOLFOX	16/4 3.68 (0.23)	76/39 1.94 (0.02)	11.9 versus 7.9/0.64 (0.39)	26.3 versus 23.9/0.93 (0.85)
Van Cutsem et al./2011 (CRYSTAL)	140 (68/72)	FOLFIRI + C versus FOLFIRI	13.2/5.5 2.38 (0.13)	70.5/44.4 1.59 (0.003)	11.8 versus 9.2/0.56 (0.04)	27.8 versus 27.7/0.85 (0.43)
Maughan et al./2011 (COIN)	178 (87/91)	XELOX or FOLFOX + C versus XELOX or FOLFOX	15/13 1.13 (0.74)	NR NR	NR/0.68 (0.03)	NR
Ye et al./2013	138 (70/68)	FOLFOX + C versus FOLFOX	25.7/7.4 3.50 (0.004)	57.1/29.4 1.94 (<0.01)	10.2 versus 5.8/0.60 (0.004)	30.9 versus 21.0/0.54 (0.013)

LCM: liver-confined metastases; RR: relative risk; HR: hazard ratio; PFS: progression-free survival; OS: overall survival; wt: wild type; pts: patients; exp: experimental; ctr: control. FOLFOX refers to folinic acid (FOL) + fluorouracil (F) + oxaliplatin (OX); FOLFIRI refers to folinic acid (FOL) + fluorouracil (F) + irinotecan (IRI); XELOX refers to capecitabine (XEL) plus oxaliplatin (OX); C refers to cetuximab.

TABLE 2: Quality of each RCT included in the meta-analysis.

Author year	Randomization	Patients blinding	Concealed allocation	Intention-to-treat analysis	Completeness to follow-up
Bokemeyer et al./2011 (OPUS)	Yes	Unclear	Unclear	Yes	Yes
Van Cutsem et al./2011 (CRYSTAL)	Yes	Unclear	Unclear	Yes	Yes
Maughan et al./2011 (COIN)	Yes	Unclear	Unclear	Yes	Yes
Ye et al./2013	Yes	Unclear	Unclear	Yes	Yes

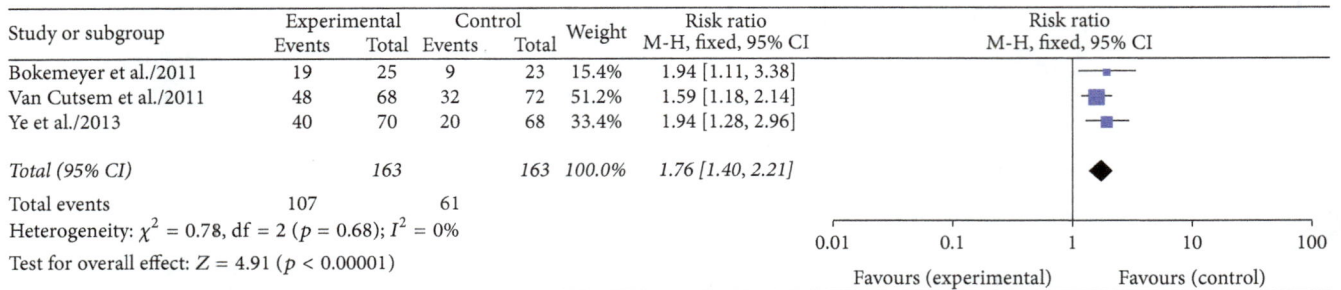

Study or subgroup	Experimental Events	Total	Control Events	Total	Weight	Risk ratio M-H, fixed, 95% CI	Risk ratio M-H, fixed, 95% CI
Bokemeyer et al./2011	19	25	9	23	15.4%	1.94 [1.11, 3.38]	
Van Cutsem et al./2011	48	68	32	72	51.2%	1.59 [1.18, 2.14]	
Ye et al./2013	40	70	20	68	33.4%	1.94 [1.28, 2.96]	
Total (95% CI)		163		163	100.0%	1.76 [1.40, 2.21]	
Total events	107		61				

Heterogeneity: $\chi^2 = 0.78$, df = 2 ($p = 0.68$); $I^2 = 0\%$
Test for overall effect: $Z = 4.91$ ($p < 0.00001$)

FIGURE 3: Meta-analysis response rate comparing chemotherapy ± cetuximab in patients with liver-limited metastases.

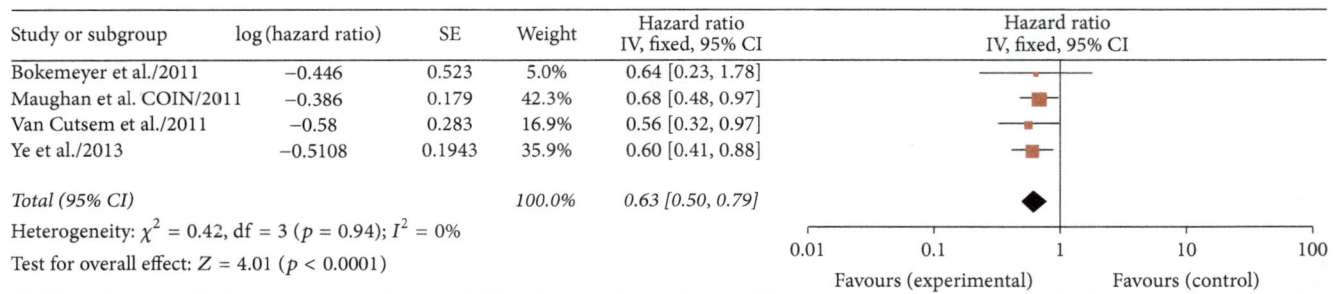

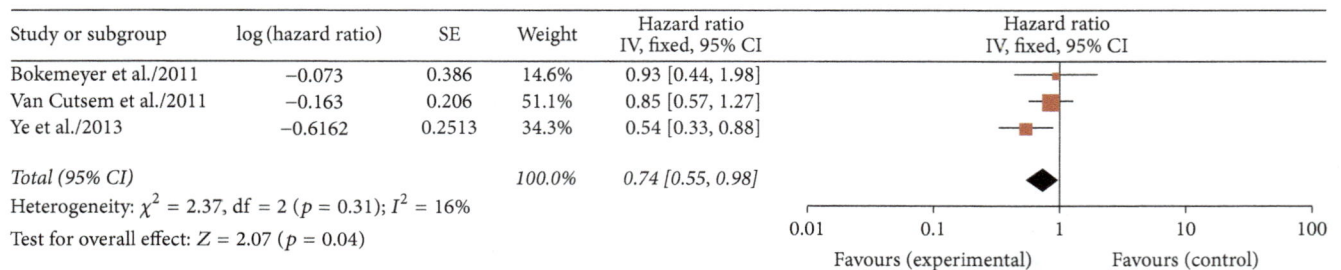

Study or subgroup	log (hazard ratio)	SE	Weight	Hazard ratio IV, fixed, 95% CI	Hazard ratio IV, fixed, 95% CI
Bokemeyer et al./2011	−0.446	0.523	5.0%	0.64 [0.23, 1.78]	
Maughan et al. COIN/2011	−0.386	0.179	42.3%	0.68 [0.48, 0.97]	
Van Cutsem et al./2011	−0.58	0.283	16.9%	0.56 [0.32, 0.97]	
Ye et al./2013	−0.5108	0.1943	35.9%	0.60 [0.41, 0.88]	
Total (95% CI)			100.0%	0.63 [0.50, 0.79]	

Heterogeneity: $\chi^2 = 0.42$, df = 3 ($p = 0.94$); $I^2 = 0\%$
Test for overall effect: $Z = 4.01$ ($p < 0.0001$)

FIGURE 4: Meta-analysis PFS comparing chemotherapy ± cetuximab in patients with liver-limited metastases.

Study or subgroup	log (hazard ratio)	SE	Weight	Hazard ratio IV, fixed, 95% CI	Hazard ratio IV, fixed, 95% CI
Bokemeyer et al./2011	−0.073	0.386	14.6%	0.93 [0.44, 1.98]	
Van Cutsem et al./2011	−0.163	0.206	51.1%	0.85 [0.57, 1.27]	
Ye et al./2013	−0.6162	0.2513	34.3%	0.54 [0.33, 0.88]	
Total (95% CI)			100.0%	0.74 [0.55, 0.98]	

Heterogeneity: $\chi^2 = 2.37$, df = 2 ($p = 0.31$); $I^2 = 16\%$
Test for overall effect: $Z = 2.07$ ($p = 0.04$)

FIGURE 5: Meta-analysis OS comparing chemotherapy ± cetuximab in patients with liver-limited metastases.

new RCT has been published. In our study, we described the outcomes of adding cetuximab in systematic chemotherapy and showed R0 resection rate, response rate, and PFS of KRAS wild type patients with CRLMs benefited from it. However, importantly, we also found that OS of KRAS wild type patients with CRLMs can also benefit from adding cetuximab; this result is quite different from the research published before, suggesting that cetuximab may be helpful for improving OS of KRAS wild type patients with CRLMs. In addition, the R0 resection rate is also higher than the results published before [13] (8.7%–17.6%, RR 2.03, $p = 0.004$ versus 11%–18%, RR 1.59, $p = 0.04$).

The reasons for such significant differences between Petrelli and Barni's study and our study perhaps ascribe to the 3 following reasons:

(1st) The studies included in each meta-analysis are different. The COIN trial, the OPUS study, and the CRYSTAL trial are the 3 RCTs included in both Petrelli and Barni's and our meta-analyses; however, our study did not include the RCT performed by Douillard et al. because this RCT mixed cetuximab and panitumumab in their study, while Petrelli and Barni's study is included. There are concerns that a lot of patients in the COIN trial go through reducing the drug dose in the period of treatment because of adverse events, so perhaps the patients in COIN trial had not gotten a full therapeutic benefit. Meanwhile, the RCT performed by Ye et al. (published in 2013, after Petrelli and Barni's study) did not reduce the drug dose in order to compromise on adverse events. So the full therapeutic benefit may not have been realized. Our study indicated adding cetuximab to potentially improve the overall survival rate.

(2nd) The drugs used in each meta-analysis are different. Petrelli and Barni's meta-analysis includes the RCT performed by Douillard et al. which mixed cetuximab and panitumumab in their study. To our knowledge, there is still not a RCT for comparing cetuximab with panitumumab, but the conclusion that panitumumab is not equally efficacious against the disease has been already reported [22]. Meanwhile, cetuximab can cause antibody dependent cellular cytotoxicity (ADCC) against tumor, but panitumumab does not have such effect because cetuximab is an IgG1 class antibody but panitumumab is an IgG2 class antibody [23].

(3rd) Racial differences existed between Petrelli and Barni's and our meta-analyses. All the patients included in Petrelli and Barni's meta-analysis are westerner, but the patients included in our study consist of westerner and Chinese. The racial differences perhaps lead to the different results between Petrelli and Barni's and our meta-analyses. As far as we know, there is not a credible evidence performed to prove that anti-EGFR does have the equal efficacy on different races yet.

However, these discussions and conclusions should be interpreted with caution due to the small sample size.

Although our meta-analysis reveals some new results, however, there are also some limitations in it. First, the number of patients analysed was limited, and the analysis of outcome as a function of KRAS status was performed retrospectively. Second, the unresectable criteria were not clearly described. Third, the patients in the former 3 RCTs included are only a subgroup of all metastatic patients rather than the last fourth RCT which enrolled solely patients with liver-limited metastases. Finally, we failed to obtain all the individual data of patients included as this is a paper-based study.

In summary, despite these defections, our study implies that the addition of cetuximab to systematic chemotherapy confers not only a significant benefit in terms of resectability, PFS, and response rate compared to systematic chemotherapy alone but also a significant benefit in terms of OS for the first time, especially for Chinese. Despite these limitations of this analysis, systematic chemotherapy plus cetuximab seems to be a promising choice for downsizing unresectable liver-confined metastases and prolonging survival time in KRAS wild type patients with CRLMs.

Competing Interests

The authors report no declarations of interest.

Authors' Contributions

W. Lv designed the study, performed the literature search, data selection and extraction, and statistical analysis, and drafted the manuscript. G. Q. Zhang searched the literature and selected and extracted the data. A. Jiao selected and extracted the data. J. L. Zhang, B. C. Zhao, Y. Shi, and B. M. Chen gave critical comments and revised the manuscript. All the authors consented to submit the manuscript and made remarkable contributions to it.

References

[1] D. Otchy, N. H. Hyman, C. Simmang et al., "Practice parameters for colon cancer," *Diseases of the Colon and Rectum*, vol. 47, no. 8, pp. 1269–1284, 2004.

[2] R. Adam, V. Delvart, G. Pascal et al., "Rescue surgery for unresectable colorectal liver metastases downstaged by chemotherapy: a model to predict long-term survival," *Annals of Surgery*, vol. 240, no. 4, pp. 644–658, 2004.

[3] E. Van Cutsem, B. Nordlinger, R. Adam et al., "Towards a pan-European consensus on the treatment of patients with colorectal liver metastases," *European Journal of Cancer*, vol. 42, no. 14, pp. 2212–2221, 2006.

[4] R. M. Goldberg, M. L. Rothenberg, E. Van Cutsem et al., "The continuum of care: a paradigm for the management of metastatic colorectal cancer," *The Oncologist*, vol. 12, no. 1, pp. 38–50, 2007.

[5] B. Chibaudel, C. Tournigand, F. Bonnetain et al., "Therapeutic strategy in unresectable metastatic colorectal cancer: an updated review," *Therapeutic Advances in Medical Oncology*, vol. 7, no. 3, pp. 153–169, 2015.

[6] F. Ciardiello and G. Tortora, "EGFR antagonists in cancer treatment," *New England Journal of Medicine*, vol. 358, no. 11, pp. 1160–1174, 2008.

[7] M. Ishida, T. Igarashi, K. Teramoto et al., "Mucinous bronchioloalveolar carcinoma with K-ras mutation arising in type 1 congenital cystic adenomatoid malformation: a case report with review of the literature," *International Journal of Clinical and Experimental Pathology*, vol. 6, no. 11, pp. 2597–2602, 2013.

[8] C. Mao, L.-X. Qiu, R.-Y. Liao et al., "KRAS mutations and resistance to EGFR-TKIs treatment in patients with non-small cell lung cancer: a meta-analysis of 22 studies," *Lung Cancer*, vol. 69, no. 3, pp. 272–278, 2010.

[9] J.-Y. Douillard, S. Siena, J. Cassidy et al., "Randomized, phase III trial of panitumumab with infusional fluorouracil, leucovorin, and oxaliplatin (FOLFOX4) versus FOLFOX4 alone as first-line treatment in patients with previously untreated metastatic colorectal cancer: the PRIME study," *Journal of Clinical Oncology*, vol. 28, no. 31, pp. 4697–4705, 2010.

[10] C. Bokemeyer, I. Bondarenko, J. T. Hartmann et al., "Efficacy according to biomarker status of cetuximab plus FOLFOX-4 as first-line treatment for metastatic colorectal cancer: the OPUS study," *Annals of Oncology*, vol. 22, no. 7, pp. 1535–1546, 2011.

[11] T. S. Maughan, R. A. Adams, C. G. Smith et al., "Addition of cetuximab to oxaliplatin-based first-line combination chemotherapy for treatment of advanced colorectal cancer: results of the randomised phase 3 MRC COIN trial," *The Lancet*, vol. 377, no. 9783, pp. 2103–1421, 2011.

[12] E. Van Cutsem, C.-H. Köhne, I. Láng et al., "Cetuximab plus irinotecan, fluorouracil, and leucovorin as first-line treatment for metastatic colorectal cancer: updated analysis of overall survival according to tumor KRAS and BRAF mutation status," *Journal of Clinical Oncology*, vol. 29, no. 15, pp. 2011–2019, 2011.

[13] F. Petrelli and S. Barni, "Resectability and outcome with anti-EGFR agents in patients with KRAS wild-type colorectal liver-limited metastases: a meta-analysis," *International Journal of Colorectal Disease*, vol. 27, no. 8, pp. 997–1004, 2012.

[14] L. Lin, L. Chen, Y. Wang, X. Meng, C. Liang, and F. Zhou, "Efficacy of cetuximab-based chemotherapy in metastatic colorectal cancer according to RAS and BRAF mutation subgroups: a meta-analysis," *Molecular and Clinical Oncology*, vol. 4, no. 6, pp. 1017–1024, 2016.

[15] L.-C. Ye, T.-S. Liu, L. Ren et al., "Randomized controlled trial of cetuximab plus chemotherapy for patients with KRAS wild-type unresectable colorectal liver-limited metastases," *Journal of Clinical Oncology*, vol. 31, no. 16, pp. 1931–1938, 2013.

[16] J. Mendelsohn and J. Baselga, "Epidermal growth factor receptor targeting in cancer," *Seminars in Oncology*, vol. 33, no. 4, pp. 369–385, 2006.

[17] J. P. T. Higgins and S. Green, *Cochrane Handbook for Systematic Reviews of Interventions Version 5.0.1*, 2008, http://onlinelibrary.wiley.com/o/cochrane/clcentral/articles/375/CN-00871375/frame.html.

[18] J. P. Higgins and S. G. Thompson, "Quantifying heterogeneity in a meta-analysis," *Statistics in Medicine*, vol. 21, no. 11, pp. 1539–1558, 2002.

[19] C. Kohne, C. Bokemeyer, S. Heeger, U. Sartorius, P. Rougier, and E. Van Cutsem, "Efficacy of chemotherapy plus cetuximab according to metastatic site in KRAS wild-type metastatic colorectal cancer (mCRC): analysis of CRYSTAL and OPUS studies," *Journal of Clinical Oncology*, vol. 29, no. 15, supplement 1, abstract 3576, 2011, Proceedings of the ASCO Annual Meeting.

[20] Y. Mise, S. Kopetz, R. J. Mehran et al., "Is complete liver resection without resection of synchronous lung metastases justified?" *Annals of Surgical Oncology*, vol. 22, no. 5, pp. 1585–1592, 2015.

[21] T. Delaunoit, S. R. Alberts, D. J. Sargent et al., "Chemotherapy permits resection of metastatic colorectal cancer: experience from Intergroup N9741," *Annals of Oncology*, vol. 16, no. 3, pp. 425–429, 2005.

[22] D. J. Jonker, C. J. O'Callaghan, C. S. Karapetis et al., "Cetuximab for the treatment of colorectal cancer," *The New England Journal of Medicine*, vol. 357, no. 20, pp. 2040–2048, 2007.

[23] P. A. Krawczyk and D. M. Kowalski, "Genetic and immune factors underlying the efficacy of cetuximab and panitumumab in the treatment of patients with metastatic colorectal cancer," *Contemporary Oncology*, vol. 18, no. 1, pp. 7–16, 2014.

10

Neurobiological Mechanism of Acupuncture for Relieving Visceral Pain of Gastrointestinal Origin

Fang Zhang,[1] Luyi Wu,[1] Jimeng Zhao,[1] Tingting Lv,[1] Zhihai Hu,[2]
Zhijun Weng,[1] Shuoshuo Wang,[2] Huangan Wu,[1] and Huirong Liu[1]

[1]*Shanghai Research Institute of Acupuncture and Meridian, Shanghai 200030, China*
[2]*Shanghai TCM-Integrated Hospital, Shanghai University of Traditional Chinese Medicine, Shanghai 200082, China*

Correspondence should be addressed to Huangan Wu; wuhuangan@126.com and Huirong Liu; lhr_tcm@139.com

Academic Editor: Agata Mulak

It is currently accepted that the neural transduction pathways of gastrointestinal (GI) visceral pain include the peripheral and central pathways. Existing research on the neurological mechanism of electroacupuncture (EA) in the treatment of GI visceral pain has primarily been concerned with the regulation of relevant transduction pathways. The generation of pain involves a series of processes, including energy transduction of stimulatory signals in the sensory nerve endings (signal transduction), subsequent conduction in primary afferent nerve fibers of dorsal root ganglia, and transmission to spinal dorsal horn neurons, the ascending transmission of sensory signals in the central nervous system, and the processing of sensory signals in the cerebral cortex. Numerous peripheral neurotransmitters, neuropeptides, and cytokines participate in the analgesic process of EA in visceral pain. Although EA has excellent efficacy in the treatment of GI visceral pain, the pathogenesis of the disease and the analgesic mechanism of the treatment have not been elucidated. In recent years, research has examined the pathogenesis of GI visceral pain and its influencing factors and has explored the neural transduction pathways of this disease.

1. Introduction

According to the International Association for the Study of Pain (IASP), "pain is an unpleasant sensory and emotional experience associated with actual or potential tissue damage." A thorough understanding of pain has not been clearly elucidated in the medical field. Research on somatic pain and neuropathic pain tends to be improved and perfect. However, the pathogenesis of visceral pain has not yet been clearly elucidated despite significant progress of relevant research. Visceral pain occurs in the interior organs (chest, abdomen, and pelvis) and is commonly observed in celiac diseases, such as gastrointestinal (GI) disorders, in the clinic. The manifestation of visceral pain is most typical in irritable bowel syndrome (IBS), and this disease is the most commonly used animal model in experimental studies of visceral pain. Visceral pain refers to pain from noxious stimuli such as painful swelling, ischemia, and inflammation that act on visceral organs via peripheral and central pathways [1]. There is a clear and unambiguous distinction between visceral pain and somatic and neuropathic pain. The characteristics of visceral pain include the following: (1) there is a vague sensation with an unclear position; (2) there is frequent accompaniment of referred pain in other areas such as the skin and muscle; (3) the generation of pain sensation is associated with motion and/or autonomic reflexes; and (4) persistent visceral pain can produce hyperalgesia in skin and deep tissues [2, 3]. Currently, the pathogenesis and influencing factors of GI visceral pain include visceral hypersensitivity, GI motility disorders, brain-gut axis abnormalities, intestinal infections, immune function changes, hereditary factors, and psychosocial factors.

Visceral pain is the most common symptom of functional bowel disorders and inflammatory bowel disease in the clinic. It is chronic in most cases and can be persistent or intermittent, which seriously affects the patient's life and work and costs substantial resources. Despite the excellent efficacy of EA in the treatment of GI visceral pain, the pathogenesis of this disease and the treatment mechanism of EA have not been investigated clearly. Over the past few years, research has examined the pathogenesis of GI visceral pain and its influencing factors and explored the neural transduction pathways of this disease. Visceral pain in IBS is a digestive disease commonly observed in clinical practice [4], but its etiology and pathogenesis have not been clarified. Epidemiological data from 2014 revealed that the worldwide prevalence rate of IBS was 3–22% [5]; this prevalence rate in China was 0.82–5.67% [6]. The clinical features of IBS cause significant inconvenience in the daily lives and work of patients and also reduce their quality of life. Therefore, the treatment methods and their efficacy for IBS are particularly critical. Modern medical treatment of GI visceral pain primarily consists of medication therapy. Despite its efficacy, long-term medication use is associated with side effects. Traditional Chinese medicine, particularly acupuncture and moxibustion therapy, has a long history and has demonstrated significant effects in pain treatment. Because it has good long-term effects without toxic side effects or recurrence, EA has been approved and recommended by the World Health Organization (WHO) as the main method of pain relief [7, 8]. According to existing studies, the possible analgesic mechanisms of EA treatment for GI visceral pain can be summarized in two aspects: the peripheral and central nervous pathways.

The neurobiological mechanism is one of the most important analgesic mechanisms of acupuncture [9]. EA stimulation of a surface acupoint activates the enteric nervous system (ENS), leading to the release of varying levels of neurochemical signaling molecules from the brain-gut axis, such as 5-HT, norepinephrine, bradykinin, histamine, and encephalin [10, 11] (Figure 1). Furthermore, these molecules inhibit inflammatory reactions or promote damage repair, interfere with the afferent peripheral sensory nerve impulses, and break the vicious noxious stimuli-pain cycle, eventually relieving the pain. In recent years, numerous scholars have made significant progress in research and discussion with respect to the mechanism of EA treatment for GI visceral pain. This paper summarizes the recent knowledge on the neurobiological mechanism of EA for relieving GI visceral pain and further discusses the new advances and directions in EA treatment of visceral pain.

2. Transduction Pathways of GI Visceral Pain

It has been accepted that the neural transduction pathways of GI visceral pain are divided into peripheral and central pathways. Existing research on the neurological mechanism of EA treatment for GI visceral pain has primarily focused on the regulation of these transduction pathways. (1) The peripheral pathway: noxious stimuli act on the receptors in the GI mucosa and are transmitted from primary afferent nerve fibers to primary sensory neurons in the dorsal root ganglia (DRG). Primary afferent nerve fibers include extrinsic and intrinsic afferent fibers that govern the GI tract. Extrinsic nerves refer to sympathetic and parasympathetic nerves, and sympathetic afferent fibers transmit signals to the spinal DRG. Parasympathetic afferent fibers include two pathways through the vagus and pelvic nerves, respectively. The afferent information from the vagus nerve is mainly relayed through the nucleus tractus solitarius (NTS) in the central nerves; the

afferent information from the pelvic organs is mainly relayed through the sacral dorsal commissural nucleus (DCN) in the central nerves. Intrinsic nerves refer to the ENS, which mainly includes the submucosal plexus and the myenteric plexus. These nerves belong to vagal afferent fibers that directly transmit signals into the NTS of the medulla [12, 13] (Figure 1). (2) The central pathway: (1) information is transduced in the primary sensory neurons of the spinal DRG and then transmitted to the spinal dorsal horn neurons (DHN), wherein nociceptive information is subject to primary central integration, followed by ascending transmission in the spinal cord through the spinothalamic tract, the spinoreticular tract, and the spinomesencephalic tract to the thalamus, the reticular formation, and the midbrain; further, the information is projected to the cerebral somatosensory cortex, the anterior cingulate cortex (ACC), and the insular cortex, resulting in visceral pain [14]. (2) NTS conduction of information: more afferent information is transmitted from the visceral portion of the NTS (caudal medial part) to the nucleus parabrachialis and then to the ventral posterior nucleus and the parvicellular part in the thalamus, finally reaching the insular cortex and constituting the main visceral afferent central pathway; part of the afferent information is transmitted along the NTS to the DCN and then to the hypothalamus and amygdala pathways, which are primarily responsible for emotional changes because of visceral sensation [15]. (3) The cingulate gyrus, amygdala, midbrain periaqueductal gray matter, and rostral ventromedial medulla (RVM) constitute the descending pathway; central signals from the nerve fibers of the RVM are projected through the ventrolateral funiculus and dorsal lateral funiculus to the spinal cord and are mainly terminated in the spinal DHN [16] (Figure 1).

3. Neurological Mechanisms of EA for Relieving GI Visceral Pain

EA analgesia has been applied in traditional Chinese medicine for thousands of years. It is now extensively used in clinical practice [18], and increasing attention has been received from clinicians and researchers in many countries. The range of treatment includes pain and inflammatory diseases. Body surface stimulation can suppress painful feelings in visceral pain. In traditional Chinese medicine, AP, moxibustion, and massage achieve this purpose by stimulating surface acupoints. These phenomena involve complex neurobiological mechanisms. It is difficult to explain them by the traditional lower center convergence-projection theory of referred pain and the classical pain transduction pathway. EA therapy and other surface physical stimulation therapies in modern medicine (e.g., lumbosacral magnetic stimulation, transcranial magnetic stimulation, and transcutaneous electrical nerve stimulation) have been applied and have been widely used in the clinic worldwide; these methods are safe and effective [18, 19]. Since the 1980s, the neurological mechanism of EA treatment for GI visceral pain began to receive sustained attention worldwide. Although the neurological mechanism of EA for relieving GI visceral pain has been partially revealed, specific transduction pathways in

Hypothalamus

μ-Opioid↑ SP↓
β-EP↑ CNF↓
PVN
AVP↑
DMH, MD
Neurons discharge (−)

Spinal dorsal horn

WDRn discharge (−)
c-fos↓ NR1↓
CRH↓ NR2B↓
CGRP↓ $P2X_2$↓
AchE↓ $P2X_3$↓
5-HT↓ $P2Y_1$↓
VIP↓ pERK↓
SP↓ pCREB↓
P38↓ β-EP↑

ST36
ST37
ST25
Acupoint (peripheral site)

Brain   MCC   Primary somatosensory cortex
pACC
ACC   Insula   Thalamus
PAG
Locus coeruleus
Amygdala   Caudal raphe nucleus
Rostral ventral medulla   Dorsal reticular nucleus

Spinal cord

Enteric nervous system

Acupuncture needle

ACC, PFC

$P2X_3$↓

DR	NTS	PTN	RVM
c-fos↓	c-fos↓	c-fos↑	c-fos↓
5-HT↓	GFAP↓		NR1↓

Neurons discharge (−)

DRG	DCN
$P2X_2$↓	GFAP↓
$P2X_3$↓	OX42↓
$P2Y_1$↓	
AchE↓	

ENS

5-HT↓	CRH↓	β-EP↑
PG↓	NGF↓	VIP↑
BK↓	TNF-α↓	ENK↑
SP/NK1R↓	c-fos↓	μ-Opioid↑
AchE↓	$P2X_2$↓	
NoS↓	$P2X_3$↓	

Surface acupoints

ATP↑
$P2X_3$↑
MC↑ (SP↑)

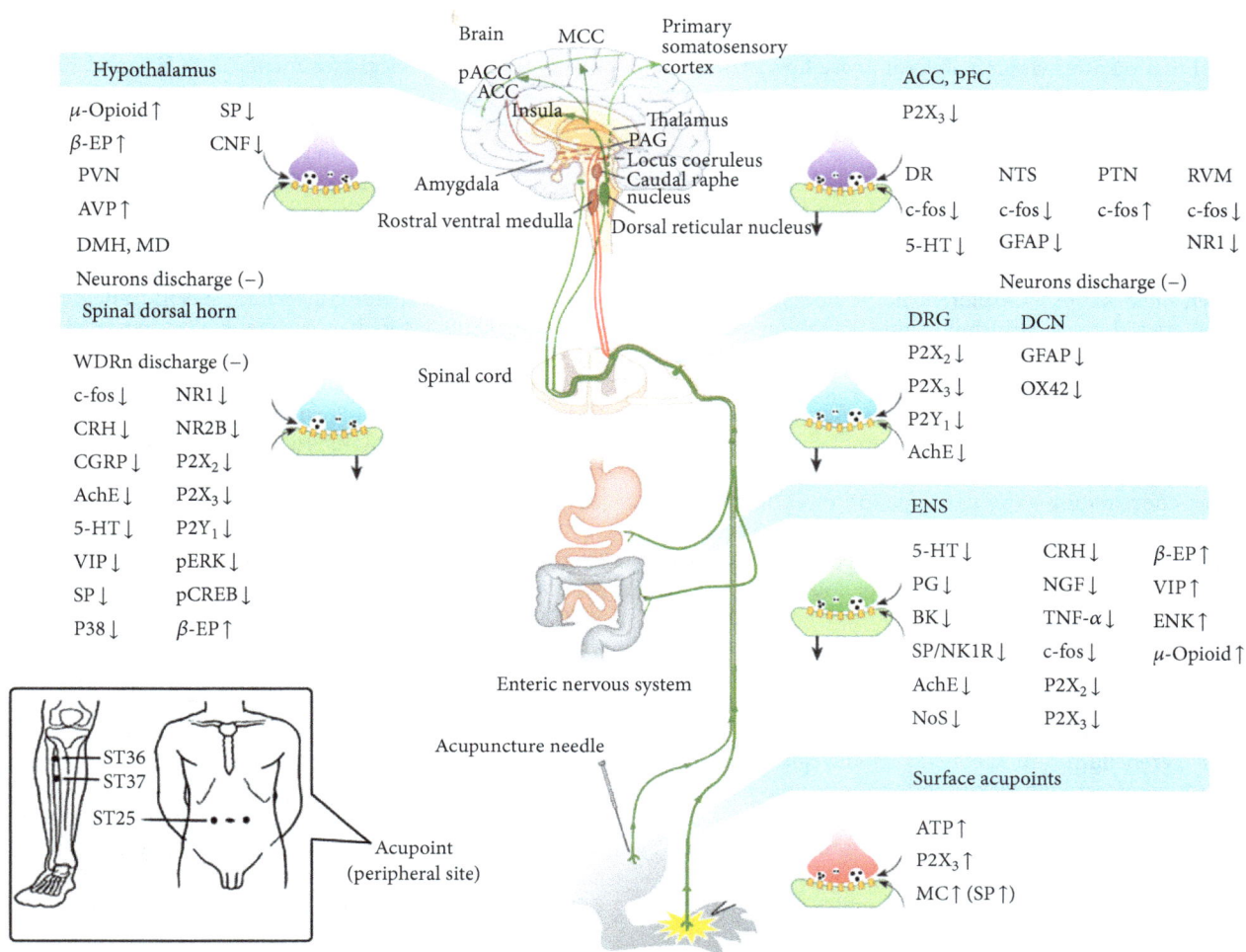

FIGURE 1: Ascending and descending pathways of the endogenous pain modulation system mediating visceral pain sensation in the brain-gut axis. Picture quoted from Zhang et al., Anesthesiology (2014) [11] and Moloney et al., Front Psychiatry (2015) [17]. RVM: rostral ventromedial medulla; MD: mediodorsal thalamic nucleus; PFC: prefrontal cortex; ACC: anterior cingulate cortex; DR: dorsal raphe nucleus; DMH: dorsomedial hypothalamic nucleus; AVP: arginine vasopressin; CNF: corticotropin releasing factor; GFAP: glial fibrillary acidic protein; WDR: wide dynamic range neurons; BK: bradykinin; PG: prostaglandins; β-EP: β-endorphin; (−): inhibition of cell discharge; NTS: nucleus of the solitary tract; TNF-α: tumor necrosis factor-α; NK1R: neuropeptide K 1R; SP: substance P; ENK: enkephalin.

EA treatment have not been found and must be determined in further study (Figure 1).

3.1. Peripheral Neurological Mechanism of EA for Relieving GI Visceral Pain.

Recent studies show that visceral hypersensitivity is one of the main pathophysiological bases of GI visceral pain. As described earlier, the pathogenesis of GI visceral pain includes the peripheral and central mechanisms. Previous research on the peripheral mechanism has primarily been concerned with how noxious stimulation acts on the receptors in the GI mucosa and activates mast cells to secrete various inflammatory mediators, such as 5-HT, prostaglandins, and bradykinin; these factors act on the corresponding receptors on the sensory nerve endings [20], thus transmitting nociceptive information to the spinal dorsal root. Research on the peripheral neurological mechanism of

EA for relieving GI visceral pain has primarily focused on neurons and associated neurotransmitters and afferent fibers.

3.1.1. Enteric Nervous System (ENS).

Over the past few years, numerous studies have found that the brain-gut axis plays a critical role in the development and progression of visceral pain. The brain-gut axis refers to the physiological and pathological phenomenon in which the central nervous system (CNS) and the GI tract mutually affect and regulate one another through neurotransmitters and chemical or electrical signals. It has a role in various functionality-, motility-, and immune-related GI disorders [21] (Figure 1). Meanwhile, the brain-gut axis forms the physiological basis of AP for regulating the GI function. The peripheral pathway of GI visceral pain mainly refers to the primary sensory neuron stage of signal transmission through primary afferent nerve fibers to the spinal DRG after noxious stimulation acting on the receptors in the GI mucosa. Presently, it is widely accepted that noxious visceral afferent nerve fibers comprise thin myelinated Aδ fibers (30–40%) and unmyelinated C fibers (60–70%) [12, 22]. During pain treatment with AP, needling sensation is a prerequisite for an analgesic effect. Electrophysiological studies found that needling sensation impulses are mainly governed by Aδ fibers (class III) and C fibers (class IV), which transmit the needling sensation to the upper spinal center, thus achieving the analgesic effect [23]. However, once AP excites afferent nerve fibers deep in the acupoint area, the pain threshold value will be increased. At the same level of nerve segment, AP in the Hegu acupoint can increase the pain threshold value deep in the acupoint itself. Such AP can achieve an obvious analgesic effect as long as it excites class II and a small amount of class III fibers deep in the acupoint area. For the distal segment, the AP analgesic effect requires the participation of C fibers. From these studies [24–26], it can be shown that the convergence of AP signals and visceral noxious afferent neurons in the spinal cord and the upper center is the neurobiological basis of AP for relieving visceral pain. AP can produce certain analgesic effects as long as it activates Aδ (class III) or C (class IV) fibers.

In the peripheral pathway of GI visceral pain, the ENS functions independently of the CNS and is also known as the "gut cerebellum." In the ENS, cholinergic neurons of the submucosal nervous plexus and the intestinal myenteric plexus can release an important neurotransmitter called acetylcholine (AchE). AchE is considered to be the primary neurotransmitter used to regulate GI motility [27] and to participate in the primary afferents of analgesic information of AP [28]. Early animal studies found that cholinergic nerves are involved in the transmission of noxious visceral pain sensation in the rat intestinal tract with acute inflammation. Electroacupuncture (EA) can reduce the AchE that has increased during inflammatory reactions to relieve visceral pain [29]. The EA stimulation (50 Hz) of rats with IBS visceral pain at acupoints ST25 and ST36 significantly reduced the visceral hypersensitivity that was induced by mechanical colorectal distension (CRD). Meanwhile, it was found that EA could downregulate the amount of mast cells, SP, vasoactive intestinal polypeptides (VIPs), neurokinin-1 receptors, and VIP receptors [30, 31] and CRH [32], NGF, and NGFR expression [33] in the descending part of the colon in the target organ, making the AWR score lower.

5-HT, as a brain-gut peptide, is widely present in the CNS and GI tract and functions as an important neurotransmitter to regulate functions of the digestive tract [34]. 5-HT_3 receptors are massively distributed in the myenteric nerve plexus (primary afferent neurons) and participate in the regulation of abdominal discomfort symptoms in IBS VP [35, 36]. Clinical studies showed that 5-HT and 5-HT_3 expression levels were markedly increased in the intestinal mucosa among patients with IBS; the application of a 5-HT3 receptor antagonist improved the threshold value of colonic CRD [37, 38]. EA stipulation of acupoint ST36 at 100 Hz downregulated colonic levels of 5-HT and 5-HT_3 expression in the brain-gut axis [39–41], further reducing

pain symptoms. Moreover, it was found that EA could regulate serum levels of 5-HT in patients with visceral hyperalgesia in clinical treatment. SP, 5-HT, and histamine released from mast cells mediated the sensitization of visceral afferent fibers [42]. Patients with irregular abdominal pain exhibited higher expression levels of colonic VIP, NK1R, and TNF-α mRNA than normal controls [43, 44]. Thus, it appears that EA downregulates peripheral chemicals to reduce the sensitivity of the splanchnic nerves, thereby achieving the effect of relieving visceral pain. However, there are no experimental designs available concerning specific antagonists and gene knockouts. Moreover, animal studies revealed that 20-Hz prestimulation of acupoint Jiaji markedly reduced the behavior response of visceral pain hyperalgesia as induced by the intestinal injection of formalin. Meanwhile, it reduced the phosphorylation of colonic mucosa P38 and downregulated fos expression but upregulated β-endorphin expression. Such effects were not observed in normal rats [45].

In the body, the epithelial cells of tubular and saclike organs (e.g., the intestines, ureter, and bladder) release ATP upon mechanical distention stimulation. P2X3 and P2X2/3 receptors act on the submucous nerve plexus in the epithelium and induce pain signals to be transmitted towards the center [46, 47]. P2X receptors (particularly the P2X2 and P2X3 subtypes) participate in the conduction and modulation of visceral nociceptive information in the peripheral and central nervous systems and are highly selectively expressed in sensory neurons [48]. Behavior, morphology, and molecular biology experiments revealed that P2X3 receptors mediate the pathogenesis of visceral pain in peripheral and central neurons in IBS rats. Fibers of P2X3 receptor-positive immunoreactive neurons are projected to spinal dorsal horn (SDH) II with the expression in these afferent nerve endings [49] being significantly positively regulated by EA [50, 51].

3.2. Spinal Neurobiological Mechanism of EA for Relieving GI Visceral Pain.
The main pathogenetic mechanism of visceral pain is visceral hypersensitivity, and the pathogenesis of visceral hypersensitivity includes the peripheral and central mechanisms. However, central sensitization has been found to be a key factor in the development and progression of visceral hypersensitivity. If central sensitization is inhibited, then chronic visceral pain can be effectively relieved [52] (Figure 1). Central sensitization is a complex process that involves various neurons, nerve nuclei or nuclei, and neurotransmitters involved in nerves. In research on the central nervous mechanism of EA for alleviating GI visceral pain, part of the mechanism was identified by functional magnetic resonance imaging [53], which may be consistent with its central conduction pathway. However, further research is still required to fully reveal the central mechanism of EA analgesia.

3.2.1. Dorsal Root Ganglion (DRG).
In the central transduction pathway of visceral pain, the spinal cord is the first level in the integration center of pain signals after entry to the central nerves. It is the relay station of afferent pain information, and it directly modulates the pain sensation

and also receives the descending regulatory signals of the upper spinal center; thus, the spinal cord is regarded as a key part in the regulation of pain stimulation [54]. The DRG, as the first level of neurons for afferent sensory information, has an extremely important role in transmitting information between peripheral and central nerves [55]. During the treatment of visceral pain, EA may inhibit the excited DRG neurons and the expression of related neurotransmitters and receptors through afferent impulses at the acupoint, thereby achieving an analgesic effect. The majority of experimental studies in rats with visceral hyperalgesia have found that the model rats presented with significant hyperalgesia to CRD, with markedly higher excitability of DRG neurons. EA stimulation of acupoint Zusanli was able to reduce the excitability of the DRG neurons and the expression of related neurotransmitters and receptors, thus remarkably relieving the symptoms of visceral hyperalgesia [56, 57]. This effect of EA was blocked by an intraperitoneal injection of naloxone. Moreover, DRG neurons can convey sensory impulses from the peripheral to the central nerves and then to the SDH, completing the transmission of primary sensory information. It was postulated that, after reducing the excitability of DRG neurons, AP may block the pathway of pain signals to a higher degree. Moreover, P2X3 receptors of DRG sensory neurons have an important role in ATP-mediated pain in IBS rats with visceral hypersensitivity [58]. The upregulated expression of P2X3 receptors was implicated in the DRG neurons of visceral pain model rats prepared by CRD, and EA was able to reduce the expression of P2X3 receptors in DRG cells [50]. The role of P2X3 receptors in the activation of nociceptors in IBS rats was further explored at the gene level by a real-time PCR analysis. Experimental evidence demonstrated that EA could relieve visceral hyperalgesia in rats with visceral pain by reducing the expression of P2X2 and P2X3 receptors in the colon and spinal cord [59] and P2Y1 receptors in DRG cells. Thus, the spinal cord and upper spinal centers have a critical role in the EA treatment of visceral pain.

3.2.2. Spinal Dorsal Horn (SDH).

The SDH plays an important role in the transmission and regulation of visceral nociceptive information. It converges visceral afferent nerves from the periphery, descending projection nerves from the senior center, and SDH neurons, thus forming a complex neural network. The SDH contains abundant neurotransmitters and associated receptors, neuromodulators, and ion channels, which not only receive and transmit nociceptive information but also preliminarily process nociceptive information [54, 60, 61]. Research of the visceral pain model in rats has found that CRD can activate the response of wide dynamic range (WDR) SDH neurons, whereas the AP stimulation of acupoints can inhibit the neuronal response activated by visceral nociceptive afferents and thus alleviate visceral pain [62]. However, SDH neurons participate in the descending transduction pathway of visceral pain. The information of AP can be conveyed through SDH neurons to the upper spinal center, thus activating the descending regulation system of pain; this mechanism contributes to the expression of SDH receptors, such as 5-HT, and further achieves an analgesic effect [63]. As stated earlier, the EA prestimulation (20 Hz) of

acupoint Jiaji markedly reduced the phosphorylation of P38, downregulated fos expression, and upregulated β-endorphin expression in colonic mucosa; a similar effect of EA was found in the SDH [45]. As described, EA can inhibit the release of algogenic neurotransmitters by regulating the activity of endogenous opioid peptides in the spinal cord and the DRG, thereby achieving the purpose of alleviating visceral pain [64]. The spinal cord of the central level has provided an important neurobiological basis for the effect of EA in alleviating visceral pain. Meanwhile, it has a critical role in regulating inflammatory and pathological pain. Recent studies have found that the EA stimulation of acupoint Shangjuxu significantly reduced visceral hypersensitivity and lowered the pain threshold in rats with IBS induced by CRD; moreover, CRH and its mRNA expression appeared abnormal in the peripheral target organs, colon, and spinal cord [32]. Thus, EA stimulation of acupoint Shangjuxu also achieves a therapeutic effect through this pathway in IBS rats with visceral hypersensitivity.

The spinal cord is the first level of the integration center for pain signals that enter the central nerves. It directly modulates pain sensation and simultaneously receives descending regulatory signals from the upper spinal center; thus, it also regulates the transmission of visceral nociceptive information. AP signals are conveyed through SDH neurons to reach the upper spinal center; once the descending modulation system of pain is activated, AP regulates the expression of SDH c-fos, p38, and 5-HT receptors to achieve an analgesic effect [65, 66]. Additionally, EA can markedly inhibit the expression of c-fos and NMDA-R1 receptors in the L6–S2 segments of the SDH and RVM [67–70] and can reduce the abnormally high excitability of visceral response neurons in the SDH and RVM. As described, the regulation of visceral pain sensation in IBS rats is achieved through multiple receptors at the spinal cord level. Experimental data have shown that EA can alleviate visceral hyperalgesia by reducing c-fos, P2X2, and P2X3 receptor expression in the colon and spinal cord [59] and P2Y1 receptor expression in the DRG cells of rats with visceral pain. Thus, the spinal cord and the upper spinal center play an important role in the analgesic mechanism of EA for visceral pain [71, 72].

3.2.3. Sacral Dorsal Commissural Nucleus (DCN).

The DCN is located in the dorsal central canal of the sacral spinal cord. It is the projection site of primary afferent signals from the pelvic organs. The DCN participates in the transmission and regulation of pain signals in the left semicolon and acts as a relay station of the brain-gut axis in the pain pathways. DCN neurons have been shown to be activated by the colonic inflammation-induced visceral pain response, and the activated neurons in turn can preliminarily integrate noxious stimuli from the colon, thereby regulating the visceral pain response [73–75]. Moreover, recent studies have shown that glial cells play an important role in pain [76]. EA stimulation of acupoint Zusanli significantly attenuated the visceral pain response induced by noxious stimulation and inhibited DCN, glial fibrillary acidic protein (GFAP), and OX42 expression, indicating that glial cells (astrocytes and microglia) in the DCN participate in the analgesic process of EA [77]; the activation time of astrocytes is earlier than that of microglia [78]. Meanwhile, there is the "exchange of information" and "conversation" between glial cells and neurons, with mutual "activation" between one another [79]. It was further postulated that AP has an inhibitory effect on the activated glial cells in the DCN of rats with visceral pain, thereby posing an inhibitory effect on the excited neurons in the DCN and further playing an analgesic effect or blocking the transmission of pain information to the upper center. This postulation must be verified in further studies.

3.3. Upper Spinal Neurobiological Mechanism of EA for Relieving GI Visceral Pain

3.3.1. Thalamic and Brainstem Reticular Neurons.
The thalamus and brainstem reticular formation are important centers for processing pain information and integrating pain sensation. Thalamic and brainstem reticular neurons are the third level of pain information transmission. AP can influence nociceptive information transmission of the thalamus and brainstem reticular formation in the upper spinal center [53, 80, 81] (Figure 1). Neurophysiological research shows that neurons that respond to noxious stimuli exist at various levels of the CNS [82]. Early studies found that hypothalamic vasopressin neurons and the paraventricular nucleus participate in the inhibitory mechanism of EA for visceral pain induced by the intraperitoneal injection of antimony potassium tartrate [83]. The EA stimulation of acupoints ST36 and ST37 EA markedly relieved visceral pain and simultaneously upregulated hypothalamus β-endorphin and SP expression [84] and CRF synthesis [32, 85] in a rat model of visceral pain induced by mechanical distension of the stomach and colon. Moreover, EA stimulation of acupoint Zusanli inhibited visceral pain; fos expression in the brainstem nucleus raphes dorsalis, shallow SDH, and colonic epithelium; and 5-HT expression in the nucleus raphes dorsalis and the SDH in a rat model of visceral pain caused by neonate-mother separation [63]. This finding suggests that the thalamic mediodorsal nucleus (MD) is involved in information transmission of not only visceral pain but also AP. EA stimulation of acupoint Zusanli markedly inhibited the discharges evoked by pain-excited neurons of the thalamic MD but increased the discharges of the pain-inhibition unit in a rat model of visceral pain, thus producing an analgesic effect [86]. Additionally, visceral pain afferent signals can cause discharge reactions in thalamic and brainstem reticular neurons and thus cause the possible convergence of two sensory afferent signals (impulses from the AP site and visceral pain) in these thalamic and brainstem reticular neurons. AP can inhibit discharge reactions in visceral pain through certain integration mechanisms of the center, thereby alleviating visceral pain [81]. The stimulation at "Zusanli-Shangjuxu" acupoints enhanced discharge activity of VPL neurons under CRD-induced visceral pain. The frequency of neuronal discharge was associated with the pressure gradient of CRD which showed that visceral noxious stimulation may intensify the body's functional response to stimulation at acupoints [87].

The electronic stimulation of skin receptive fields and acupoint Zusanli can inhibit the response of somatic and visceral convergence neurons of the thalamic ventrobasal nucleus to the CRD [88]. The skin receptive fields of thalamic neurons that are responsive to visceral nociceptive sensations are mainly located on the stomach meridian in traditional Chinese medicine. Therefore, stimulation of the receptive fields will generate a stronger inhibitory effect compared to acupoint Zusanli.

3.3.2. Nucleus Tractus Solitarius (NTS).
The NTS is located in the dorsal medial part of the medulla oblongata. It acts as the relay nuclei of the visceral primary afferent fibers, which receive afferent information from the peripheral nerves and the spinal cord or medulla oblongata. Meanwhile, the NTS participates in the transmission of visceral nociceptive pain information and is an important central passageway for nociceptive afferent fibers and integration and regulation of visceral pain sensation [89]. The c-fos serves as a marker of active neurons [90], and the expression of glial fibrillary acidic protein (GFAP) is a sign of active glial cells [76]. Both c-fos and GFAP participate in the regulation of GI visceral pain. Research on the mechanism of EA for relieving GI visceral pain found that AP pretreatment markedly reduced c-fos positive neurons and GFAP expression in the NTS in model rats with GI visceral pain; these results suggest that the regulatory process of AP in visceral pain is closely related to the NTS [91]. Meanwhile, CRD can induce an excitatory response in related neurons in the NTS whereas EA stimulation poses an inhibitory effect on these neurons; these findings provide electrophysiological evidence that the NTS receives the afferent information of CRD-induced visceral pain and participates in the analgesic process of AP [92, 93] (Figure 1).

3.3.3. Rostral Ventromedial Medulla (RVM).
The RVM is located at the central junction of the pontine reticular formation. It plays a critical role in the central regulation of pain and additionally serves as a common pathway of the upper spinal center for descending regulation of visceral noxious stimuli. The RVM has a dual role in regulating visceral pain, and it may inhibit or facilitate the input of noxious stimuli [94, 95]. The RVM can induce analgesia when receiving high intensity electrical stimulation and high concentrations of certain excitatory neurotransmitter microinjections; however, it will promote the pain response when receiving low intensity electrical stimulation or low concentrations of certain excitatory neurotransmitters [54]. Experimental studies found that, after CRD stimulation, model rats presented with increased excitability of visceral responsive neurons in the RVM, with an abnormal increase in c-fos positive neurons; EA treatment markedly inhibited the expression of c-fos positive neurons in the RVM of model rats with IBS and thus reduced the abnormally high excitability of visceral responsive neurons in the RVM. This may be one mechanism by which AP alleviates chronic visceral hyperalgesia. EA stimulation (5–100 Hz) of acupoint Zusanli can reduce the AWR score and IBS-induced glutamate N1 and fos overexpression in the RVM [72]. Application of the NMDAR antagonist in the RVM could inhibit visceral pain

[70, 96], indicating that EA inhibits the activation of NMDA in the RVM to alleviate visceral pain.

3.3.4. ACC and Prefrontal Cortex (PFC). Nerve nuclei such as the PFC, ACC, thalamic medial nuclei, amygdala, midbrain periaqueductal gray matter, and caudate nucleus that participate in pain sensation and modulation have extensive fiber links and are important centers of pain sensation [97–99]. After being transmitted through the ascending pathways such as the pelvic and splanchnic nerves, visceral pain is integrated in the ACC. PET revealed the activation of the ACC in IBS patients after CRD [100]. In situ hybridization and immunohistochemical studies indicated that P2X3 receptors are expressed at certain levels in the PFC and ACC of adult rats; mechanical CRD could upregulate P2X3 expression in the PFC and ACC; moreover, EA stimulation of acupoint Shangjuxu could regulate the P2X3 receptors in the PFC and ACC [57], with an excellent modulatory effect on the degree of central sensitization and visceral hyperalgesia.

4. Others

Under the rectal balloon distension plus electroacupuncture condition, stimulation by electroacupuncture at Tianshu (ST 25) manifested a decreased regional cerebral metabolic rate of glucose in the left cingulate gyrus, right insula, right caudate nucleus, fusiform gyrus, and hippocampal gyrus. Electroacupuncture therapy relieved abdominal pain, distension, or discomfort by decreasing glucose metabolism in the brain [101]. A few studies recently published in Nature Medicine have shown that EA excites vagus nerves by surface stimulation of acupoint Zusanli, further leading to a strong systemic anti-inflammatory effect [102, 103]. This anti-inflammatory effect is achieved through dopamine, and its pathophysiological process typically reflects the function of the nerve-endocrine-immune network. It remains unclear whether this anti-inflammatory effect plays a role in the mechanism of EA for relieving inflammatory visceral pain (e.g., IBD). Nonetheless, all of these findings provide a good basis for revealing the mechanism of EA treatment for inflammatory visceral pain.

5. Conclusion and Outlook

Under physiological and pathological conditions, the processing of pain information by the body generally has cross-level features. Although research has been conducted on both the cellular and the molecular levels (e.g., chemical transmission mechanism of signals), there is also a higher level of exploration including serial and parallel processing of signals that eventually form sensory perception. With the continuous development of science and technology, research on EA analgesia has entered the molecular neurobiology level. This paper systematically discusses the major neurobiological mechanisms of EA analgesia for GI visceral pain from the aspects of the peripheral and central pathways. Various pathways and substances are involved in the mechanism of EA for alleviating visceral pain. Although both peripheral and central nerves participate in the analgesic mechanism, most of our information has been derived from elucidation of in vitro animal experiments. There remains a lack of verification by in vivo functional experiments and clinical trials. Further clarification is necessary to understand how these structures jointly function during the analgesic process of EA. Additionally, most existing studies have observed the regulatory effect of EA on neurotransmitters at the peripheral and central levels to discuss the possible mechanism of EA analgesia. However, relatively accurate neural pathways of EA analgesia have not yet been revealed because of the high complexity and diversity of nerve distribution in the transmission and modulation of visceral pain. Meanwhile, experimental research on EA for alleviating visceral pain is often focused on functional GI disorders, particularly IBS, as a model to investigate the underlying mechanism. Thus far, research has been lacking on AP analgesia of visceral pain in inflammatory GI disorders. Therefore, continuous investigation of the neural pathways of EA analgesia will be the priority of future research.

Competing Interests

The authors declare that there are no competing interests regarding the publication of this paper.

Authors' Contributions

Revision of the manuscript was done by Fang Zhang, Luyi Wu, Jimeng Zhao, and Tingting Lv. Acquisition and analysis of references were carried out by Zhihai Hu, Zhijun Weng, and Shuoshuo Wang. Study concept and design were the responsibility of Huirong Liu and Huangan Wu. Fang Zhang, Luyi Wu, and Jimeng Zhao contributed equally to this work.

Acknowledgments

This work was supported by the National Natural Science Foundation of China, (81403474); the National Key Basic Research Program of China (973 Program) (2015CB554500); Shanghai Municipal Commission of Health and Family Planning (20144Y0227).

References

[1] M. Chichlowski and C. Rudolph, "Visceral pain and gastrointestinal microbiome," *Journal of Neurogastroenterology and Motility*, vol. 21, no. 2, pp. 172–181, 2015.

[2] T. J. Ness and G. F. Gebhart, "Visceral pain: a review of experimental studies," *Pain*, vol. 41, no. 2, pp. 167–234, 1990.

[3] M. A. Giamberardino and L. Vecchiet, "Visceral pain, referred hyperalgesia and outcome: new concepts," *European journal of anaesthesiology. Supplement*, vol. 10, pp. 61–66, 1995.

[4] G. Barbara, C. Cremon, V. Annese et al., "Randomised controlled trial of mesalazine in IBS," *Gut*, vol. 65, no. 1, pp. 82–90, 2014.

[5] S. Basandra and D. Baja, "Epidemiology of dyspepsia and irritable bowel syndrome (IBS) in medical students of Northern

India," *Journal of Clinical and Diagnostic Research*, vol. 8, no. 12, pp. JC13–JC16, 2014.

[6] X. Q. Li, M. Chang, D. Xu et al., "The current status of the epidemiological study of irritable bowel syndrome in China," *Chinese Journal of Gastroenterology and Hepatology*, vol. 22, no. 8, pp. 734–739, 2013.

[7] A. Owen-Smith, C. Sterk, F. Mccarty, D. Hankerson-Dyson, and R. Diclemente, "Development and evaluation of a complementary and alternative medicine use survey in African-Americans with acquired immune deficiency syndrome," *Journal of Alternative and Complementary Medicine*, vol. 16, no. 5, pp. 569–577, 2010.

[8] R. Sadeghi, M. A. Heidarnia, M. Zagheri Tafreshi, M. Rassouli, and H. Soori, "The reasons for using acupuncture for pain relief," *Iranian Red Crescent Medical Journal*, vol. 16, no. 9, Article ID e15435, 2014.

[9] J. S. Han, "Acupuncture analgesia: areas of consensus and controversy," *Pain*, vol. 152, no. 3, supplement, pp. S41–S48, 2011.

[10] D. Gupta, D. Dalai, S. Swapnadeep et al., "Acupuncture (Zhēn Jiǔ)—an emerging adjunct in routine oral care," *Journal of Traditional and Complementary Medicine*, vol. 4, no. 4, pp. 218–223, 2014.

[11] R. Zhang, L. Lao, K. Ren, and B. M. Berman, "Mechanisms of acupuncture-electroacupuncture on persistent pain," *Anesthesiology*, vol. 120, no. 2, pp. 482–503, 2014.

[12] G. F. Gebhart, "Visceral pain—peripheral sensitisation," *Gut*, vol. 47, S4, pp. iv54–iv55, 2000.

[13] S. Sikandar and A. H. Dickenson, "Visceral pain: the ins and outs, the ups and downs," *Current Opinion in Supportive and Palliative Care*, vol. 6, no. 1, pp. 17–26, 2012.

[14] S. Elsenbruch, C. Rosenberger, U. Bingel, M. Forsting, M. Schedlowski, and E. R. Gizewski, "Patients with irritable bowel syndrome have altered emotional modulation of neural responses to visceral stimuli," *Gastroenterology*, vol. 139, no. 4, pp. 1310–1319, 2010.

[15] E. J. Baik, Y. Jeong, T. S. Nam, W. K. Kim, and K. S. Paik, "Mechanism of transmission and modulation of renal pain in cats; effect of nucleus raphe magnus stimulation on renal pain," *Yonsei Medical Journal*, vol. 36, no. 4, pp. 348–360, 1995.

[16] C. H. T. Kwok, I. M. Devonshire, A. J. Bennett, and G. J. Hathway, "Postnatal maturation of endogenous opioid systems within the periaqueductal grey and spinal dorsal horn of the rat," *Pain*, vol. 155, no. 1, pp. 168–178, 2014.

[17] R. D. Moloney, S. M. O'Mahony, T. G. Dinan, and J. F. Cryan, "Stress-induced visceral pain: toward animal models of irritable-bowel syndrome and associated comorbidities," *Frontiers in Psychiatry*, vol. 6, article no. 15, 2015.

[18] H. Zheng, Y. Li, W. Zhang et al., "Electroacupuncture for patients with diarrhea-predominant irritable bowel syndrome or functional diarrhea: a randomized controlled trial," *Medicine*, vol. 95, no. 24, Article ID e3884, 2016.

[19] T. Algladi, M. Harris, P. J. Whorwell, P. Paine, and S. Hamdy, "Modulation of human visceral sensitivity by noninvasive magnetoelectrical neural stimulation in health and irritable bowel syndrome," *Pain*, vol. 156, no. 7, pp. 1348–1356, 2015.

[20] E. A. Mayer and K. Tillisch, "The brain-gut axis in abdominal pain syndromes," *Annual Review of Medicine*, vol. 62, pp. 381–396, 2011.

[21] E. A. Mayer, D. Padua, and K. Tillisch, "Altered brain-gut axis in autism: comorbidity or causative mechanisms?" *BioEssays*, vol. 36, no. 10, pp. 933–939, 2014.

[22] J. N. Sengupta and G. F. Gebhart, "Mechanosensitive afferent fibers in the gastrointestinal and lower urinary tracts," in *Visceral Pain. Progress in Pain Research and Management*, G. F. Gebhart, Ed., vol. 5, pp. 75–98, IASP Press, Seattle, Wash, USA, 1995.

[23] X. Liu, P. Huang, and M. Jiang, "The effects of capsaicin blocking C fibers of nervi peroneus communis and its influence on analgesia of EA at 'Zusanli'," *Acupuncture Research*, vol. 22, no. 4, pp. 295–301, 1997.

[24] G. W. Lu, R. Z. Liang, J. Q. Xie et al., "Analysis of the analgesic effect of 'Zusanli' acupuncture on peripheral afferent nerve fibers," *Chinese Sciences*, vol. 22, no. 5, pp. 495–503, 1979.

[25] L. X. Zhu, C. Y. Li, B. Yang et al., "The effect of neonatal capsaicin on acupuncture analgesia," *Acupuncture Research*, vol. 4, pp. 285–291, 1990.

[26] P. J. Rong, *Convergence and Interaction between the Inputs of Visceral Nociception and Acupuncture*, Beijing University of Chinese Medicine, 2004.

[27] K. McConalogue and J. B. Furness, "3 Gastrointestinal neurotransmitters," *Bailliere's Clinical Endocrinology and Metabolism*, vol. 8, no. 1, pp. 51–76, 1994.

[28] X. M. Guan, M. K. Ai, L. Q. Ru et al., "Action of acetylcholine in the primary input of acupuncture analgesic information," *Acupuncture Research*, vol. 19, no. 3-4, p. 97, 1994.

[29] H. J. Wu, L. Zhou, L. Q. Ru et al., "Study on the enteric nervous mechanism of electro-acupuncture anti-acute inflammatory visceral pain in rats," *Acupuncture Research*, vol. 24, no. 2, pp. 138–142, 1999.

[30] M. Xiao-Peng, L.-Y. Tan, Y. Yang et al., "Effect of electro-acupuncture on substance P, its receptor and corticotropin-releasing hormone in rats with irritable bowel syndrome," *World Journal of Gastroenterology*, vol. 15, no. 41, pp. 5211–5217, 2009.

[31] H.-G. Wu, B. Jiang, E.-H. Zhou et al., "Regulatory mechanism of electroacupuncture in irritable bowel syndrome: preventing MC activation and decreasing SP VIP secretion," *Digestive Diseases and Sciences*, vol. 53, no. 6, pp. 1644–1651, 2008.

[32] H.-R. Liu, X.-Y. Fang, H.-G. Wu et al., "Effects of electroacupuncture on corticotropin-releasing hormone in rats with chronic visceral hypersensitivity," *World Journal of Gastroenterology*, vol. 21, no. 23, pp. 7181–7190, 2015.

[33] Y.-N. Liu, H.-G. Wu, X.-M. Wang et al., "Electroacupuncture down-regulates the expressions of colonic NGF and NGFR in visceral hypersensitivity rats," *Journal of Acupuncture and Tuina Science*, vol. 13, no. 2, pp. 67–73, 2015.

[34] R. Huang, J. Zhao, L. Wu et al., "Mechanisms underlying the analgesic effect of moxibustion on visceral pain in irritable bowel syndrome: a review," *Evidence-based Complementary and Alternative Medicine*, vol. 2014, Article ID 895914, 7 pages, 2014.

[35] X.-P. Ma, J. Hong, C.-P. An et al., "Acupuncture-moxibustion in treating irritable bowel syndrome: how does it work?" *World Journal of Gastroenterology*, vol. 20, no. 20, pp. 6044–6054, 2014.

[36] G. M. Mawe and J. M. Hoffman, "Serotonin signalling in the gut-functions, dysfunctions and therapeutic targets," *Nature Reviews Gastroenterology and Hepatology*, vol. 10, no. 8, pp. 473–486, 2013.

[37] M. Delvaux, D. Louvel, J.-P. Mamet, R. Campos-Oriola, and J. Frexinos, "Effect of alosetron on responses to colonic distension in patients with irritable bowel syndrome," *Alimentary Pharmacology and Therapeutics*, vol. 12, no. 9, pp. 849–855, 1998.

[38] C.-C. Feng, X.-J. Yan, X. Chen et al., "Vagal anandamide signaling via cannabinoid receptor 1 contributes to luminal 5-HT

modulation of visceral nociception in rats," *Pain*, vol. 155, no. 8, pp. 1591–1604, 2014.

[39] D. Chu, P. Cheng, H. Xiong, J. Zhang, S. Liu, and X. Hou, "Electroacupuncture at ST-36 relieves visceral hypersensitivity and decreases 5-HT3 receptor level in the colon in chronic visceral hypersensitivity rats," *International Journal of Colorectal Disease*, vol. 26, no. 5, pp. 569–574, 2011.

[40] X. Zhu, Z. Liu, W. Niu et al., "Effects of electroacupuncture at ST25 and BL25 in a *Sennae*-induced rat model of diarrhoea-predominant irritable bowel syndrome," *Acupuncture in Medicine*, 2016.

[41] J. Zhao, L. Chen, C. Zhou et al., "Comparison of electroacupuncture and moxibustion for relieving visceral hypersensitivity in rats with constipation-predominant irritable bowel syndrome," *Evidence-Based Complementary and Alternative Medicine*, vol. 2016, Article ID 9410505, 8 pages, 2016.

[42] D. Keszthelyi, F. J. Troost, M. Simrén et al., "Revisiting concepts of visceral nociception in irritable bowel syndrome," *European Journal of Pain*, vol. 16, no. 10, pp. 1444–1454, 2012.

[43] J. Simpson, F. Sundler, D. J. Humes, D. Jenkins, J. H. Scholefield, and R. C. Spiller, "Post inflammatory damage to the enteric nervous system in diverticular disease and its relationship to symptoms," *Neurogastroenterology and Motility*, vol. 21, no. 8, pp. 847–e58, 2009.

[44] D. J. Humes, J. Simpson, J. Smith et al., "Visceral hypersensitivity in symptomatic diverticular disease and the role of neuropeptides and low grade inflammation," *Neurogastroenterology and Motility*, vol. 24, no. 4, pp. 318–e163, 2012.

[45] C. Li, J. Yang, J. Sun et al., "Brain responses to acupuncture are probably dependent on the brain functional status," *Evidence-Based Complementary and Alternative Medicine*, vol. 2013, Article ID 175278, 14 pages, 2013.

[46] G. Burnstock and C. Kennedy, "P2X receptors in health and disease," *Advances in Pharmacology*, vol. 61, pp. 333–372, 2011.

[47] G. Burnstock, "Purinergic signalling in the gastrointestinal tract and related organs in health and disease," *Purinergic Signalling*, vol. 10, no. 1, pp. 3–50, 2014.

[48] C.-C. Chen, A. N. Akopian, L. Sivilotti, D. Colquhoun, G. Burnstock, and J. N. Wood, "A P2X purinoceptor expressed by a subset of sensory neurons," *Nature*, vol. 377, no. 6548, pp. 428–431, 1995.

[49] R. A. North, "Molecular physiology of P2X receptors," *Physiological Reviews*, vol. 82, no. 4, pp. 1013–1067, 2002.

[50] Z. J. Weng, L. Y. Wu, Y. Lu et al., "Electroacupuncture diminishes p2x2 and p2x3 purinergic receptor expression in dorsal root ganglia of rats with visceral hypersensitivity," *Neural Regeneration Research*, vol. 8, no. 9, pp. 802–808, 2013.

[51] X. X. Guo, J. F. Chen, Y. Lu et al., "Electroacupuncture at He-Mu points reduces P2X4 receptor expression in visceral hypersensitivity," *Neural Regeneration Research*, vol. 8, no. 22, pp. 2069–2077, 2013.

[52] S. Sarkar, A. R. Hobson, P. L. Furlong, C. J. Woolf, D. G. Thompson, and Q. Aziz, "Central neural mechanisms mediating human visceral hypersensitivity," *American Journal of Physiology—Gastrointestinal and Liver Physiology*, vol. 281, no. 5, pp. G1196–G1202, 2001.

[53] R. E. Harris, J.-K. Zubieta, D. J. Scott, V. Napadow, R. H. Gracely, and D. J. Clauw, "Traditional Chinese acupuncture and placebo (sham) acupuncture are differentiated by their effects on μ-opioid receptors (MORs)," *NeuroImage*, vol. 47, no. 3, pp. 1077–1085, 2009.

[54] D. P. Qi, *Chronic Visceral Hyperalgesia and Neurobiological Mechanism of Acupuncture in Relieving Visceral Pain*, Fudan University, 2011.

[55] J. H. Winston, G.-Y. Xu, and S. K. Sarna, "Adrenergic stimulation mediates visceral hypersensitivity to colorectal distension following heterotypic chronic stress," *Gastroenterology*, vol. 138, no. 1, pp. 294–304, 2010.

[56] G.-Y. Xu, J. H. Winston, and J. D. Z. Chen, "Electroacupuncture attenuates visceral hyperalgesia and inhibits the enhanced excitability of colon specific sensory neurons in a rat model of irritable bowel syndrome," *Neurogastroenterology and Motility*, vol. 21, no. 12, pp. 1302–e125, 2009.

[57] Z. J. Weng, L. Y. Wu, C. L. Zhou et al., "Effect of electroacupuncture on P2X3 receptor regulation in the peripheral and central nervous systems of rats with visceral pain caused by irritable bowel syndrome," *Purinergic Signalling*, vol. 11, no. 3, pp. 321–329, 2015.

[58] M. Shinoda, J.-H. La, K. Bielefeldt, and G. F. Gebhart, "Altered purinergic signaling in colorectal dorsal root ganglion neurons contributes to colorectal hypersensitivity," *Journal of Neurophysiology*, vol. 104, no. 6, pp. 3113–3123, 2010.

[59] M. Dong, *Regulatory effects of electroacupuncture on P2X2, 3 receptor and c-fos of rats with irritable bowel syndrome visceral sensitivity [M.S. thesis]*, Shanghai University of Traditional Chinese Medicine, 2011.

[60] A. J. Todd, "Neuronal circuitry for pain processing in the dorsal horn," *Nature Reviews Neuroscience*, vol. 11, no. 12, pp. 823–836, 2010.

[61] X.-Q. Luo, Q.-Y. Cai, Y. Chen et al., "Tyrosine phosphorylation of the NR2B subunit of the NMDA receptor in the spinal cord contributes to chronic visceral pain in rats," *Brain Research*, vol. 1542, pp. 167–175, 2014.

[62] L.-L. Yu, L. Li, P.-J. Rong et al., "Changes in responses of neurons in spinal and medullary subnucleus reticularis dorsalis to acupoint stimulation in rats with visceral hyperalgesia," *Evidence-Based Complementary and Alternative Medicine*, vol. 2014, Article ID 768634, 8 pages, 2014.

[63] J. C. Wu, E. T. Ziea, L. Lao et al., "Effect of electroacupuncture on visceral hyperalgesia, serotonin and fos expression in an animal model of irritable bowel syndrome," *Journal of Neurogastroenterology and Motility*, vol. 16, no. 3, pp. 306–314, 2010.

[64] D. Qi, S. Wu, Y. Zhang, and W. Li, "Electroacupuncture analgesia with different frequencies is mediated via different opioid pathways in acute visceral hyperalgesia rats," *Life Sciences*, vol. 160, pp. 64–71, 2016.

[65] K.-D. Xu, T. Liang, K. Wang, and D.-A. Tian, "Effect of pre-electroacupuncture on p38 and c-Fos expression in the spinal dorsal horn of rats suffering from visceral pain," *Chinese Medical Journal*, vol. 123, no. 9, pp. 1176–1181, 2010.

[66] W.-C. Yu, G.-Y. Huang, M.-M. Zhang, and W. Wang, "Effect of connexin 43 knockout on acupuncture-induced down-regulation of c-fos expression in spinal dorsal horn in visceral pain mice," *Acupuncture Research*, vol. 33, no. 3, pp. 179–182, 2008.

[67] K. M. Cui, W. M. Li, X. Gao, K. Chung, J. M. Chung, and G. C. Wu, "Electro-acupuncture relieves chronic visceral hyperalgesia in rats," *Neuroscience Letters*, vol. 376, no. 1, pp. 20–23, 2005.

[68] J. Zhou and W. M. Li, "Influence of electroacupuncture on expression of NMDA receptors in the spinal cord of irritable bowel syndrome rat," *Shanghai Journal of Acupuncture and Moxibustion*, vol. 27, no. 6, pp. 38–40, 2008.

[69] D. B. Qi and W. M. Li, "Effect of electroacupuncture on expression of NMDA-R1 receptor in the rostral ventromedial medulla of rats with chronic visceral hyperalgesia," *Shanghai Journal of Acupuncture and Moxibustion*, vol. 30, no. 7, pp. 491–494, 2011.

[70] L. D. Wang, *Regulation mechanism of moxibustion on PKCε and NR1, NR2B subunit of the NMDA receptor in the spinal cord on irritable bowel syndrome rats with visceral hyperalgesia [M.S. thesis]*, Shanghai University of Traditional Chinese Medicine, 2014.

[71] P.-J. Rong, B. Zhu, Q.-F. Huang, X.-Y. Gao, H. Ben, and Y.-H. Li, "Acupuncture inhibition on neuronal activity of spinal dorsal horn induced by noxious colorectal distention in rat," *World Journal of Gastroenterology*, vol. 11, no. 7, pp. 1011–1017, 2005.

[72] D.-B. Qi and W.-M. Li, "Effects of electroacupuncture on expression of c-fos protein and N-methyl-D-aspartate receptor 1 in the rostral ventromedia medulla of rats with chronic visceral hyperalgesia," *Journal of Chinese Integrative Medicine*, vol. 10, no. 4, pp. 416–423, 2012.

[73] J. Shanxue, Z. Hua, Q. Bingzhi et al., "Visceral and somatic primary afferent inputs convergence onto the neurons of the sacral dorsal commissural nucleus in the cat," *Chinese Journal of Neuroanatomy*, vol. 13, no. 1, pp. 29–35, 1997.

[74] M.-M. Zhang, W. Ji, L.-Y. Pei et al., "Acute colitis induces neurokinin 1 receptor internalization in the rat lumbosacral spinal cord," *PLoS ONE*, vol. 8, no. 3, Article ID e59234, 2013.

[75] Q. Ming, R. Zhiren, Y. Qi et al., "Effects of electroacupuncture at Tsusanli acupoint on morphological changes in neurons and glia cells in sacral dorsal commissual nudeus of rats with ulcerative colitis," *Medical Journal of Chinese People's Liberation Army*, vol. 33, no. 12, pp. 1454–1456, 2008.

[76] R.-R. Ji, T. Berta, and M. Nedergaard, "Glia and pain: is chronic pain a gliopathy?" *Pain*, vol. 154, no. 1, pp. S10–S28, 2013.

[77] W. Jingjie, Q. Ming, Q. Jianyong et al., "Effect of electroacupuncture at Tsusanli on visceral pain behavior and the expression of GFAP and OX42 in dorsal commissural nucleus in visceralgia rats," *Chinese Journal of Neuroanatomy*, vol. 22, no. 3, pp. 337–341, 2006.

[78] D. Y. Xia, J. J. Wang, S. H. Lu et al., "The changes of ethology and the neuron and glia of dorsal commissural nucleus induced by distended the colon of rats with IBS," *Chinese Journal of Gastroenterology and Hepatology*, vol. 16, no. 6, pp. 589–597, 2007.

[79] P. Bezzi and A. Volterra, "A neuron-glia signalling network in the active brain," *Current Opinion in Neurobiology*, vol. 11, no. 3, pp. 387–394, 2001.

[80] X. Tian, S. Chen, and Z. Cao, "Mechanism of CaMK II in the modulation of visceral hyperalgesia," *Chinese Journal of Gastroenterology*, vol. 16, no. 4, pp. 235–237, 2011.

[81] Acupuncture Anesthesia Principle Cooperative Research Group in Sichuan Medical School, "Effect of acupuncture on neurons of thalamus and brainstem reticular formation due to human visceral pain," *Acupuncture Research*, pp. 40–46, 1978.

[82] C. J. Woolf, "Central sensitization: implications for the diagnosis and treatment of pain," *Pain*, vol. 152, no. 3, pp. S2–S15, 2011.

[83] S. Gong, W.-P. Yin, and Q.-Z. Yin, "Involvement of vasopressinergic neurons of paraventricular nucleus in the electroacupuncture-induced inhibition of experimental visceral pain in rats," *Acta Physiologica Sinica*, vol. 44, no. 5, pp. 434–441, 1992.

[84] Y.-P. Lin, Y. Peng, S.-X. Yi, and S. Tang, "Effect of different frequency electroacupuncture on the expression of substance P and beta-endorphin in the hypothalamus in rats with gastric distension-induced pain," *Zhen ci yan jiu = Acupuncture research / [Zhongguo yi xue ke xue yuan Yi xue qing bao yan jiu suo bian ji]*, vol. 34, no. 4, pp. 252–257, 2009.

[85] H.-G. Wu, H.-R. Liu, Z.-A. Zhang et al., "Electro-acupuncture relieves visceral sensitivity and decreases hypothalamic corticotropin-releasing hormone levels in a rat model of irritable bowel syndrome," *Neuroscience Letters*, vol. 465, no. 3, pp. 235–237, 2009.

[86] L. P. Run, C. Ma, X. R. Xiang et al., "Electro-acupuncture can inhibit the unit discharges in mediodorsal thalamic nucleus of rats induced by visceral pain," *Chinese Journal of Pain Medicine*, vol. 10, no. 3, pp. 177–180, 2004.

[87] P.-J. Rong, J.-J. Zhao, L.-L. Yu et al., "Function of nucleus ventralis posterior lateralis thalami in acupoint sensitization phenomena," *Evidence-based Complementary and Alternative Medicine*, vol. 2015, Article ID 516851, 6 pages, 2015.

[88] J.-L. Zhang, S.-P. Zhang, and H.-Q. Zhang, "Effect of electroacupuncture on thalamic neuronal response to visceral nociception," *European Journal of Pain*, vol. 13, no. 4, pp. 366–372, 2009.

[89] P. P. J. Van Der Veek, C. A. Swenne, H. Van De Vooren, A. L. Schoneveld, R. Maestri, and A. A. M. Masclee, "Viscerosensory-cardiovascular reflexes: altered baroreflex sensitivity in irritable bowel syndrome," *American Journal of Physiology - Regulatory Integrative and Comparative Physiology*, vol. 289, no. 4, pp. R970–R976, 2005.

[90] Y. Ji, B. Tang, D.-Y. Cao, G. Wang, and R. J. Traub, "Sex differences in spinal processing of transient and inflammatory colorectal stimuli in the rat," *Pain*, vol. 153, no. 9, pp. 1965–1973, 2012.

[91] Q. Ming, H. Yu-Xin, W. Jing-Jie et al., "Effects of Electroacupuncture at 'Zusanli' (ST 36) on the expression of c-fos and glial fibril-lary acidic protein in the medullary visceral zone in visceral pain rats," *Acupuncture Research*, vol. 31, no. 3, pp. 136–139, 2006.

[92] K. Liu, *The Role of NTS in Acupuncture Regulating Blood Pressure, Gastrointestinal Sensation and Motility in Anesthetized Rats*, China Academy of Traditional Chinese Medicine, 2012.

[93] K. Liu, X.-Y. Gao, L. Li et al., "Neurons in the nucleus tractus solitarius mediate the acupuncture analgesia in visceral pain rats," *Autonomic Neuroscience: Basic and Clinical*, vol. 186, pp. 91–94, 2014.

[94] S. Sikandar and A. H. Dickenson, "Pregabalin modulation of spinal and brainstem visceral nociceptive processing," *Pain*, vol. 152, no. 10, pp. 2312–2322, 2011.

[95] F. Porreca, M. H. Ossipov, and G. F. Gebhart, "Chronic pain and medullary descending facilitation," *Trends in Neurosciences*, vol. 25, no. 6, pp. 319–325, 2002.

[96] R. Sanoja, V. Tortorici, C. Fernandez, T. J. Price, and F. Cervero, "Role of RVM neurons in capsaicin-evoked visceral nociception and referred hyperalgesia," *European Journal of Pain*, vol. 14, no. 2, pp. 120.e1–120.e9, 2010.

[97] B.-C. Shyu, R. W. Sikes, L. J. Vogt, and B. A. Vogt, "Nociceptive processing by anterior cingulate pyramidal neurons," *Journal of Neurophysiology*, vol. 103, no. 6, pp. 3287–3301, 2010.

[98] N. Yan, B. Cao, J. Xu, C. Hao, X. Zhang, and Y. Li, "Glutamatergic activation of anterior cingulate cortex mediates the affective component of visceral pain memory in rats," *Neurobiology of Learning and Memory*, vol. 97, no. 1, pp. 156–164, 2012.

[99] R. W. Sikes, L. J. Vogt, and B. A. Vogt, "Distribution and properties of visceral nociceptive neurons in rabbit cingulate cortex," *Pain*, vol. 135, no. 1-2, pp. 160–174, 2008.

[100] B. D. Naliboff, S. Berman, B. Suyenobu et al., "Longitudinal change in perceptual and brain activation response to visceral stimuli in irritable bowel syndrome patients," *Gastroenterology*, vol. 131, no. 2, pp. 352–365, 2006.

[101] H. Liu, L. Qi, X. Wang et al., "Electroacupuncture at Tianshu (ST 25) for diarrhea-predominant irritable bowel syndrome using positron emission tomography changes in visceral sensation center," *Neural Regeneration Research*, vol. 5, no. 16, pp. 1220–1225, 2010.

[102] S. S. Chavan and K. J. Tracey, "Regulating innate immunity with dopamine and electroacupuncture," *Nature Medicine*, vol. 20, no. 3, pp. 239–241, 2014.

[103] R. Torres-Rosas, G. Yehia, G. Peña et al., "Dopamine mediates vagal modulation of the immune system by electroacupuncture," *Nature Medicine*, vol. 20, no. 3, pp. 291–295, 2014.

11

Multidisciplinary Treatment for Colorectal Peritoneal Metastases: Review of the Literature

Shaobo Mo[1,2] and Guoxiang Cai[1,2]

[1]Department of Colorectal Surgery, Fudan University Shanghai Cancer Center, Shanghai 200032, China
[2]Department of Oncology, Shanghai Medical College, Fudan University, Shanghai 200032, China

Correspondence should be addressed to Guoxiang Cai; gxcai@fudan.edu.cn

Academic Editor: Amosy M'Koma

Peritoneum is one of the common sites of metastasis in advanced stage colorectal cancer patients. Colorectal cancer patients with peritoneal metastases (PM) are traditionally believed to have poor prognosis, which indicates it is of no value to adopt surgical treatment. With the advancement of surgical techniques, hyperthermic intraperitoneal chemotherapy (HIPEC), and multidisciplinary treatment in recent years, the cognition and treatment strategies of colorectal peritoneal metastases (CPM) have changed dramatically. In terms of prognosis, CPM under the palliative systemic treatment shows an inferior outcome compared with nonperitoneal metastasis. Nevertheless, some CPM patients amenable to the complete peritoneal cytoreductive surgery (CRS) combined with HIPEC may achieve long-term survival. The prognostic factors of CPM comprise peritoneal carcinomatosis index (PCI), completeness of cytoreduction score (CC score), the presence of extraperitoneal metastasis (liver, etc.), Peritoneal Surface Disease Severity Score (PSDSS), Japanese peritoneal staging, and so forth. Taken together, literature data suggest that a multimodality approach combining complete peritoneal CRS plus HIPEC, systemic chemotherapy, and targeted therapy may be the best treatment option for PM from colorectal cancer.

1. Introduction

Peritoneal spread is common in advanced stage colorectal cancer patients and was reported in the past to be associated with a poor prognosis [1–3]. Approximately 5.0% of colorectal cancer patients present synchronous peritoneal metastases (PM) and about 19.0% may manifest metachronous disease [4, 5]. PM is often accompanied by distant metastasis of other organs, such as the liver and lungs. It has been reported that 88% of colorectal peritoneal metastases (CPM) had other concomitant distant metastases [6]. PM is traditionally perceived as the advanced manifestation of colorectal cancer, with a median survival of 5–7 months, which hardly has the healing possibility and the value of surgical treatment [1, 7, 8].

With the purpose of seeking more effective treatments for CPM, myriads of approaches have been undertaken over the past decades. Recently, with the accumulation of massive researches on CPM, there is a better understanding of the prognosis of CPM and prognostic influence factors [9]. Moreover, the attitude towards the therapeutic strategies for

CPM has changed tremendously with the update of the concept of multidisciplinary treatment and advances in surgical techniques and hyperthermic intraperitoneal chemotherapy (HIPEC) [10, 11]. Therefore, the therapeutic efficacy of PM has been greatly improved, achieving better long-term survival in patients with PM from colorectal carcinoma [12].

In this review we commit to exploring the recent advances in multidisciplinary treatment for CPM.

2. Risks for Development of CPM

Defining risk factors for the development of CPM is needed to better select patients at high risk for developing PM, which consequently might benefit from intensified adjuvant treatment regimens.

In the population-based study by Segelman et al. [3], independent predictors for developing metachronous CPM were colonic cancer, in particular right-sided, stages T3-T4 tumor, lymph node statuses N1-N2, fewer than 12 lymph nodes harvested, emergency procedures, and nonradical resection of the primary tumor (R1 or R2). From a prospectively expanded single-institutional database with 2406 consecutive patients with colorectal cancer (CRC), clinical and histological data were analyzed for independent risk factors, the results of which demonstrated that age <62 years, N2-status, T4-status, and location of the primary in the left colon or appendix were independent risk factors for the development of metachronous CPM [13].

The results of study by Lemmens et al. [2] showed that the risk of synchronous CPM was increased in case of advanced T stage, advanced N stage, poor differentiation grade, younger age, mucinous adenocarcinoma, and right-sided localization of primary tumor. In the study by Jayne and coworkers [1], 53% of the patients with synchronous PM had a rectal cancer and as for the remaining patients, the primary tumor was located in the left, transverse, and right colon in 25%, 7%, and 16%, respectively. According to the study by Sadahiro et al. [14], the primary tumor was most often located in the right colon ($p = 0.02$), with significantly more lymph node metastases in patients with synchronous PM ($p < 0.001$), while the primary tumor was mostly located in the left colon (34%) in the study of Mulsow et al. [15].

3. The Prognosis and Prognostic Factors of CPM

Recent clinical studies show that, receiving palliative systemic treatment alone, patients with CPM have poorer prognosis than those diagnosed with nonperitoneal metastasis. However, the therapeutic approach combining cytoreductive surgery with HIPEC and systemic treatment can achieve long-term survival in appropriate patients with PM from colorectal origin. Furthermore, peritoneal carcinomatosis index (PCI), completeness of cytoreduction score (CC score), liver metastasis, and other related factors are the prognostic influence factors of CPM patients.

3.1. The Prognosis of CPM. A pooled analysis of North Central Cancer Treatment Group Phase III Trials N9741 and N9841 enrolled 2,095 patients with metastatic colorectal cancer (mCRC) and 364 patients with CPM included, receiving palliative chemotherapy (5-fluorouracil, oxaliplatin, or irinotecan). The results of the research showed that patients with CPM shared a significantly shorter median overall survival (OS) (12.7 versus 17.6 months, $p < 0.001$) and progression-free survival (PFS) (5.8 versus 7.2 months, $p = 0.001$) compared with nonperitoneal mCRC patients [6]. Similar conclusion can also be drawn in the CAIRO study (previously untreated mCRC patients were treated with chemotherapy) and the CAIRO2 study (previously untreated mCRC patients were treated with chemotherapy and targeted therapy). Klaver et al. [16] reported that no matter how chemotherapy is used alone or combined with targeted therapy, the median OS in patients undergoing CPM were markedly lower than that in patients with mCRC without peritoneal involvement.

CPM patients under the palliative systemic treatment were reported to be connected with poor outcomes, but the prognosis of CPM patients will change noticeably with effective surgical therapy combined with HIPEC. Elias et al. [17] reported the results of their research conducted in French Gustave Roussy Hospital. This research recruited 287 colorectal cancer patients with liver metastases on whom a complete (R0) hepatic lesions resection was performed and 119 cases with PM undergoing peritoneal cytoreductive surgery (CRS) plus HIPEC between 1993 and 2009, excluding patients presenting both liver metastases and PM. The results showed that there were no statistical differences between the liver metastases group and the PM group in 5-year OS rates (38.5% and 36.5%, resp.; $p > 0.05$). A study from Australia has also come to the similar conclusion, whose results revealed that the 5-year OS rates of colorectal cancer patients with liver metastases or PM treated with R0 resection of the liver disease or CRS plus HIPEC, respectively, were 33.3% and 32.1% ($p > 0.05$) [18].

3.2. The Prognostic Factors of CPM

3.2.1. Peritoneal Carcinomatosis Index. Peritoneal carcinomatosis index (PCI), a scoring system that quantifies the extent of carcinomatosis, has been recognized as one of the most important prognostic indicators for the long-term outcomes of CPM patients [19–22]. The size and distribution of peritoneal deposits were recorded using the PCI system as described by Glehen et al. [12]. The abdomen is divided into thirteen regions: central region (0), right upper region (1), epigastrium region (2), left upper region (3), left blank region (4), left lower region (5), pelvis region (6), right lower region (7), and right blank region (8), and the small bowel is divided into four: upper jejunum region (9), lower jejunum region (10), upper ileum region (11), and lower ileum region (12) [12, 23]. Each one is assigned a lesion-size (LS) score of 0 to 3, which would be representative of the largest implant lesion visualized. LS-0 stands for no tumor seen, LS-1 indicates implants <0.25 cm, LS-2 indicates implants between 0.25 and 5 cm, and LS-3 indicates implants >5 cm or a confluence of disease [12, 23]. PCI score is a final numerical score of 0–39 [12, 24]. One recent study conducted by Faron et al. (2016) demonstrated a perfect linear relationship between the PCI and OS [25]. A survival analysis according to the PCI indicated that the 5-year OS rate was prominently higher in CPM patients with a low PCI (<10) than in patients with a PCI ranging from 10 to 20 or a PCI of more than 20 (53%, 23%, and 12%, resp.; $p < 0.001$) [26]. Besides, Elias et al. [10] reported a 44% of 5-year OS rate with a PCI score of 6 or less and 7% with a score greater than 19. PCI also influences the likelihood of complete cytoreduction. Most scholars assert that CPM patients with PCI >20 have poor oncological outcomes, thus unsuitable for the extensive peritoneal CRS.

3.2.2. Completeness of Cytoreduction Score. Completeness of cytoreduction score (CC score) reflects the thoroughness degree of peritoneal CRS. CC score is calculated according to the maximum diameter of residual tumor after surgery: CC-0 indicates no residual tumor, CC-1 stands for the maximum diameter of residual tumor <2.5 mm, CC-2 stands for the maximum diameter of residual tumor between 2.5 mm and 2.5 cm, and CC-3 stands for the maximum diameter of residual tumor > 2.5 cm [27]. For colorectal cancer, a complete cytoreduction score includes both CC-0 and CC-1: CC-0 indicates that all visible tumors are removed completely, and CC-1 presents that only a very small amount of residual tumors that are expected to be eradicated by the HIPEC remain not resected [28]. Complete CRS is not only an important prognostic influence factor but also a necessary requirement for long-term benefit in the management of PM. A French multicentre trial included 523 patients who had undergone operation from 23 centers in four French-speaking countries between 1990 and 2007, the results of which showed remarkably better survival in patients with complete CRS than in those with incomplete CRS [10]. Huang et al. [29] found that CRS plus perioperative intraperitoneal chemotherapy can be safely performed to provide encouraging survival benefits for patients with CPM. Hence, CC-0 and CC-1 have been recommended to be the standard for CRS by most researches. Conversely, CC-2 and CC-3 surgery should not be recommended presently.

3.2.3. Liver Metastasis.

It is still controversial when it comes to the prognosis of CPM patients with liver metastasis. On the one hand, the concomitant liver metastasis is a poor prognostic factor. Related researches showed that the prognosis of CPM patients with liver metastasis was conspicuously worse than that of patients with CPM [30]. Elias et al. [10] reported in a multivariate analysis that even if a complete CRS could be obtained with effort, a resectable liver metastasis during the CRS was still a negative prognostic indicator for CPM patients. Glehen et al. [12] confirmed that CPM patients with simultaneous liver metastasis were linked with worse outcomes. On the other hand, a systematic review analyzed the prognosis of colorectal liver metastasis patients with extrahepatic metastasis undergoing surgical resection, the result of which showed that, with the liver resection plus peritoneal CRS for the CPM patients, the 5-year OS rate of 25% can be materialized [31]. Kianmanesh et al. [32] reported that there were no distinct discrepancies as for the survival rate between patients who underwent CRS plus HIPEC for PM alone (including the primary resection) and those who had liver metastasis resection (median survival, 35.3 versus 36.0 months, $p = 0.73$). Some studies have shown that CPM patients with localized PM (PCI < 12) and limited liver metastases (less than 3 metastatic lesions) may benefit from liver metastasis resection and peritoneal CRS [30]. Thus, some authors propose to consider intensive therapy only in patients with PCI <12 and <3 liver metastases [30, 33, 34].

3.2.4. Other Related Factors.

The Peritoneal Surface Disease Severity Score (PSDSS) was put forward by The American Society of Peritoneal Surface Malignancies [35]. PSDSS consists of 3 prognostic categories: (1) clinical symptoms, (2) extent of peritoneal dissemination (PCI determined on a computed tomographic scan), and (3) primary tumor histology, each of which is subcategorized according to severity [36, 37]. PSDSS can be performed when patients are diagnosed with CPM without the need for intraoperative staging [35]. Clinical analyses testified that PSDSS was an independent

prognostic indicator concerning survival not only for patients who underwent a complete CRS and HIPEC, but also for patients treated with systemic chemotherapy without CRS [36, 38–40]. However, although PSDSS is a very interesting system as a recent proposition, it is not used in a common practice and not a rule to be as equivalent as PCI.

The Japanese Society for Cancer of the Colon and Rectum (JSCCR) classifies PM into three subgroups: P1 indicates metastases only to adjacent peritoneum, P2 stands for a few metastases to distant peritoneum, and P3 represents numerous metastases to distant peritoneum. Relevant researches certified that different P stage was significantly associated with different prognosis [5, 41].

4. Treatment for CPM

4.1. Peritoneal CRS.

Colorectal peritoneal metastatic lesions and organs involved should be surgically removed during CRS. Apart from peritoneum, greater omentum, lesser omentum, gallbladder, appendix, and ovaries may often be resected, sometimes part of small intestines, rectum and sigmoid colon, uterus, spleen and distal stomach, and so forth as well. Surgeons should attempt to remove all the visible tumors to obtain a complete cytoreduction during peritoneal CRS [34]. Based on current literature, the principle of the CPM resection should meet both the criteria of oncology and the criteria of organ function. The criteria of oncology consist of 3 aspects: (1) PCI < 20, (2) surgical resection of all the peritoneal metastases or the maximum diameter of residual tumor <2.5 mm (CC-0 and CC-1), and (3) R0 resection of the primary tumor and nonperitoneal metastases (liver, lung, or ovary). The criteria of organ function encompass 2 facets: (1) age < 75 and KPS > 70 and (2) small intestinal mesentery without severe contracture and no severe small intestinal obstruction. The preoperative assessment of the CPM surgery should include the oncology and the functional evaluation. The oncology evaluations are as follows: (1) tumor antigen (CEA, CA19-9, and CA125), (2) imaging evaluation of peritoneal metastases (enhanced multislice computed tomography (CT) scans plus multiplanar reconstruction, enhanced magnetic resonance imaging (MRI), or positron emission tomography-computed tomography (PET-CT) of abdomen and pelvis), and (3) imaging evaluation of primary tumor and extraperitoneal metastasis. The functional evaluations include gastrointestinal dynamic contrast examination or enhanced CT of the abdomen and pelvis performed to figure out whether there are multisegmental small intestinal obstructions due to small intestinal mesentery contracture.

4.2. HIPEC.

HIPEC refers to intraoperative delivery of chemotherapic agents in a recirculating perfusion of the abdominal cavity under hyperthermic conditions [42]. In addition to the traditional superiority of intraperitoneal chemotherapy (abdominal local high concentration, low concentration of peripheral blood, and mild systemic toxicity), HIPEC also has the following advantages: (1) the direct killing effect of hyperthermia, (2) the chemotherapy enhancement effect of hyperthermia, and (3) mechanical flushing effect of irrigation. It can be performed in a closed or open method, before or after surgery. The open method makes it more uniform in distribution of heat and chemotherapy drugs, but the operation is relatively inconvenient and heat emission exists. For the closed method, it can reduce the exposure of the medical personnel to chemotherapy; its performance is relatively simple; and the increased abdominal pressure may contribute to the peritoneal permeation of the chemotherapy drugs, whereas the problem is that heat and drugs are not uniformly allocated. At present, there is no gold standard for the chemotherapy drugs used in HIPEC. The American Society of Peritoneal Surface Malignancies (ASPSM) recommends patients to undergo 40 mg mitomycin intraperitoneal perfusion during 90 min at 42°C [43]. Elias et al. [44] from French Gustave Roussy Cancer Campus also reported a series of patients treated with oxaliplatin in the perfusate at $460 \, mg/m^2$ in $2 \, L/m^2$ during 30 minutes at 43°C and later reported another protocol with oxaliplatin $360 \, mg/m^2$ plus irinotecan $360 \, mg/m^2$ in $2 \, L/m^2$ of dextrose 5%. During the same time, patients received an intravenous administration of 5-fluorouracil ($400 \, mg/m^2$) and leucovorin ($20 \, mg/m^2$).

4.3. Systemic Chemotherapy. CPM patients have a poor prognosis, and the median survival without chemotherapy is about 6 months [1, 7]. In terms of systemic chemotherapy, there is no difference between CRPC patients and other nonperitoneal metastasis patients, but the effect of systemic chemotherapy is worse in the former compared with that in the latter. In the past few years, new drugs have been introduced into systemic chemotherapy. The application of targeted therapy drugs such as bevacizumab and cetuximab further improves the efficacy of peritoneal metastatic carcinoma. In the retrospective study, receiving chemotherapy in combination with targeted therapy could significantly prolong the OS of CPM patients to 18.2 months, the effect of which is still worse than that of the patients with liver or lung metastases yet [45].

5. Multidisciplinary Treatment Strategy for CPM

Complete peritoneal CRS plus HIPEC and systemic treatment (including chemotherapy and targeted therapy) are currently the best modality of multidisciplinary treatment for CPM patients. During CRS, all the visible tumors should be removed to obtain a complete peritoneal CRS. In addition to the cytoreductive surgery, HIPEC is administered to eradicate the tiny and microscopic peritoneal diseases. Systemic chemotherapy is always significant since PM is often part of systemic metastasis. The combined application of these three aspects will probably improve the prognosis of colorectal peritoneal metastatic carcinoma.

According to the National Comprehensive Cancer Network (NCCN) guidelines, combined peritoneal CRS and HIPEC have not been routinely recommended for CPM patients. Nonetheless, the NCCN guidelines also recommend to carry out more well-designed clinical trials. In contrast, the European Society for Medical Oncology (ESMO) guidelines hold more positive attitude towards it. The ESMO guidelines

recommend that CPM patients with low PCI should be treated with surgery plus HIPEC when a complete CRS can be obtained. In Japan, a complete CRS has been recommended for patients with P1 phase CPM as well as P2 phase CPM if technically possible [5]. In China, combined peritoneal CRS and HIPEC have also been recommended by experts for CPM patients with PCI <20.

Randomized clinical trials have confirmed that combined peritoneal CRS and HIPEC plus systemic chemotherapy is superior to palliative systemic therapy for CPM patients (the median survival, 22.3 and 12.6 months, resp., $p = 0.032$) [19]. The 5-year survival was 45% for those patients in whom a complete CRS was achieved [46]. The superiority of combined peritoneal CRS and HIPEC plus systemic chemotherapy can also be clarified in a retrospective study which compared patients undergoing CRS plus HIPEC with comparable controls treated with palliative chemotherapy during the same period but who did not benefit from CRS plus HIPEC because the technique was unavailable in the center at that time. The 5-year OS rates of patients undergoing combined peritoneal CRS and HIPEC plus systemic chemotherapy were significantly higher than that of the patients with palliative systemic therapy (51% versus 13%, resp.) [47].

For CPM patients with PCI >20, peritoneal CRS is not suitable for them currently. However, with the appearance of more effective chemotherapeutic and targeted drugs, it is possible to achieve the reduction of PCI by effective chemotherapy, thereby creating the possibility for further surgery. Because of the high risk of postoperative recurrence of peritoneal metastasis, it is held that CPM patients with PCI <20 may benefit from the modality of perioperative chemotherapy.

6. Controversial Issues and Latest Progress

6.1. Diffusion-Weighted MRI. Preoperative MRI and CT of the abdomen and pelvis play a critical role in the assessment of the extent of peritoneal and visceral disease in patients being considered for CRS and HIPEC for CPM [48]. In comparison with CT, MRI uses different types of image contrast to create images that are more sensitive for detection of peritoneal lesions [49–51]. With major refinements in hardware and software, functional MRI such as diffusion-weighted MRI (DWI) has become technically possible. Various tumors actuate restricted diffusion of water protons which can be evaluated by DWI, resulting in an area of altered signal on DWI [48]. The sensitivity of DWI for depicting peritoneal tumor has opened the gate to potential advancements in detecting disseminated peritoneal metastatic disease. Recently, there have been several very interesting researches regarding DWI [52]. In 2012, Low and Barone [53] calculated the PCI based on DWI before surgery in 35 patients with peritoneal metastatic disease. Compared to surgical-site findings, the overall sensitivity and specificity were 88% and 74%. Besides, Espada et al. [54] developed a scoring system with a diagnostic accuracy of 91% by evaluating DWI for detection of PM in 34 patients. In a more recent report [48], preoperative DWI and CT scanning to determine the PCI were performed in 22 patients with PM undergoing CRS, where DWI demonstrated predictive accuracy of 91%, 83%, and 94% in overall category, low to moderate tumor burden (PCI ≤ 20), and large tumor burden (PCI > 20), compared with CT with a corresponding predictive accuracy of 50%, 50%, and 44%. Of note, it has been reported in 2012 that DWI and 18 fluoro-deoxy-glucose positron emission tomography-computed tomography (18FDG-PET/CT) showed similar high accuracy in diagnosing peritoneal metastatic carcinoma [55]. Furthermore, DWI appears more sensitive than PET/CT in the supramesocolic area; nevertheless, the limitation of lower sensitivity in the detection of small implants still exists in DWI [55]. Interestingly, a prospective comparison of CT, PET/CT, and whole body DWI in 32 patients conducted by Michielsen et al. [56] in 2014 noted an accuracy for detection of peritoneal disease of 91% on DWI compared with 75% on CT and 71% on FDG-PET/CT, with surgical reference standard in all cases. It is desirable to improve the detection and characterization of peritoneal implants by the simultaneous use of 18FDG-PET and DWI, which remains to be confirmed by future studies [57, 58].

6.2. Fluorescence Imaging. Intraoperative fluorescence imaging- (FI-) guided surgery is an emerging technology in the war against cancer that has been proved to improve tumor detection in different tumor types [59–61]. Among the different probes used in identifying neoplasm, indocyanine green (ICG) has been introduced as a safe and useful indicator [61]. Until now, only a few clinical studies have analyzed the potential role of FI taking in PM [62]. Liberale et al. [62] demonstrated in a pilot study that sensitivity and specificity of ICG-FI in patients with nonmucinous CPM were 87.5% and 100%; contrarily, among the mucinous tumors, the sensitivity of ICG-FI was 0%. Unexpectedly, in 4 out of 14 patients (29%), additional PM that were not found using visualization and palpation were detected in the surgery modified by intraoperative ICG-FI [62].

6.3. Catumaxomab. Catumaxomab is a trifunctional monoclonal antibody with a mouse-derived anti-EpCAM Fab (fragment antigen-binding) region and a rat anti-CD3 Fab [63]. Catumaxomab antineoplastic activity has been confirmed in vitro, notably in malignant ascites, resulting in a decreased rate of EpCAM plus cells and the release of proinflammatory cytokines (interferon-γ, tumor necrosis factor-α, interleukin- (IL-) 2, and IL-6), which enables tumor cells of PM to be specifically identified by catumaxomab via the anti-EpCAM-binding site [64, 65]. Therefore, intraperitoneal catumaxomab therapy represents a targeted immunotherapy against PM [66]. A randomized phase II/III trial was carried out in 258 patients with symptomatic malignant ascites secondary to EpCAM + carcinomas, to assess the efficacy and safety of intraperitoneal catumaxomab treatment [67]. In this study, patients were randomly assigned to paracentesis plus intraperitoneal catumaxomab or paracentesis alone. The primary endpoint was puncture-free survival used to evaluate the efficacy of intraperitoneal administration of catumaxomab. Puncture-free survival was significantly longer in the group treated with catumaxomab than the control group (46

versus 11 days, $p < 0.0001$). Median overall survival was similar between the two groups (72 versus 68 days, $p = 0.0846$).

6.4. Systematic Second-Look Surgery and HIPEC. Systematic second-look surgery and HIPEC for CRC patients considered to be at high risk of developing PM have aroused a growing interest among the scientific community. CPM is generally diagnosed in its advanced phase because of the late symptoms onset, low sensitive imaging techniques, and tumor markers. Therefore, the concept of early intervention has emerged. Second-look surgery and HIPEC in patient with a high risk of developing PM treated with curative surgery for CRC have been proposed, but again this would be limited to a small group of patients [68]. In the prospective study, Elias and colleagues reported 29 selected patients at high risk of developing PM without any sign of recurrence on imaging studies who underwent second-look surgery 13 months after resection of the primary tumor. In 55% of patients, persistent adenocarcinoma was documented. In patients with documented disease at second look 9 of 16 patients were disease-free at 27 months of median follow-up [69]. Besides, patient with or without macroscopic PM at second-look surgery treated with CRS and HIPEC developed a low rate of peritoneal recurrences (17% at a median follow-up of 30 months) [70]. One ongoing prospective randomized clinical trial is designed in France. All patients at risk will receive the gold standard adjuvant systemic chemotherapy with FOLFOX 6 over 6 months. Patients with a negative follow-up will be randomly assigned to surveillance or second-look laparotomy and HIPEC. The object of the clinical trial is to evaluate the peritoneal recurrence rate for 3 years.

6.5. The Necessity of HIPEC. CRS plus HIPEC is increasingly being used for the treatment of PM of colorectal origin. However, it is still controversial whether HIPEC is the indispensable cornerstone of the best modality of multidisciplinary treatment for CPM [71]. It is not yet possible to evaluate the morbidity and mortality rates related to HIPEC alone independently of CRS, as both procedures are performed jointly during the same surgery. Only those patients who undergo CRS can receive HIPEC. The published mortality rates in CRS + HIPEC range from 0 to 11% (mean 4–6%) [71]. Survival rates are reported better in patients who undergo CRS + HIPEC versus those who receive systemic chemotherapy [72]. Seeking to elucidate the true role of HIPEC in the context of radical combined therapy, a multicentre, randomized, open-label study currently in phase III (PRODIGE 7) was designed with parallel groups and two treatment arms comparing CRS + HIPEC + systemic chemotherapy before or after surgery versus CRS + systemic chemotherapy before or after surgery. The final collection date for primary outcome measure was completed in December 2015. Once the results of this study are achieved, we should have considerably more evidence regarding the efficacy of this treatment modality [71].

7. Conclusion

Complete peritoneal CRS plus HIPEC and systemic treatment (including chemotherapy and targeted therapy) might be the best modality of multidisciplinary treatment for CPM. Patients appropriate for aggressive therapy undergoing complete peritoneal CRS plus HIPEC and systemic treatment can get better long-term outcome. PCI and CC score are important prognostic indicators of CPM patients. More well-designed clinical trials are in terrible need to figure out the best multidisciplinary treatment modality for CPM.

Competing Interests

The authors declare that there is no conflict of interests regarding the publication of this paper.

Acknowledgments

This work was supported by Department of Colorectal Surgery, Fudan University Shanghai Cancer Center.

References

[1] D. G. Jayne, S. Fook, C. Loi, and F. Seow-Choen, "Peritoneal carcinomatosis from colorectal cancer," *British Journal of Surgery*, vol. 89, no. 12, pp. 1545–1550, 2002.

[2] V. E. Lemmens, Y. L. Klaver, V. J. Verwaal, H. J. Rutten, J. W. W. Coebergh, and I. H. de Hingh, "Predictors and survival of synchronous peritoneal carcinomatosis of colorectal origin: a population-based study," *International Journal of Cancer*, vol. 128, no. 11, pp. 2717–2725, 2011.

[3] J. Segelman, F. Granath, T. Holm, M. MacHado, H. Mahteme, and A. Martling, "Incidence, prevalence and risk factors for peritoneal carcinomatosis from colorectal cancer," *British Journal of Surgery*, vol. 99, no. 5, pp. 699–705, 2012.

[4] Y. R. B. M. van Gestel, I. H. J. T. de Hingh, M. P. P. van Herk-Sukel et al., "Patterns of metachronous metastases after curative treatment of colorectal cancer," *Cancer Epidemiology*, vol. 38, no. 4, pp. 448–454, 2014.

[5] T. Watanabe, M. Itabashi, Y. Shimada et al., "Japanese Society for Cancer of the Colon and Rectum (JSCCR) guidelines 2010 for the treatment of colorectal cancer," *International Journal of Clinical Oncology*, vol. 17, no. 1, pp. 1–29, 2012.

[6] J. Franko, Q. Shi, C. D. Goldman et al., "Treatment of colorectal peritoneal carcinomatosis with systemic chemotherapy: a pooled analysis of north central cancer treatment group phase III trials N9741 and N9841," *Journal of Clinical Oncology*, vol. 30, no. 3, pp. 263–267, 2012.

[7] B. Sadeghi, C. Arvieux, O. Glehen et al., "Peritoneal carcinomatosis from non-gynecologic malignancies: results of the EVOCAPE 1 multicentric prospective study," *Cancer*, vol. 88, no. 2, pp. 358–363, 2000.

[8] D. Z. J. Chu, N. P. Lang, C. Thompson, P. K. Osteen, and K. C. Westbrook, "Peritoneal carcinomatosis in nongynecologic malignancy. A prospective study of prognostic factors," *Cancer*, vol. 63, no. 2, pp. 364–367, 1989.

[9] I. Thomassen, Y. R. Van Gestel, V. E. Lemmens, and I. H. De Hingh, "Incidence, prognosis, and treatment options for patients with synchronous peritoneal carcinomatosis and liver metastases from colorectal origin," *Diseases of the Colon and Rectum*, vol. 56, no. 12, pp. 1373–1380, 2013.

[10] D. Elias, F. Gilly, F. Boutitie et al., "Peritoneal colorectal carcinomatosis treated with surgery and perioperative intraperitoneal chemotherapy: Retrospective Analysis of 523 Patients From a Multicentric French Study," *Journal of Clinical Oncology*, vol. 28, no. 1, pp. 63–68, 2010.

[11] A. Bhatt and D. Goéré, "Cytoreductive surgery plus HIPEC for peritoneal metastases from colorectal cancer," *Indian Journal of Surgical Oncology*, vol. 7, no. 2, pp. 177–187, 2016.

[12] O. Glehen, F. Kwiatkowski, P. H. Sugarbaker et al., "Cytoreductive surgery combined with perioperative intraperitoneal chemotherapy for the management of peritoneal carcinomatosis from colorectal cancer: a multi-institutional study," *Journal of Clinical Oncology*, vol. 22, no. 16, pp. 3284–3292, 2004.

[13] A. G. Kerscher, T. C. Chua, M. Gasser et al., "Impact of peritoneal carcinomatosis in the disease history of colorectal cancer management: a longitudinal experience of 2406 patients over two decades," *British Journal of Cancer*, vol. 108, no. 7, pp. 1432–1439, 2013.

[14] S. Sadahiro, T. Suzuki, Y. Maeda et al., "Prognostic factors in patients with synchronous peritoneal carcinomatosis (PC) caused by a primary cancer of the colon," *Journal of Gastrointestinal Surgery*, vol. 13, no. 9, pp. 1593–1598, 2009.

[15] J. Mulsow, S. Merkel, A. Agaimy, and W. Hohenberger, "Outcomes following surgery for colorectal cancer with synchronous peritoneal metastases," *British Journal of Surgery*, vol. 98, no. 12, pp. 1785–1791, 2011.

[16] Y. L. B. Klaver, L. H. J. Simkens, V. E. P. P. Lemmens et al., "Outcomes of colorectal cancer patients with peritoneal carcinomatosis treated with chemotherapy with and without targeted therapy," *European Journal of Surgical Oncology*, vol. 38, no. 7, pp. 617–623, 2012.

[17] D. Elias, M. Faron, B. S. Iuga et al., "Prognostic similarities and differences in optimally resected liver metastases and peritoneal metastases from colorectal cancers," *Annals of Surgery*, vol. 261, no. 1, pp. 157–163, 2015.

[18] C. Q. Cao, T. D. Yan, W. Liauw, and D. L. Morris, "Comparison of optimally resected hepatectomy and peritonectomy patients with colorectal cancer metastasis," *Journal of Surgical Oncology*, vol. 100, no. 7, pp. 529–533, 2009.

[19] V. J. Verwaal, S. van Ruth, E. de Bree et al., "Randomized trial of cytoreduction and hyperthermic intraperitoneal chemotherapy versus systemic chemotherapy and palliative surgery in patients with peritoneal carcinomatosis of colorectal cancer," *Journal of Clinical Oncology*, vol. 21, no. 20, pp. 3737–3743, 2003.

[20] R. G. da Silva and P. H. Sugarbaker, "Analysis of prognostic factors in seventy patients having a complete cytoreduction plus perioperative intraperitoneal chemotherapy for carcinomatosis from colorectal cancer," *Journal of the American College of Surgeons*, vol. 203, no. 6, pp. 878–886, 2006.

[21] D. Elias, F. Blot, A. El Otmany et al., "Curative treatment of peritoneal carcinomatosis arising from colorectal cancer by complete resection and intraperitoneal chemotherapy," *Cancer*, vol. 92, no. 1, pp. 71–76, 2001.

[22] T. D. Yan, F. Chu, M. Links, P. C. Kam, D. Glenn, and D. L. Morris, "Cytoreductive surgery and perioperative intraperitoneal chemotherapy for peritoneal carcinomatosis from colorectal carcinoma: non-mucinous tumour associated with an improved survival," *European Journal of Surgical Oncology*, vol. 32, no. 10, pp. 1119–1124, 2006.

[23] P. H. Sugarbaker, "Peritoneal surface oncology: review of a personal experience with colorectal and appendiceal malignancy," *Techniques in Coloproctology*, vol. 9, no. 2, pp. 95–103, 2005.

[24] J.-L. Koh, T. D. Yan, D. Glenn, and D. L. Morris, "Evaluation of preoperative computed tomography in estimating peritoneal

cancer index in colorectal peritoneal carcinomatosis," *Annals of Surgical Oncology*, vol. 16, no. 2, pp. 327–333, 2009.

[25] M. Faron, R. Macovei, D. Goéré, C. Honoré, L. Benhaim, and D. Elias, "Linear relationship of peritoneal cancer index and survival in patients with peritoneal metastases from colorectal cancer," *Annals of Surgical Oncology*, vol. 23, no. 1, pp. 114–119, 2016.

[26] D. Goéré, D. Malka, D. Tzanis et al., "Is there a possibility of a cure in patients with colorectal peritoneal carcinomatosis amenable to complete cytoreductive surgery and intraperitoneal chemotherapy?" *Annals of Surgery*, vol. 257, no. 6, pp. 1065–1071, 2013.

[27] A. A. K. Tentes, "The management of peritoneal surface malignancy of colorectal cancer origin," *Techniques in Coloproctology*, vol. 8, no. 1, pp. S39–S42, 2004.

[28] P. H. Sugarbaker and D. P. Ryan, "Cytoreductive surgery plus hyperthermic perioperative chemotherapy to treat peritoneal metastases from colorectal cancer: standard of care or an experimental approach?" *The Lancet Oncology*, vol. 13, no. 8, pp. e362–e369, 2012.

[29] Y. Huang, N. A. Alzahrani, T. C. Chua, W. Liauw, and D. L. Morris, "Impacts of low peritoneal cancer index on the survival outcomes of patient with peritoneal carcinomatosis of colorectal origin," *International Journal of Surgery*, vol. 23, pp. 181–185, 2015.

[30] L. Maggiori, D. Goéré, B. Viana et al., "Should patients with peritoneal carcinomatosis of colorectal origin with synchronous liver metastases be treated with a curative intent? A Case-control Study," *Annals of Surgery*, vol. 258, no. 1, pp. 116–121, 2013.

[31] M. Hwang, T. T. Jayakrishnan, D. E. Green et al., "Systematic review of outcomes of patients undergoing resection for colorectal liver metastases in the setting of extra hepatic disease," *European Journal of Cancer*, vol. 50, no. 10, pp. 1747–1757, 2014.

[32] R. Kianmanesh, S. Scaringi, J.-M. Sabate et al., "Iterative cytoreductive surgery associated with hyperthermic intraperitoneal chemotherapy for treatment of peritoneal carcinomatosis of colorectal origin with or without liver metastases," *Annals of Surgery*, vol. 245, no. 4, pp. 597–603, 2007.

[33] D. Elias, E. Benizri, M. Pocard, M. Ducreux, V. Boige, and P. Lasser, "Treatment of synchronous peritoneal carcinomatosis and liver metastases from colorectal cancer," *European Journal of Surgical Oncology*, vol. 32, no. 6, pp. 632–636, 2006.

[34] C. Vallicelli, D. Cavaliere, F. Catena et al., "Management of peritoneal carcinomatosis from colorectal cancer: review of the literature," *International Journal of Colorectal Disease*, vol. 29, no. 8, pp. 895–898, 2014.

[35] J. Esquivel, A. M. Lowy, M. Markman et al., "The American Society of Peritoneal Surface Malignancies (ASPSM) Multiinstitution Evaluation of the Peritoneal Surface Disease Severity Score (PSDSS) in 1,013 Patients with Colorectal Cancer with Peritoneal Carcinomatosis," *Annals of Surgical Oncology*, vol. 21, no. 13, pp. 4195–4201, 2014.

[36] J. O. W. Pelz, A. Stojadinovic, A. Nissan, W. Hohenberger, and J. Esquivel, "Evaluation of a peritoneal surface disease severity score in patients with colon cancer with peritoneal carcinomatosis," *Journal of Surgical Oncology*, vol. 99, no. 1, pp. 9–15, 2009.

[37] J. L. Ng, W. S. Ong, C. S. Chia, G. H. Tan, K. Soo, and M. C. Teo, "Prognostic relevance of the Peritoneal Surface Disease Severity Score compared to the peritoneal cancer index for

colorectal peritoneal carcinomatosis," *International Journal of Surgical Oncology*, vol. 2016, Article ID 2495131, 7 pages, 2016.

[38] T. C. Chua, D. L. Morris, and J. Esquivel, "Impact of the peritoneal surface disease severity score on survival in patients with colorectal cancer peritoneal carcinomatosis undergoing complete cytoreduction and hyperthermic intraperitoneal chemotherapy," *Annals of Surgical Oncology*, vol. 17, no. 5, pp. 1330–1336, 2010.

[39] J. O. W. Pelz, T. C. Chua, J. Esquivel et al., "Evaluation of best supportive care and systemic chemotherapy as treatment stratified according to the retrospective peritoneal surface disease severity score (PSDSS) for peritoneal carcinomatosis of colorectal origin," *BMC Cancer*, vol. 10, article 689, 2010.

[40] J. Esquivel, T. C. Chua, A. Stojadinovic et al., "Accuracy and clinical relevance of computed tomography scan interpretation of peritoneal cancer index in colorectal cancer peritoneal carcinomatosis: A Multi-institutional Study," *Journal of Surgical Oncology*, vol. 102, no. 6, pp. 565–570, 2010.

[41] H. Kobayashi, K. Kotake, K. Funahashi et al., "Clinical benefit of surgery for stage IV colorectal cancer with synchronous peritoneal metastasis," *Journal of Gastroenterology*, vol. 49, no. 4, pp. 646–654, 2014.

[42] J. S. Spratt, R. A. Adcock, M. Muskovin, W. Sherrill, and J. McKeown, "Clinical delivery system for intraperitoneal hyperthermic chemotherapy," *Cancer Research*, vol. 40, no. 2, pp. 256–260, 1980.

[43] K. Turaga, E. Levine, R. Barone et al., "Consensus guidelines from the American Society of Peritoneal Surface Malignancies on standardizing the delivery of hyperthermic intraperitoneal chemotherapy (HIPEC) in colorectal cancer patients in the United States," *Annals of Surgical Oncology*, vol. 21, no. 5, pp. 1501–1505, 2014.

[44] D. Elias, L. Sideris, M. Pocard et al., "Efficacy of intraperitoneal chemohyperthermia with oxaliplatin in colorectal peritoneal carcinomatosis. Preliminary results in 24 patients," *Annals of Oncology*, vol. 15, no. 5, pp. 781–785, 2004.

[45] Y. L. B. Klaver, B. J. M. Leenders, G.-J. Creemers et al., "Addition of biological therapies to palliative chemotherapy prolongs survival in patients with peritoneal carcinomatosis of colorectal origin," *American Journal of Clinical Oncology*, vol. 36, no. 2, pp. 157–161, 2013.

[46] V. J. Verwaal, S. Bruin, H. Boot, G. Van Slooten, and H. Van Tinteren, "8-Year follow-up of randomized trial: cytoreduction and hyperthermic intraperitoneal chemotherapy versus systemic chemotherapy in patients with peritoneal carcinomatosis of colorectal cancer," *Annals of Surgical Oncology*, vol. 15, no. 9, pp. 2426–2432, 2008.

[47] D. Elias, J. H. Lefevre, J. Chevalier et al., "Complete cytoreductive surgery plus intraperitoneal chemohyperthermia with oxaliplatin for peritoneal carcinomatosis of colorectal origin," *Journal of Clinical Oncology*, vol. 27, no. 5, pp. 681–685, 2009.

[48] R. N. Low, R. M. Barone, and J. Lucero, "Comparison of MRI and CT for predicting the Peritoneal Cancer Index (PCI) preoperatively in patients being considered for cytoreductive surgical procedures," *Annals of Surgical Oncology*, vol. 22, no. 5, pp. 1708–1715, 2015.

[49] R. N. Low, R. M. Barone, J. M. Gurney, and W. D. Muller, "Mucinous appendiceal neoplasms: preoperative MR staging and classification compared with surgical and histopathologic findings," *American Journal of Roentgenology*, vol. 190, no. 3, pp. 656–665, 2008.

[50] R. N. Low, C. P. Sebrechts, R. M. Barone, and W. Muller, "Diffusion-weighted MRI of peritoneal tumors: comparison with conventional MRI and surgical and histopathologic findings—a feasibility study," *American Journal of Roentgenology*, vol. 193, no. 2, pp. 461–470, 2009.

[51] S. Kyriazi, D. J. Collins, V. A. Morgan, S. L. Giles, and N. M. deSouza, "Diffusion-weighted imaging of peritoneal disease for noninvasive staging of advanced ovarian cancer," *Radiographics*, vol. 30, no. 5, pp. 1269–1285, 2010.

[52] A. G. Rockall, "Diffusion weighted MRI in ovarian cancer," *Current Opinion in Oncology*, vol. 26, no. 5, pp. 529–535, 2014.

[53] R. N. Low and R. M. Barone, "Combined diffusion-weighted and gadolinium-enhanced MRI can accurately predict the peritoneal cancer index preoperatively in patients being considered for cytoreductive surgical procedures," *Annals of Surgical Oncology*, vol. 19, no. 5, pp. 1394–1401, 2012.

[54] M. Espada, J. R. Garcia-Flores, M. Jimenez et al., "Diffusion-weighted magnetic resonance imaging evaluation of intra-abdominal sites of implants to predict likelihood of suboptimal cytoreductive surgery in patients with ovarian carcinoma," *European Radiology*, vol. 23, no. 9, pp. 2636–2642, 2013.

[55] M. Soussan, G. Des Guetz, V. Barrau et al., "Comparison of FDG-PET/CT and MR with diffusion-weighted imaging for assessing peritoneal carcinomatosis from gastrointestinal malignancy," *European Radiology*, vol. 22, no. 7, pp. 1479–1487, 2012.

[56] K. Michielsen, I. Vergote, K. Op De Beeck et al., "Whole-body MRI with diffusion-weighted sequence for staging of patients with suspected ovarian cancer: a clinical feasibility study in comparison to CT and FDG-PET/CT," *European Radiology*, vol. 24, no. 4, pp. 889–901, 2014.

[57] M. Barral, C. Eveno, C. Hoeffel et al., "Diffusion-weighted magnetic resonance imaging in colorectal cancer," *Journal of Visceral Surgery*, vol. 153, no. 5, pp. 361–369, 2016.

[58] N. F. Schwenzer, H. Schmidt, S. Gatidis et al., "Measurement of apparent diffusion coefficient with simultaneous MR/positron emission tomography in patients with peritoneal carcinomatosis: comparison with 18F-FDG-PET," *Journal of Magnetic Resonance Imaging*, vol. 40, no. 5, pp. 1121–1128, 2014.

[59] K. Polom, D. Murawa, Y. S. Rho, P. Nowaczyk, M. Hünerbein, and P. Murawa, "Current trends and emerging future of indocyanine green usage in surgery and oncology: a literature review," *Cancer*, vol. 117, no. 21, pp. 4812–4822, 2011.

[60] B. E. Schaafsma, J. S. D. Mieog, M. Hutteman et al., "The clinical use of indocyanine green as a near-infrared fluorescent contrast agent for image-guided oncologic surgery," *Journal of Surgical Oncology*, vol. 104, no. 3, pp. 323–332, 2011.

[61] J. A. Zelken and A. P. Tufaro, "Current trends and emerging future of indocyanine green usage in surgery and oncology: an update," *Annals of Surgical Oncology*, vol. 22, no. 3, pp. 1271–1283, 2015.

[62] G. Liberale, S. Vankerckhove, M. G. Caldon et al., "Fluorescence imaging after indocyanine green injection for detection of peritoneal metastases in patients undergoing cytoreductive surgery for peritoneal carcinomatosis from colorectal cancer: a pilot study," *Annals of Surgery*, vol. 264, no. 6, pp. 1110–1115, 2016.

[63] P. Ruf and H. Lindhofer, "Induction of a long-lasting antitumor immunity by a trifunctional bispecific antibody," *Blood*, vol. 98, no. 8, pp. 2526–2534, 2001.

[64] M. Jäger, A. Schoberth, P. Ruf et al., "Immunomonitoring results of a phase II/III study of malignant ascites patients treated with the trifunctional antibody catumaxomab (Anti-EpCAM x anti-CD3)," *Cancer Research*, vol. 72, no. 1, pp. 24–32, 2012.

[65] M. A. Ströhlein and M. M. Heiss, "Intraperitoneal immunotherapy to prevent peritoneal carcinomatosis in patients with advanced gastrointestinal malignancies," *Journal of Surgical Oncology*, vol. 100, no. 4, pp. 329–330, 2009.

[66] M. A. Ströhlein and M. M. Heiss, "Immunotherapy of peritoneal carcinomatosis," *Cancer treatment and research*, vol. 134, pp. 483–491, 2007.

[67] M. M. Heiss, P. Murawa, P. Koralewski et al., "The trifunctional antibody catumaxomab for the treatment of malignant ascites due to epithelial cancer: results of a prospective randomized phase II/III trial," *International Journal of Cancer*, vol. 127, no. 9, pp. 2209–2221, 2010.

[68] P. H. Sugarbaker, "Second-look surgery for colorectal cancer: revised selection factors and new treatment options for greater success," *International Journal of Surgical Oncology*, vol. 2011, Article ID 915078, 8 pages, 2011.

[69] D. Elias, D. Goéré, D. Di Pietrantonio et al., "Results of systematic second-look surgery in patients at high risk of developing colorectal peritoneal carcinomatosis," *Annals of Surgery*, vol. 247, no. 3, pp. 445–450, 2008.

[70] D. Elias, C. Honoré, F. Dumont et al., "Results of systematic second-look surgery plus hipec in asymptomatic patients presenting a high risk of developing colorectal peritoneal carcinomatosis," *Annals of Surgery*, vol. 254, no. 2, pp. 289–293, 2011.

[71] F. Losa, P. Barrios, R. Salazar et al., "Cytoreductive surgery and intraperitoneal chemotherapy for treatment of peritoneal carcinomatosis from colorectal origin," *Clinical and Translational Oncology*, vol. 16, no. 2, pp. 128–140, 2014.

[72] J. Franko, Z. Ibrahim, N. J. Gusani, M. P. Holtzman, D. L. Bartlett, and H. J. Zeh III, "Cytoreductive surgery and hyperthermic intraperitoneal chemoperfusion versus systemic chemotherapy alone for colorectal peritoneal carcinomatosis," *Cancer*, vol. 116, no. 16, pp. 3756–3762, 2010.

12

Metformin and Diammonium Glycyrrhizinate Enteric-Coated Capsule versus Metformin Alone versus Diammonium Glycyrrhizinate Enteric-Coated Capsule Alone in Patients with Nonalcoholic Fatty Liver Disease and Type 2 Diabetes Mellitus

Rong Zhang,[1,2] **Keran Cheng,**[1,3] **Shizan Xu,**[1,2] **Sainan Li,**[1] **Yuqing Zhou,**[1,3]
Shunfeng Zhou,[1,3] **Rui Kong,**[1,3] **Linqiang Li,**[1,3] **Jingjing Li,**[1] **Jiao Feng,**[1] **Liwei Wu,**[1]
Tong Liu,[1] **Yujing Xia,**[1] **Jie Lu,**[1] **Chuanyong Guo,**[1] **and Yingqun Zhou**[1]

[1]*Department of Gastroenterology, Shanghai Tenth People's Hospital, Tongji University, School of Medicine, Shanghai 200072, China*
[2]*The First Clinical Medical College of Nanjing Medical University, Nanjing 210029, China*
[3]*The School of Medicine of Soochow University, Suzhou 215006, China*

Correspondence should be addressed to Chuanyong Guo; guochuanyong@hotmail.com and Yingqun Zhou; yqzh02@163.com

Academic Editor: Amosy M'Koma

Objective. The present study was conducted to compare the efficacy of metformin combined with diammonium glycyrrhizinate enteric-coated capsule (DGEC) versus metformin alone versus DGEC alone for the treatment of nonalcoholic fatty liver disease (NAFLD) in patients with type 2 diabetes mellitus (T2DM). *Subjects and Methods.* 163 patients with NAFLD and T2DM were enrolled in this 24-week study and were randomized to one of three groups: group 1 was treated with metformin alone; group 2 was treated with DGEC alone; group 3 received metformin plus DGEC combination therapy. Anthropometric parameters, liver function, lipid profile, serum ferritin (SF), metabolic parameters, liver/spleen computed tomography (CT) ratio, and fibroscan value were evaluated at baseline and after 8, 16, and 24 weeks of treatment. *Results.* After 24 weeks, significant improvements in all measured parameters were observed in three groups ($P < 0.05$) except for the improvements in low density lipoprotein cholesterol (LDL-C) and metabolic parameters in group 2 which did not reach statistical significance ($P > 0.05$). Compared with group 1 and group 2, the patients in group 3 had greater reductions in observed parameters apart from CB and TB ($P < 0.05$). *Conclusions.* This study showed that metformin plus DGEC was more effective than metformin alone or DGEC alone in reducing liver enzymes, lipid levels, and metabolic parameters and ameliorating the degree of hepatic fibrosis in patients with NAFLD and T2DM.

1. Introduction

Nonalcoholic fatty liver disease (NAFLD) is currently the most common comorbidity and cause of chronic liver disease in adults. The magnitude of the epidemic has indicated that NAFLD is an increasingly recognized public health issue worldwide.

The majority of patients with NAFLD are asymptomatic or have slightly elevated liver enzymes [mild to moderate increase in alanine aminotransferase (ALT) and gamma glutamine transpeptidase (GGT)] or vague upper abdominal pain. NAFLD is characterized by hepatic steatosis during imaging and/or histology and is defined as ≥5%–10% of hepatocytes exhibiting macroscopic steatosis [1, 2] and is diagnosed by no alcohol history or ethanol intake ≤70 g per week in women and ≤140 g per week in men and excludes other etiologies of steatosis, such as virus hepatitis and steatogenic drug administration [3–5]. NAFLD encompasses a clinicopathologic spectrum of conditions ranging from NAFL (simple steatosis, a benign process) to nonalcoholic steatohepatitis (NASH) [2]. Although the pathology of NAFL is usually nonprogressive, some cases may then develop NASH, which is an important risk factor for cerebrovascular disease, cardiovascular disease, and liver fibrosis, and can ultimately progress to liver cirrhosis and even hepatocellular carcinoma [6]. Epidemiological studies have revealed that the prevalence of NAFLD is 20%–40% in western countries, 12%–30% in Asian countries [5], and 20.9% in mainland China [7]. Generally, NAFLD is accompanied by a range of metabolic comorbidities such as visceral obesity, hyperlipidemia, insulin resistance (IR)/diabetes mellitus, and hypertension and is considered a manifestation of the metabolic syndrome (MS) in liver [2, 8]. The prevalence of type 2 diabetes mellitus (T2DM) in patients with NAFLD can reach 70%, and in turn, T2DM increases the risk of NAFLD [9]. With an increase in the rate of urbanization and inappropriate lifestyle changes in modern society, people have a high risk of developing NAFLD due to the growing prevalence of obesity and T2DM [10]. IR is prevalent in NAFLD [11] and is, therefore, a therapeutic target in NAFLD. In addition to treatments aimed at the liver (antioxidants and hepatocyte protective agents), other treatment strategies to ameliorate MS such as improvements in lifestyle, weight loss, and insulin-sensitizing agents (metformin or thiazolidinediones) are necessary [12, 13]. Metformin prescribed in patients with NAFLD and T2DM causes weight loss, reduces liver transaminases, and improves hepatomegaly and IR or insulin secretion [14–16], whereas improvements in histology remain controversial [17, 18]. Thiazolidinediones (rosiglitazone or pioglitazone) have been shown to improve steatosis and liver enzyme levels and regulate glucolipid metabolism. However, the use of thiazolidinediones is restricted due to side effects (ischemic heart disease, heart failure, potential hepatotoxicity, liver failure, weight gain, edema, low bone mineral density, and an increased risk of bladder cancer) [19].

Diammonium glycyrrhizinate enteric-coated capsule (DGEC) is the lipid ligand complex of 18-α-diammonium glycyrrhizinate and phosphatidylcholine and has therapeutic effects including a hepatocytic membrane-protective effect, improves liver function, and has a steroid hormone-like effect [20, 21]. However, the steroid hormone-like effect is commonly associated with side effects, especially IR and weight gain. As metformin improves resistance to insulin sensitivity and glucose metabolism, we wondered if metformin combined with DGEC would have a synergistic effect in the amelioration of NAFLD and T2DM. Thus, the present study was designed to assess whether the therapeutic effect of metformin combined with DGEC in NAFLD and T2DM was better than each of these agents alone in patients also treated with diet and exercise.

2. Subjects and Methods

2.1. Subjects. The study was carried out in Shanghai Tenth People's Hospital (Tongji University, School of Medicine, Shanghai, China), where a cohort of 163 patients aged 18–65 years were recruited from January 2013 to December 2015. Patients diagnosed with NAFLD at ultrasonography (US)/computed tomography (CT) who also had T2DM were eligible for the study. The diagnostic criteria for NAFLD were in accordance with the 2010 Chinese guidelines for the diagnosis and management of NAFLD [3]. The criteria for T2DM were in accordance with the 2013 China guideline for

T2DM [22]. Fatty liver was diagnosed by CT before the study, and all patients with a liver/spleen CT ratio <1 were diagnosed with fatty liver. A liver/spleen CT ratio <1.0 and >0.7 was considered mild fatty liver, a liver/spleen CT ratio ≤0.7 and >0.5 was considered moderate fatty liver, and a liver/spleen CT ratio ≤0.5 was considered severe fatty liver.

Exclusion criteria were as follows: (1) Signs of hepatic virus infection (hepatitis B antigen or hepatitis C antibodies), drug-induced hepatic disease, Wilson's disease, cytomegalovirus infection, hemochromatosis, autoimmune liver disease, liver cirrhosis, or liver diseases other than NAFLD; (2) connective tissue diseases or hereditary disorders related to obesity (such as Prader-Willi syndrome) and pathological obesity (such as Cushing syndrome); (3) severe heart disease and/or severe hypertension, severe hepatic and renal dysfunction, cancer, or other severe diseases; (4) history of taking medicine which would disturb observations or the absorption of therapeutic drugs (such as hypotensive drugs, prednisone, amiodarone, and statins); (5) diseases affecting blood glucose levels (such as hyperthyroidism and hypercortisolism) or acute diabetic complications such as ketoacidosis and hyperosmolar coma; (6) poor compliance/adherence to treatment; (7) excessive alcohol intake (ethanol intake >140 g per week in males, >70 g per week in females).

2.2. Randomization. Patients (163) were randomly assigned to three groups, and 146 patients completed the study. Group 1 ($n = 50$) was treated with metformin 500 mg three times a day; group 2 ($n = 50$) was treated with DGEC 450 mg three times a day; group 3 ($n = 46$) received metformin (500 mg, three times a day) plus DGEC (450 mg, three times a day). All groups received treatment for 24 weeks, and all enrolled patients were prescribed the same lifestyle modification program (hypocaloric diet in conjunction with regular aerobic exercise; dietary composition: 20% protein, carbohydrate > 50%, and fat < 30% per day; exercise: moderate aerobic physical exercise 60 min per day, at least 5 days a week) during the treatment period. To reduce gastrointestinal side effects, metformin was initially administered at 500 mg per day and was progressively increased to a final dose of 500 mg three times per day. All therapeutic agents were kept stable to prevent possible effects on the study variables.

2.3. Observations. At baseline and after 24 weeks of treatment, demographic and anthropometric data (social and family history, physical exam, body weight, and height) were measured in all patients. A blood sample collected after overnight fasting was used to assess liver function [ALT, aspartate aminotransferase (AST), GGT, conjugated bilirubin (CB), and total bilirubin (TB)], lipid metabolism [total cholesterol (TC), triacylglycerol (TG), high-density lipoprotein cholesterol (HDL-C), and low density lipoprotein cholesterol (LDL-C)], serum ferritin (SF), glucose metabolism [fasting blood glucose (FBG), fasting insulin (FINS), homeostasis model assessment of insulin resistance (HOMA-IR)], liver/spleen CT ratio, and the fibroscan value. All patients received CT to measure liver density before and after 24 weeks of treatment. The lipid profile was determined at 4-weekly intervals during treatment. Patients were instructed to limit their alcohol intake during the treatment period, and daily consumption and side effects were reported during follow-up visits. BMI was calculated according to the formula: BMI = weight (in kilograms)/height (in meters) [2]. The homeostatic model assessment of IR (HOMA-IR) was calculated as follows: HOMA-IR = fasting plasma insulin (in mU/L) × FBG (in mmol/L)/22.5. Liver enzymes and lipid profile were measured by a Roche automatic biochemical analyzer (Hitachi Modular P/D, Can 433, Hoffmann-La Roche Inc., Geneva, Switzerland). HbA1c was determined using an automatic glycosylated hemoglobin analyzer (HLC-723G8, TOSOH corporation, Tokyo, Japan). Plasma glucose was measured by an automated glucose oxidase method (Glucose Analyzer 2, Beckman Coulter Inc., Fullerton, California, USA) and insulin was assessed using Roche automatic immunoassay analyzer (Cobas 6000 e601, Hoffmann-La Roche Inc., Geneva, Switzerland). Liver ultrasound was performed in all patients by a single experienced radiologist, blinded to the study, using a 5 MHz Siemens Sonoline Omnia instrument (Siemens Medical Solutions Inc., MountainView, California, USA). The CT value was measured using Siemens Somatom and GE Medical Systems (MX8000, Philips, Cleveland, Ohio, USA). Transient ultrasound elastography (Fibroscan) is a well validated noninvasive tool which measures liver stiffness to quantify liver fibrosis in chronic liver diseases [23]. The fibroscan value was measured using a Fibroscan 502 diasonograph (Echosens, Paris, France). Metformin was produced by the Sino-American Shanghai Squibb Company (Shanghai, China, 500 mg/tablet). DGEC was produced by Jiangsu Chia Tai-Tianqing Pharmaceutical Co., Ltd. (Jiangsu, China, 150 mg/tablet).

2.4. Statistical Analysis. All data were analyzed using SPSS version 20.0 software (SPSS, Inc., Chicago, IL, USA) and Prism 6.0 (GraphPad Software Inc., La Jolla, CA, USA) for Windows. Quantitative data were reported as means ± standard deviation (SD). Categorical variables were described using frequency distributions and presented as frequency (%). The Kolmogorov–Smirnov test was used to determine whether the sample data were derived from a normal distribution population. The results, with normal distribution before and after treatment in each group, were evaluated by the paired *t*-test or rank sum test. Intergroup differences between the three groups at baseline and at 24 weeks were compared using one-way analysis of variance or the rank sum test. The Chi-square test was used to compare qualitative variables. All tests were two-sided and a *P* value less than 0.05 was considered statistically significant.

3. Results

3.1. Patient Characteristics at Baseline. All demographic and biochemical parameters at baseline were similar in the three groups in terms of gender, age, liver function, and metabolic parameters. One hundred and sixty-three patients with NAFLD and T2DM were screened for study participation, and 146 patients (85 males and 61 females) completed the 24-week treatment period. In group 1, 50 completed the study, 31 males (62.0%) and 19 females (38.0%), aged 26–77

years with an average age of 56.30 ± 12.47 years. In group 2, 50 patients completed treatment, 29 males (58.0%) and 21 females (42.0%), aged 29–68 years with an average age of 54.64 ± 9.71 years. In group 3, 4 patients were lost to follow-up and the remaining 25 males (54.3%) and 21 females (45.7%), aged 25–66 years with a mean age of 54.17 ± 10.42 years, completed treatment. The distribution of baseline data was assessed to determine whether the samples followed a normal distribution. At baseline, no statistically significant differences were observed between the three groups with respect to anthropometric parameters (sex, age, weight, and height), BMI, liver function (ALT, AST, and GGT), lipid profile (HbA1c, FBG, and FINS), SF, liver/spleen CT ratio, and fibroscan value (Table 1). The proportion of patients with mild fatty liver at baseline was 29.5% (43 patients; 13 in group 1, 16 in group 2, and 14 in group 3). The proportion of patients with moderate fatty liver at baseline was 44.5% (65 patients; 22 in group 1, 21 in group 2, and 22 in group 3). The proportion of patients with severe fatty liver at baseline was 26.0% (38 patients; 15 in group 1, 13 in group 2, and 10 in group 3) (Table 2).

3.2. Anthropometric Parameters after Treatment. Metformin treatment was associated with a significant reduction in weight and BMI before and after 24 weeks of treatment in group 1 (from 76.43 ± 10.16 to 71.27 ± 10.50 kg, *P* < 0.001; from 28.17 ± 2.60 to 26.24 ± 3.52, *P* < 0.001, resp.). Similar results were observed in group 2 (from 75.93 ± 11.17 to 73.28 ± 10.82 kg, *P* < 0.001; from 27.53 ± 2.81 to 26.59 ± 2.95, *P* < 0.001, resp.). Furthermore, compared with group 1 and group 2, group 3 tended to show a more favorable improvement in weight and BMI (*P* < 0.05) (Tables 1 and 3).

3.3. Liver Function after Treatment. A downward trend in liver function was seen in the three groups (Figure 1). From baseline to the end of the 24-week treatment period, significant reductions in liver enzymes (ALT, AST, and GGT) were observed in the metformin-treated group (*P* < 0.001, *P* = 0.016, and *P* < 0.001, resp.) and in the DGEC-treated group (*P* < 0.001), whereas in the metformin plus DGEC combination group, lower liver enzyme (ALT, AST, and GGT) levels than either the metformin-treated group or the DGEC-treated group were observed at 24 weeks (*P* < 0.001 for group 3 versus group 1 and *P* < 0.05 for group 3 versus group 2). Furthermore, compared with group 1, the mean serum concentrations of liver enzymes in group 2 decreased markedly (*P* < 0.05) (Table 3). As summarized in Table 4 and illustrated in Figure 1, changes in liver enzymes in all three groups were maximal during the first 8 weeks and then gradually declined during the remaining treatment period.

3.4. Lipid Parameters after Treatment. As shown in Table 3 and Figures 1 and 2, the mean values of TG, TC, and LDL-C declined and HDL-C increased in the three groups. In the metformin-diet-exercise group, despite a significant decrease in the levels of TG (*P* < 0.001), TC (*P* < 0.001), and LDL-C (*P* = 0.047) at 24 weeks, patients had an elevated HDL-C concentration compared with baseline data (*P* < 0.001). The DGEC-diet-exercise group had a reduction in

TABLE 1: Parameters of patients with T2DM and NAFLD at baseline.

	Group 1 ($n = 50$)		Group 2 ($n = 50$)		Group 3 ($n = 46$)		P value*
	Baseline	24 weeks	Baseline	24 weeks	Baseline	24 weeks	
Age (yr)	53.46 ± 11.25		54.64 ± 9.71		54.17 ± 10.42		0.85
Gender (M/F)	31/19		29/21		25/21		0.75
Weight (kg)	76.43 ± 10.16	71.27 ± 10.50	75.93 ± 11.17	73.28 ± 10.82	75.92 ± 11.54	66.59 ± 10.28	0.97
Height (m)	1.65 ± 0.08		1.66 ± 0.07		1.65 ± 0.08		0.63
BMI (kg/m²)	28.17 ± 2.60	26.34 ± 3.52	27.53 ± 2.81	26.59 ± 2.95	27.96 ± 2.97	24.56 ± 3.03	0.52
ALT (U/L)	86.75 ± 27.59	63.04 ± 26.80	90.79 ± 28.13	40.45 ± 16.30	91.64 ± 28.61	32.23 ± 16.18	0.66
AST (U/L)	67.28 ± 34.68	53.38 ± 29.81	69.38 ± 35.79	32.06 ± 10.41	69.60 ± 36.00	25.91 ± 13.82	0.94
GGT (U/L)	88.96 ± 43.02	59.53 ± 32.38	90.29 ± 37.12	43.32 ± 22.63	93.27 ± 34.98	33.57 ± 16.07	0.86
CB (umol/L)	5.14 ± 3.10	3.07 ± 1.80	6.52 ± 4.18	3.60 ± 2.36	6.45 ± 3.40	4.09 ± 3.12	0.10
TB (umol/L)	15.77 ± 6.29	9.81 ± 4.87	15.31 ± 6.79	12.16 ± 4.83	17.25 ± 7.72	11.04 ± 4.92	0.37
TG (mmol/L)	2.97 ± 1.21	1.82 ± 0.96	3.07 ± 1.04	1.80 ± 0.78	3.24 ± 1.21	1.33 ± 0.57	0.52
TC (mmol/L)	6.57 ± 1.71	5.22 ± 1.22	6.39 ± 1.73	5.44 ± 1.19	6.62 ± 1.71	4.38 ± 1.47	0.79
HDL (mmol/L)	0.91 ± 0.30	1.14 ± 0.39	0.94 ± 0.28	1.09 ± 0.39	0.95 ± 0.28	1.32 ± 0.35	0.80
LDL (mmol/L)	4.09 ± 1.34	3.59 ± 1.50	3.95 ± 1.02	3.66 ± 1.50	4.15 ± 0.87	2.80 ± 1.35	0.68
SF (µg/L)	216.85 ± 81.06	160.18 ± 66.23	223.02 ± 78.37	177.47 ± 67.09	227.50 ± 87.31	130.19 ± 63.63	0.82
HbA1c (%)	8.82 ± 1.79	6.84 ± 1.42	8.70 ± 1.74	8.20 ± 1.90	9.09 ± 1.80	6.23 ± 0.93	0.55
FBG (mmol/L)	9.10 ± 3.02	7.23 ± 1.92	9.27 ± 2.35	8.51 ± 2.22	9.35 ± 2.41	6.38 ± 1.29	0.89
FINS (mU/L)	14.63 ± 3.89	12.04 ± 4.28	15.06 ± 3.71	13.96 ± 3.94	14.84 ± 4.58	9.87 ± 3.39	0.87
HOMA-IR	6.02 ± 3.04	4.16 ± 2.46	6.34 ± 2.51	5.50 ± 2.65	6.56 ± 3.55	2.93 ± 1.51	0.68
CT ratio	0.62 ± 0.16	0.74 ± 0.20	0.62 ± 0.16	0.73 ± 0.21	0.64 ± 0.15	0.89 ± 0.21	0.81
Fibroscan	10.83 ± 2.91	8.54 ± 2.73	11.08 ± 2.33	8.68 ± 2.46	9.94 ± 2.47	6.72 ± 2.02	0.08

P values* were calculated by one-factor analysis of variance or the Wilcoxon signed rank test for intergroup comparisons at baseline.
Group 1: metformin-diet-exercise-treated group; group 2: DGEC-diet-exercise-treated group; group 3: drugs combination-diet-exercise-treated group.

TABLE 2: Classification of steatosis in NAFLD before and after treatment.

	Mild		Moderate		Severe		Total
	Before	After	Before	After	Before	After	
Group 1	13 (26.0%)	27 (54.0%)	22 (44.0%)	16 (32.0%)	15 (30.0%)	7 (14.0%)	50 (100%)
Group 2	16 (32.0%)	26 (52.0%)	21 (42.0%)	14 (28.0%)	13 (26.0%)	10 (20.0%)	50 (100%)
Group 3	14 (30.4%)	37 (80.4%)	22 (47.8%)	7 (15.2%)	10 (21.7%)	2 (4.3%)	50 (100%)

TG ($P < 0.001$), TC ($P = 0.013$), and HDL-C ($P = 0.004$), but a nonsignificant mild reduction in LDL-C ($P = 0.288$) after 24 weeks of treatment. As shown in Table 3, changes in the levels of circulating serum lipids at the final evaluation reached statistical significance in the groups ($P = 0.004$ for TG, $P < 0.001$ for TC, $P = 0.01$ for HDL-C, and $P = 0.007$ for LDL-C). Compared with the metformin-diet-exercise group, statistically significant differences were observed for TG ($P = 0.009$), TC ($P = 0.002$), HDL-C ($P = 0.024$), and LDL-C ($P = 0.009$). In addition, the mean plasma concentrations of TG, TC, HDL-C, and LDL-C were significantly lower in patients in the metformin plus DGEC combination-diet-exercise group than in the DGEC-diet-exercise group ($P = 0.003$, $P < 0.001$, $P = 0.004$, and $P = 0.004$, resp.).

3.5. Metabolic Parameters after Treatment. At the end of the 24-week treatment period, HbA1c, FPG, FINS, and HOMA-IR improved in the three groups; however, the changes were significantly different between the groups ($P < 0.001$) (Table 3). In group 1, the patients had decreased mean values of HbA1c ($P < 0.001$), FPG ($P < 0.001$), FINS ($P = 0.006$),

and HOMA-IR ($P = 0.001$) after 24 weeks of treatment compared with baseline data. Patients in group 2 had no significant within-group differences in HbA1c, FPG, FINS, and HOMA-IR compared with baseline ($P = 0.09$, $P = 0.071$, $P = 0.114$, and $P = 0.098$, resp.). When the groups were compared at 24 weeks, patients who received metformin plus DGEC had lower HbA1c ($P = 0.039$ for group 3 versus group 1, $P < 0.001$ for group 3 versus group 2, resp.), FPG ($P = 0.034$ for group 3 versus group 1, $P < 0.001$ for group 3 versus group 2), FINS ($P = 0.007$ for group 3 versus group 1, $P < 0.001$ for group 3 versus group 2), and HOMA-IR ($P = 0.011$ for group 3 versus group 1, $P < 0.001$ for group 3 versus group 2) levels than those who received metformin alone or DGEC alone (Table 3).

3.6. Other Clinical Characteristics after Treatment. In the metformin-treated group and the DGEC-treated group, reduced levels of SF, liver/spleen CT ratio, and fibroscan value ($P < 0.001$) were observed after 24 weeks of treatment. When the entire cohort at the end of the treatment period was assessed for intergroup comparisons, significant differences

TABLE 3: Comparisons within groups and between groups in patients with T2DM and NAFLD at 24 weeks.

	Group 1 (n = 50) P1 value	Group 2 (n = 50) P2 value	Group 3 (n = 46) P3 value	P value#	P1 value+	P2 value+	P3 value+
Weight (kg)	<0.001	<0.001	<0.001	0.008	0.341	0.032	0.002
BMI (kg/m^2)	<0.001	<0.001	<0.001	0.004	0.689	0.007	0.002
ALT (U/L)	<0.001	<0.001	<0.001	<0.001	<0.001	<0.001	0.044
AST (U/L)	0.016	<0.001	<0.001	<0.001	<0.001	<0.001	0.049
GGT (U/L)	<0.001	<0.001	<0.001	<0.001	0.014	<0.001	0.048
CB (μmol/L)	<0.001	<0.001	<0.001	0.131	0.495	0.158	0.777
TB (μmol/L)	<0.001	0.008	<0.001	0.058	0.017	0.219	0.261
TG (mmol/L)	<0.001	<0.001	<0.001	0.004	0.999	0.009	0.003
TC (mmol/L)	<0.001	0.013	<0.001	<0.001	0.402	0.002	<0.001
HDL (mmol/L)	<0.001	0.004	<0.001	0.01	0.492	0.024	0.004
LDL (mmol/L)	0.047	0.288	<0.001	0.007	0.804	0.009	0.004
SF (μg/L)	<0.001	<0.001	<0.001	0.002	0.191	0.027	0.001
HbA1c (%)	<0.001	0.09	<0.001	<0.001	<0.001	0.039	<0.001
FBG (mmol/L)	<0.001	0.071	<0.001	<0.001	0.008	0.034	<0.001
FINS (mU/L)	0.006	0.114	<0.001	<0.001	0.015	0.007	<0.001
HOMA-IR	0.001	0.098	<0.001	<0.001	0.030	0.011	<0.001
CT ratio	<0.001	<0.001	<0.001	<0.001	0.912	0.001	<0.001
Fibroscan	<0.001	<0.001	<0.001	<0.001	0.990	0.001	<0.001

P value# was calculated by one-factor analysis of variance or the Wilcoxon signed rank test for intergroup comparisons at 24 weeks.
P1 value, P2 value, and P3 value were calculated by the paired t-test or the Wilcoxon signed rank test for within groups.
P1 value+ for comparisons between group 2 and group 1, P2 value+ for comparisons between group 3 and group 1, and P3 value+ for comparisons between group 3 and group 2.

were observed for SF, liver/spleen CT ratio, and fibroscan value ($P < 0.001$). At 24 weeks, patients in the drug combination group showed marked improvements in SF, liver/spleen CT ratio, and fibroscan value ($P < 0.001$) compared to the metformin-treated group and DGEC-treated group (Table 3).

3.7. Therapeutic Effectiveness. Table 2 shows the number of subjects (percent relative to the baseline, which was considered 100%) in whom improvements were observed after 24 weeks of treatment. Following 24 weeks of treatment, mild fatty liver increased by 28.0% (13 versus 27 patients, before versus after treatment) in group 1, increased by 20.0% (16 versus 26 patients, before versus after treatment) in group 2, and increased by 50.0% (14 versus 37 patients, before versus after treatment) in group 3. Moderate fatty liver was lower in the three groups compared with baseline data (44.0% versus 32.0% in group 1, 42.0% versus 28.0% in group 2, and 47.8% versus 15.2% in group 3). At the end of the study, the number of patients with severe fatty liver in group 3 (4.3%) was lower than that in group 1 (14%) and group 2 (20%).

In general, significant improvements in liver steatosis were observed in the three groups at 24 weeks ($P < 0.001$). Significant improvements, demonstrated by CT, from baseline to 24 weeks, were seen in eight patients (16.0%) in group 1, in seven patients in group 2 (14.0%), and in twelve patients in group 3 (26.1%). A mild improvement in steatosis was observed in 20 patients (40.0%) in the metformin-treated group and in 16 patients (32.0%) in the DGEC-treated group, and significant improvements were seen in 28 patients (60.9%) in the drug combination group. The overall

remission rate of fatty liver (including slight and significant improvements) was 87% (40 patients) in group 3 over 24 weeks of treatment, whereas the overall remission rate was 56% and 46% in group 1 and group 2, respectively (Table 5).

3.8. Side Effects. No severe side effects were noted during the treatment period, with the exception of a few episodes of mild gastrointestinal disorders (nausea, abdominal pain, and/or diarrhea), fatigue, and an increase in lactate level, which were usually observed early after starting metformin therapy. A marginal increase in lactate level was observed in three patients over the 24-week treatment period, but there were no episodes of acidosis. All patients were able to tolerate treatment with the exception of three patients who discontinued treatment due to a fluctuation in lactate level.

4. Discussion

NAFLD is the commonest cause of chronic liver disease worldwide, and NAFLD-associated mortality is rising at an alarming rate, which has attracted worldwide attention. NAFLD is reported to have a high prevalence in subjects with T2DM [2]. NAFLD and T2DM regularly coexist as they share a common pathophysiology, synergistically augment the risk of diabetic complications, and increase the incidence of NAFLD progression to diseases such as cirrhosis and hepatocellular carcinoma [24, 25]. The molecular mechanisms of NAFLD have not yet been entirely clarified but involve the interaction of multiple complex mechanisms. It is currently

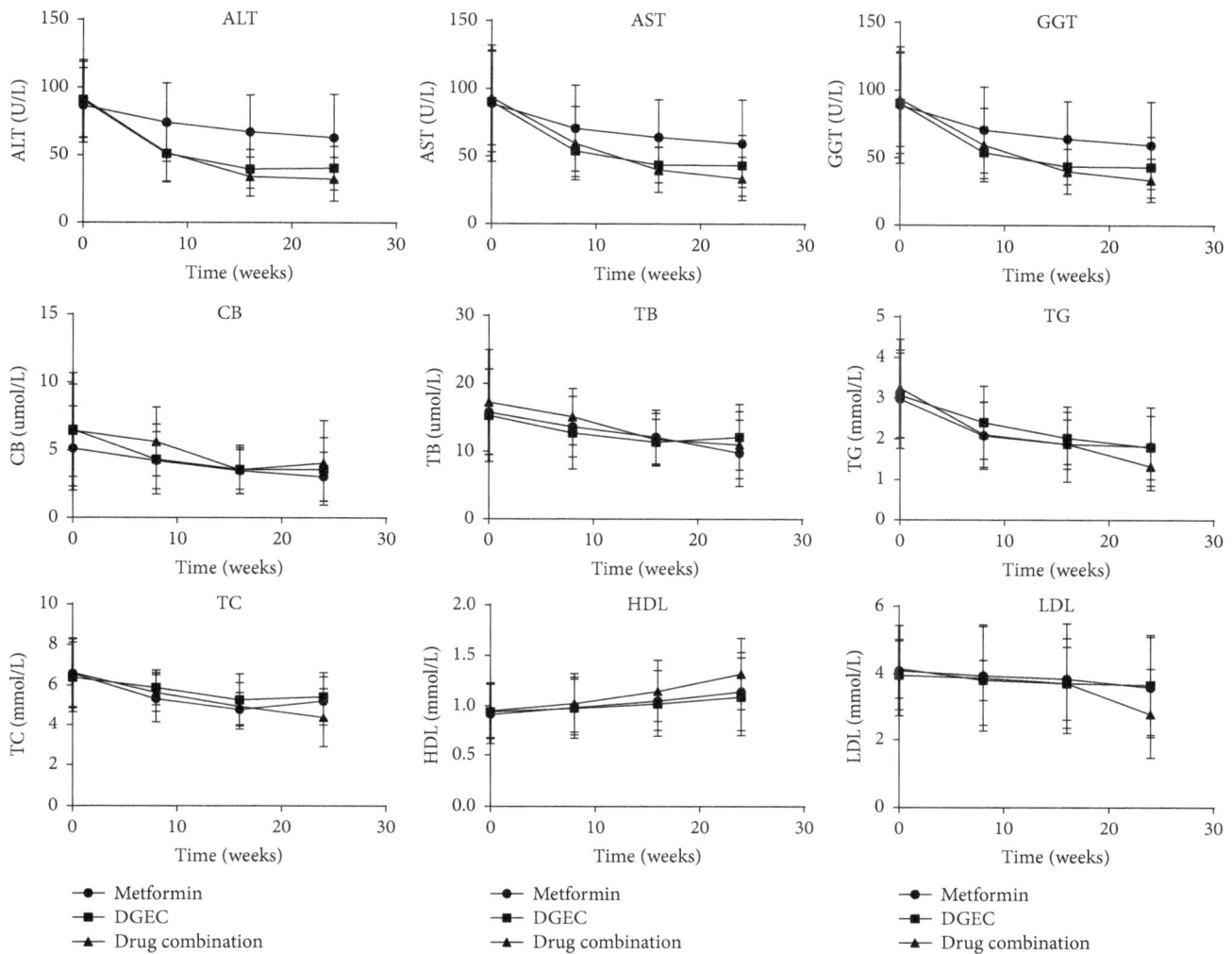

FIGURE 1: Changes in liver enzymes and lipid parameters over the 24-week treatment period (line chart).

well recognized that the pathogenesis of NAFLD is due to the so-called two-hit hypothesis, which was initially proposed in 1988 [26]. The first hit refers to hepatic steatosis (the accumulation of triglycerides). Inflammation and oxidative stress caused by oxide metabolites within the hepatocytes are recognized as the second hit [27]. The "multihit" theory has been reported in recent years, which is not in accordance with previous theories, and includes genetic factors, inflammation (especially derived from the gut and adipose tissue), insulin resistance, adipocytokine imbalance, and endoplasmic reticulum stress [6]. However, systemic insulin resistance is still a major determinant in the development of NAFLD independent of coexisting factors [28, 29]. Insulin resistance may compromise the ability of insulin to regulate glucose metabolism. Insulin resistance (adipose tissue and liver) and the associated hyperinsulinemia accelerate the degradation of peripheral adipose tissue and elevate fatty acid level in patients with T2DM. Furthermore, hepatic rather than peripheral insulin sensitivity is independently related to liver fat content [28]. An increase in fatty acid level

contributes to more lipoylation to triglycerides, which are deposited in the liver, leading to fatty liver.

Previous studies have indicated that weight loss may have beneficial effects in patients with NAFLD, which may serve as a first-line approach in NAFLD. Exercise was reported to alter the liver mitochondria phospholipidomic profile and maintain mitochondrial function in NASH [30]. A meta-analysis showed that weight loss ≥5% was related to an improvement in hepatic steatosis and weight loss ≥7% improved the NAFLD activity score [31]. However, lifestyle modifications are limited due to difficulties regarding adherence. No treatment strategies targeting patients with NAFLD and T2DM have been established, indicating that etiological treatments (aimed at ameliorating visceral obesity, hyperlipidemia, and diabetes mellitus/insulin resistance) have a high priority. Therefore, insulin-sensitizing agents have been evaluated for the treatment of NAFLD and T2DM, and metformin is an attractive treatment due to its favorable safety profile and potential therapeutic effect [13, 32–34]. It is reported in the literature [35] that metformin not

TABLE 4: Liver function and lipid Profile in the three groups at baseline and during treatment.

	Baseline	8 weeks	16 weeks	24 weeks
ALT (U/L)				
Group 1	86.75 ± 27.59	74.22 ± 29.09	67.19 ± 27.40	63.04 ± 26.80
Group 2	90.79 ± 28.13	51.03 ± 21.18	39.70 ± 14.37	40.45 ± 16.30
Group 3	91.64 ± 28.61	51.80 ± 21.22	34.07 ± 14.55	32.23 ± 16.18
AST (U/L)				
Group 1	67.28 ± 34.68	60.19 ± 25.57	56.16 ± 22.66	53.38 ± 29.81
Group 2	69.38 ± 35.79	41.64 ± 15.20	32.98 ± 11.78	32.06 ± 10.41
Group 3	69.60 ± 36.00	43.72 ± 16.35	31.33 ± 13.68	25.91 ± 13.82
GGT (U/L)				
Group 1	88.96 ± 43.02	70.71 ± 31.81	64.23 ± 27.85	59.53 ± 32.38
Group 2	90.29 ± 37.12	53.92 ± 19.09	43.68 ± 13.24	43.32 ± 22.63
Group 3	93.27 ± 34.98	59.70 ± 27.20	40.02 ± 116.75	33.57 ± 16.07
CB (μmol/L)				
Group 1	5.14 ± 3.10	4.26 ± 2.11	3.51 ± 1.70	3.07 ± 1.80
Group 2	6.52 ± 4.18	4.35 ± 2.58	3.59 ± 1.46	3.60 ± 2.36
Group 3	6.45 ± 3.40	5.63 ± 2.54	3.57 ± 1.79	4.09 ± 3.12
TB (μmol/L)				
Group 1	15.77 ± 6.29	13.66 ± 4.46	12.17 ± 3.95	9.81 ± 4.87
Group 2	15.31 ± 6.79	12.76 ± 5.35	11.40 ± 3.36	12.16 ± 4.83
Group 3	17.25 ± 7.72	15.12 ± 4.14	11.78 ± 3.89	11.04 ± 4.92
TG (mmol/L)				
Group 1	2.97 ± 1.21	2.08 ± 0.82	1.87 ± 0.92	1.82 ± 0.96
Group 2	3.07 ± 1.04	2.40 ± 0.90	2.02 ± 0.64	1.80 ± 0.78
Group 3	3.24 ± 1.21	2.12 ± 0.80	1.88 ± 0.61	1.33 ± 0.57
TC (mmol/L)				
Group 1	6.57 ± 1.71	5.33 ± 1.19	4.79 ± 0.85	5.22 ± 1.22
Group 2	6.39 ± 1.73	5.89 ± 0.87	5.28 ± 1.28	5.44 ± 1.19
Group 3	6.62 ± 1.71	5.65 ± 0.96	4.95 ± 1.18	4.38 ± 1.47
HDL-C (mmol/L)				
Group 1	0.91 ± 0.30	0.98 ± 0.28	1.05 ± 0.30	1.14 ± 0.39
Group 2	0.94 ± 0.28	0.98 ± 0.31	1.02 ± 0.33	1.09 ± 0.39
Group 3	0.95 ± 0.28	1.03 ± 0.29	1.15 ± 0.31	1.32 ± 0.35
LDL-C (mmol/L)				
Group 1	4.09 ± 1.34	3.94 ± 1.47	3.85 ± 1.64	3.59 ± 1.50
Group 2	3.95 ± 1.02	3.87 ± 1.59	3.72 ± 1.34	3.66 ± 1.50
Group 3	4.15 ± 0.87	3.81 ± 0.59	3.71 ± 1.09	2.80 ± 1.35

only increases glucose utilization in peripheral tissues, but also inhibits the production of glucose, triglycerides, and cholesterol and stimulates fatty acid oxidation, preventing the progression of NAFLD [18, 36]. However, further studies are needed to determine the exact mechanism of action of metformin in NAFLD.

The dominant effective constituent in DGEC is phosphatidylcholine and glycyrrhizic acid (GA). Phosphatidylcholine is an essential component in cellular membranes and is reported to reduce serum cholesterol level, improve obese status and obesity-related complications, which further decrease the morbidity of NAFLD, and promote the recovery of liver function [37, 38]. GA, a triterpenoid saponin, which is derived from the traditional Chinese medicine, Gancao, was found to modify fatty acids and improve lipid metabolism [39, 40]. Moreover, GA also promotes cell regeneration and

was reported to significantly improve hepatocyte steatosis, hepatocyte necrosis, and interstitial inflammation [41, 42]. GA can be hydrolyzed to glycyrrhetinic acid in the human body. It has been reported that the chemical structure of glycyrrhetinic acid is similar to the steroid ring of aldosterone and thereby elevates serum hydrocortisone level and exerts steroid hormone-like effects such as inhibition of synthesis and the release of inflammatory mediators (prostacyclin E2, histamine) [43]. The steroid hormone-like effects of GA and glycyrrhetinic acid also cause some side effects, such as insulin resistance, glucose metabolism disturbance, electrolyte imbalance (hypernatremia and hypokalemia), edema, and weight gain [39].

The present study was undertaken to evaluate the efficacy of metformin plus DGEC in patients with NAFLD and T2DM compared with metformin alone and DGEC alone. Following

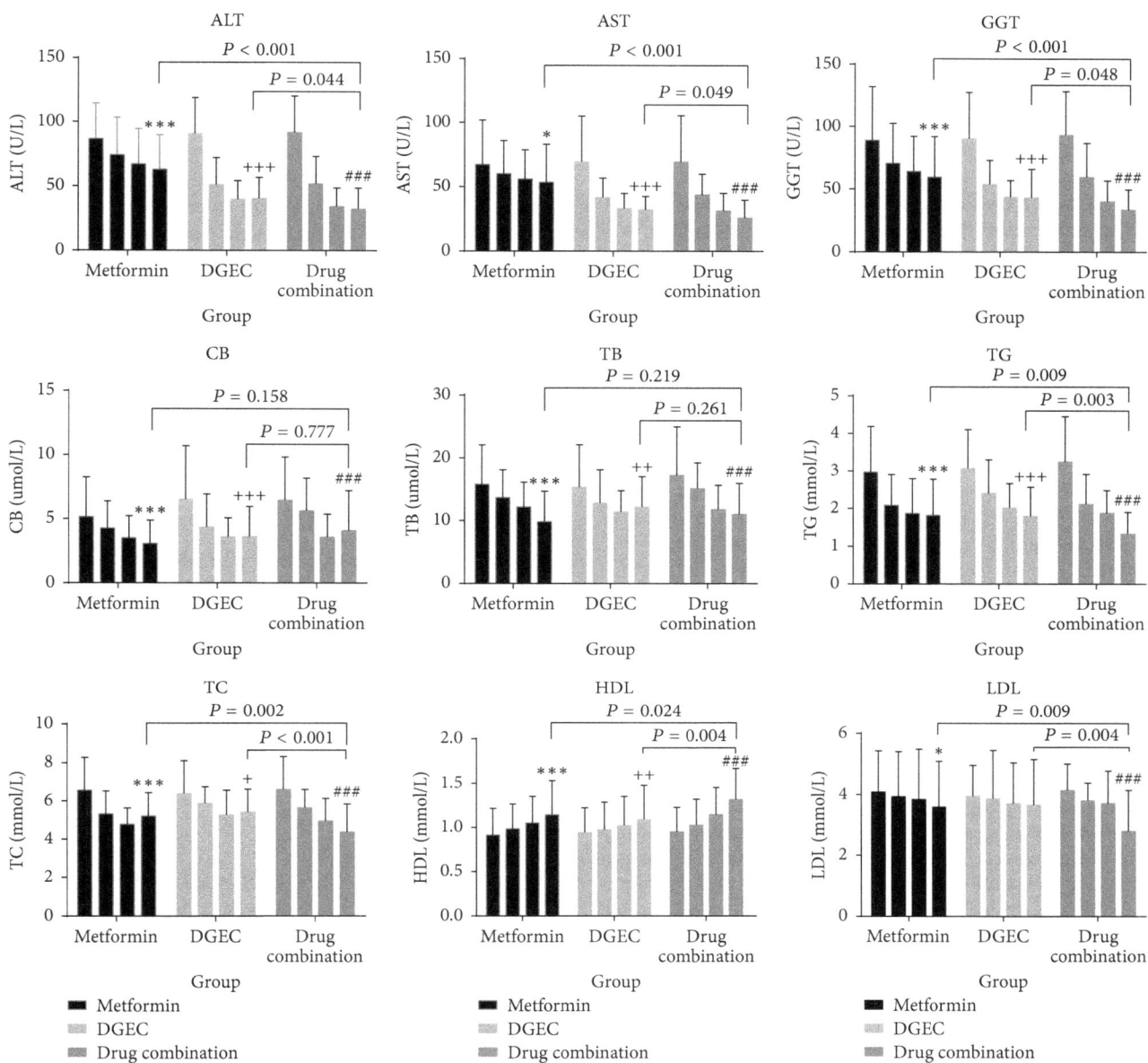

FIGURE 2: Changes in liver enzymes and lipid parameters over the 24-week treatment period (histogram). ∗ ∗ ∗ refer to $P < 0.001$ for comparisons within metformin group. + + + refer to $P < 0.001$ for comparisons within DGEC group. ### refer to $P < 0.001$ for comparisons within drug combination group. ∗ refers to $P < 0.05$ for comparisons within metformin group. ++ refer to $P < 0.01$ for comparisons within DGEC group. + refer to $P < 0.05$ for comparisons within DGEC group.

TABLE 5: Therapeutic effectiveness in the three groups.

	Ineffective	Mild efficacy	Significant efficacy	Total
Group 1	22 (44.0%)	20 (40.0%)	8 (16.0%)	50 (100%)
Group 2	27 (54.0%)	16 (32.0%)	7 (14.0%)	50 (100%)
Group 3	6 (13.0%)	28 (60.9%)	12 (26.1%)	46 (100%)

6 months of treatment, the overall remission rate in the metformin plus DGEC combination group was better (87%) than that in the metformin-treated group (56%) and the DGEC-treated group (50.9%). Furthermore, the proportion of patients with severe fatty liver decreased from 21.7% to 4.3% in the drug combination group, from 30% to 14% in the metformin-treated group, and from 26% to 20% in the DGEC-treated group. The outcomes in our study indicated that patients treated with metformin plus DGEC may have a more favorable prognosis, and this may be of

clinical significance considering the high risk of severe fatty liver progression to NASH, liver fibrosis, and even liver carcinoma. In our study, all treatment groups showed an improvement in anthropometric parameters, liver function, circulating lipid concentrations, metabolic parameters, SF, and fibroscan value. The metformin-treated group tended to have a greater decrease in the lipid profile and metabolic indices compared with the DGEC-treated group, whereas the latter group seemed to have greater improvement in liver enzymes. After 6 months of treatment, patients treated with metformin plus DGEC had greater improvements in weight, liver function, glucolipid metabolism, SF, and liver steatosis than either the metformin alone or DGEC alone group. The findings in the metformin-treated group were generally similar to those observed in previous studies [14, 18, 36, 44], which reported significant improvements in weight loss, glucose and lipid metabolism, and insulin sensitivity. Loomba et al. [18] and Nadeau et al. [14] observed a significant decrease in liver enzymes at 48 weeks and 6 months, respectively. However, the observations for liver enzymes in NAFLD are conflicting. Nair et al. [45] reported that, during the initial 3 months, there was an improvement in ALT, whereas after 3 months of treatment, the concentrations of ALT increased gradually to pretreatment levels. Kazemi et al. [46] attributed the improvements in liver enzymes to weight loss, and metformin had no significant effect on liver enzyme levels. Our outcomes in the DGEC-treated group partly conformed with the results seen in the study by Eu et al. [47] who indicated that GA resulted in statistically significant improvements in FBG, insulin sensitivity, serum free fatty acids, and lipid metabolism in high-fat diet-induced obese rats. Lim et al. [43] also reported similar observations where GA improved dyslipidemia via the selective induction of tissue lipoprotein lipase (a key regulator of lipoprotein metabolism) expression and inhibited the development of insulin sensitivity associated with tissue steatosis. However, we found only a slight decrease in glucose metabolism and insulin sensitivity with no statistical significance, which seemed to contradict previously published studies. Although this result is disheartening, it does not rule out DGEC being potentially efficacious in ameliorating glycolipid metabolism. The inconsistencies in results may be attributed to the weight gain caused by the steroid hormone-like effects, which partly counteracted the benefits of DGEC treatment. However, promising results were obtained when metformin was combined with DGEC, which was more effective than either treatment alone in the management of patients with NAFLD and T2DM. This indicated that metformin may alleviate insulin resistance caused by the steroid hormone-like effects of DGEC, and the combination of metformin and DGEC could have a synergistic effect in ameliorating NAFLD and T2DM.

Our study had the following limitations: (1) In the metformin-diet-exercise-treated group, we could not exclude the benefits of weight loss due to the lack of placebo with lifestyle intervention alone and the lack of an open-label design. (2) Histological data were not available in these patients. (3) It is also possible that 6 months was insufficient time to assess changes in liver function. (4) Sample size was small. (5) Drug dosage was not sufficient to achieve significant effects.

5. Conclusions

This study demonstrated that the administration of metformin combined with DGEC was more effective than metformin alone or DGEC alone in improving liver enzymes, glucolipid metabolism, and hepatic steatosis in patients with NAFLD and T2DM. Further randomized, controlled studies with a longer follow-up period are warranted to definitively determine the therapeutic effect of metformin combined with DGEC in patients with NAFLD and T2DM.

Competing Interests

The authors declare that they have no competing interests.

Authors' Contributions

Rong Zhang and Keran Cheng contributed equally to this work and share first authorship.

Acknowledgments

The authors thank all participants in this study. This study was supported by Chinese foundation for hepatitis prevention and control, Tianqing liver disease research fund subject (no. 20120005).

References

[1] Z. M. Younossi, A. B. Koenig, D. Abdelatif, Y. Fazel, L. Henry, and M. Wymer, "Global epidemiology of nonalcoholic fatty liver disease-Meta-analytic assessment of prevalence, incidence, and outcomes," *Hepatology*, vol. 64, no. 1, pp. 73–84, 2016.

[2] H. Yki-Järvinen, "Diagnosis of non-alcoholic fatty liver disease (NAFLD)," *Diabetologia*, vol. 59, no. 6, pp. 1104–1111, 2016.

[3] J. G. Fan, "Guidelines for management of nonalcoholic fatty liver disease: an updated and revised Edition," *Chinese Journal of the Frontiers of Medical Science (Electronic Version)*, vol. 18, no. 3, pp. 163–166, 2012.

[4] N. Chalasani, Z. Younossi, J. E. Lavine et al., "The diagnosis and management of non-alcoholic fatty liver disease: Practice Guideline by the American Association for the Study of Liver Diseases, American College of Gastroenterology, and the American Gastroenterological Association," *Hepatology*, vol. 55, no. 6, pp. 2005–2023, 2012.

[5] S. Watanabe, E. Hashimoto, K. Ikejima et al., "Evidence-based clinical practice guidelines for nonalcoholic fatty liver disease/nonalcoholic steatohepatitis," *Journal of Gastroenterology*, vol. 50, no. 4, pp. 364–377, 2015.

[6] H. Tilg and A. R. Moschen, "Evolution of inflammation in nonalcoholic fatty liver disease: the multiple parallel hits hypothesis," *Hepatology*, vol. 52, no. 5, pp. 1836–1846, 2010.

[7] Z. Li, J. Xue, P. Chen, L. Chen, S. Yan, and L. Liu, "Prevalence of nonalcoholic fatty liver disease in mainland of China: a meta-analysis of published studies," *Journal of Gastroenterology and Hepatology*, vol. 29, no. 1, pp. 42–51, 2014.

[8] K. Hassan, V. Bhalla, M. E. El Regal, and H. Hesham A-Kader, "Nonalcoholic fatty liver disease: a comprehensive review of a growing epidemic," *World Journal of Gastroenterology*, vol. 20, no. 34, pp. 12082–12101, 2014.

[9] Y. Liu and T. Hong, "The pathogenesis and management of non-alcoholic fatty liver disease coexisted with type 2 diabetes," *Zhonghua Yi Xue Za Zhi*, vol. 95, no. 44, pp. 3565–3567, 2015.

[10] Y. Eguchi, H. Hyogo, M. Ono et al., "Prevalence and associated metabolic factors of nonalcoholic fatty liver disease in the general population from 2009 to 2010 in Japan: a multicenter large retrospective study," *Journal of Gastroenterology*, vol. 47, no. 5, pp. 586–595, 2012.

[11] E. Bugianesi, A. Gastaldelli, E. Vanni et al., "Insulin resistance in non-diabetic patients with non-alcoholic fatty liver disease: sites and mechanisms," *Diabetologia*, vol. 48, no. 4, pp. 634–642, 2005.

[12] K. Cusi, "Treatment of patients with type 2 diabetes and non-alcoholic fatty liver disease: current approaches and future directions," *Diabetologia*, vol. 59, no. 6, pp. 1112–1120, 2016.

[13] I. Doycheva and R. Loomba, "Effect of metformin on ballooning degeneration in nonalcoholic steatohepatitis (NASH): when to use metformin in nonalcoholic fatty liver disease (NAFLD)," *Advances in Therapy*, vol. 31, no. 1, pp. 30–43, 2014.

[14] K. J. Nadeau, L. B. Ehlers, P. S. Zeitler, and K. Love-Osborne, "Treatment of non-alcoholic fatty liver disease with metformin versus lifestyle intervention in insulin-resistant adolescents," *Pediatric Diabetes*, vol. 10, no. 1, pp. 5–13, 2009.

[15] S. Rouabhia, N. Milic, and L. Abenavoli, "Metformin in the treatment of non-alcoholic fatty liver disease: safety, efficacy and mechanism," *Expert Review of Gastroenterology and Hepatology*, vol. 8, no. 4, pp. 343–349, 2014.

[16] A. Nar and O. Gedik, "The effect of metformin on leptin in obese patients with type 2 diabetes mellitus and nonalcoholic fatty liver disease," *Acta Diabetologica*, vol. 46, no. 2, pp. 113–118, 2009.

[17] M. O. Rakoski, A. G. Singal, M. A. M. Rogers, and H. Conjeevaram, "Meta-analysis: insulin sensitizers for the treatment of non-alcoholic steatohepatitis," *Alimentary Pharmacology & Therapeutics*, vol. 32, no. 10, pp. 1211–1221, 2010.

[18] R. Loomba, G. Lutchman, D. E. Kleiner et al., "Clinical trial: pilot study of metformin for the treatment of non-alcoholic steatohepatitis," *Alimentary Pharmacology and Therapeutics*, vol. 29, no. 2, pp. 172–182, 2009.

[19] Y. Takahashi, K. Sugimoto, H. Inui, and T. Fukusato, "Current pharmacological therapies for nonalcoholic fatty liver disease/nonalcoholic steatohepatitis," *World Journal of Gastroenterology*, vol. 21, no. 13, pp. 3777–3785, 2015.

[20] Y. Cheng and F. Yu, "Effects of diammonium glycyrrhizinate phosphatidylcholine complex treatment on rat nonalcoholic fatty liver disease," *Chinese Journal of Clinical Pharmacology and Therapeutics*, no. 1, pp. 15–19, 2012.

[21] Q. Huo and S. Gu, "Diammonium glycyrrhizinate enteric-coated capsules in treatment of patients with fatty liver disease: a meta-analysis," *Journal of Practical Hepatology*, no. 4, pp. 371–374, 2015.

[22] Chinese Diabetes Society, "2013 China guideline for type 2 diabetes," *Chinese Journal of Diabetes Mellitus*, 2014.

[23] D. H. Kaswala, M. Lai, and N. H. Afdhal, "Fibrosis assessment in Nonalcoholic Fatty Liver Disease (NAFLD) in 2016," *Digestive Diseases and Sciences*, vol. 61, no. 5, pp. 1356–1364, 2016.

[24] M. Noureddin and M. E. Rinella, "Nonalcoholic fatty liver disease, diabetes, obesity, and hepatocellular carcinoma," *Clinics in Liver Disease*, vol. 19, no. 2, pp. 361–379, 2015.

[25] J. M. Hazlehurst, C. Woods, T. Marjot, J. F. Cobbold, and J. W. Tomlinson, "Non-alcoholic fatty liver disease and diabetes," *Metabolism*, vol. 65, no. 8, pp. 1096–1108, 2016.

[26] C. P. Day and O. F. W. James, "Steatohepatitis: a tale of two 'hits'?" *Gastroenterology*, vol. 114, no. 4, pp. 842–845, 1998.

[27] K. Tziomalos, V. G. Athyros, and A. Karagiannis, "Non-alcoholic fatty liver disease in type 2 diabetes: pathogenesis and treatment options," *Current Vascular Pharmacology*, vol. 10, no. 2, pp. 162–172, 2012.

[28] A. Kotronen, L. Juurinen, M. Tiikkainen, S. Vehkavaara, and H. Yki-Järvinen, "Increased liver fat, impaired insulin clearance, and hepatic and adipose tissue insulin resistance in type 2 diabetes," *Gastroenterology*, vol. 135, no. 1, pp. 122–130, 2008.

[29] P. Dongiovanni, R. Rametta, M. Meroni, and L. Valenti, "The role of insulin resistance in nonalcoholic steatohepatitis and liver disease development—a potential therapeutic target?" *Expert Review of Gastroenterology and Hepatology*, vol. 10, no. 2, pp. 229–242, 2016.

[30] I. O. Gonçalves, E. Maciel, E. Passos et al., "Exercise alters liver mitochondria phospholipidomic profile and mitochondrial activity in non-alcoholic steatohepatitis," *International Journal of Biochemistry and Cell Biology*, vol. 54, pp. 163–173, 2014.

[31] G. Musso, M. Cassader, F. Rosina, and R. Gambino, "Impact of current treatments on liver disease, glucose metabolism and cardiovascular risk in non-alcoholic fatty liver disease (NAFLD): a systematic review and meta-analysis of randomised trials," *Diabetologia*, vol. 55, no. 4, pp. 885–904, 2012.

[32] D. L. R. L. Conde, T. E. Vrenken, M. Buist-Homan, K. N. Faber, and H. Moshage, "Metformin protects primary rat hepatocytes against oxidative stress-induced apoptosis," *Pharmacology Research & Perspectives*, vol. 3, no. 2, Article ID e00125, 2015.

[33] K. Tajima, A. Nakamura, J. Shirakawa et al., "Metformin prevents liver tumorigenesis induced by high-fat diet in C57Bl/6 mice," *American Journal of Physiology—Endocrinology and Metabolism*, vol. 305, no. 8, pp. E987–E998, 2013.

[34] B. Fruci, S. Giuliano, A. Mazza, R. Malaguarnera, and A. Belfiore, "Nonalcoholic fatty liver: a possible new target for type 2 diabetes prevention and treatment," *International Journal of Molecular Sciences*, vol. 14, no. 11, pp. 22933–22966, 2013.

[35] G. Schimmack, R. A. DeFronzo, and N. Musi, "AMP-activated protein kinase: role in metabolism and therapeutic implications," *Diabetes, Obesity and Metabolism*, vol. 8, no. 6, pp. 591–602, 2006.

[36] G. A. Garinis, B. Fruci, A. Mazza et al., "Metformin versus dietary treatment in nonalcoholic hepatic steatosis: a randomized study," *International Journal of Obesity*, vol. 34, no. 8, pp. 1255–1264, 2010.

[37] A. Al Rajabi, G. S. F. Castro, R. P. da Silva et al., "Choline supplementation protects against liver damage by normalizing cholesterol metabolism in Pemt/Ldlr knockout mice fed a high-fat diet," *Journal of Nutrition*, vol. 144, no. 3, pp. 252–257, 2014.

[38] H. S. Lee, Y. Nam, Y. Chung et al., "Beneficial effects of phosphatidylcholine on high-fat diet-induced obesity, hyperlipidemia and fatty liver in mice," *Life Sciences*, vol. 118, no. 1, pp. 7–14, 2014.

[39] H. Takii, T. Kometani, T. Nishimura, T. Nakae, S. Okada, and T. Fushiki, "Antidiabetic effect of glycyrrhizin in genetically diabetic KK-Ay mice," *Biological and Pharmaceutical Bulletin*, vol. 24, no. 5, pp. 484–487, 2001.

[40] H. P. Yaw, S. H. Ton, H.-F. Chin, M. K. Abdul Karim, H. A. Fernando, and K. A. Kadir, "Modulation of lipid metabolism in glycyrrhizic acid-treated rats fed on a high-calorie diet and exposed to short or long-term stress," *International Journal of Physiology, Pathophysiology and Pharmacology*, vol. 7, no. 1, pp. 61–75, 2015.

[41] J.-Y. Li, H.-Y. Cao, P. Liu, G.-H. Cheng, and M.-Y. Sun, "Glycyrrhizic acid in the treatment of liver diseases: literature review," *BioMed Research International*, vol. 2014, Article ID 872139, 15 pages, 2014.

[42] C.-Y. Hsiang, L.-J. Lin, S.-T. Kao, H.-Y. Lo, S.-T. Chou, and T.-Y. Ho, "Glycyrrhizin, silymarin, and ursodeoxycholic acid regulate a common hepatoprotective pathway in HepG2 cells," *Phytomedicine*, vol. 22, no. 7-8, pp. 768–777, 2015.

[43] W. Y. A. Lim, Y. Y. Chia, S. Y. Liong, S. Ha Ton, K. A. Kadir, and S. N. A. Syed Husain, "Lipoprotein lipase expression, serum lipid and tissue lipid deposition in orally-administered glycyrrhizic acid-treated rats," *Lipids in Health and Disease*, vol. 8, article no. 31, 2009.

[44] E. Bugianesi, E. Gentilcore, R. Manini et al., "A randomized controlled trial of metformin versus vitamin E or prescriptive diet in nonalcoholic fatty liver disease," *American Journal of Gastroenterology*, vol. 100, no. 5, pp. 1082–1090, 2005.

[45] S. Nair, A. M. Diehl, M. Wiseman, G. H. Farr Jr., and R. P. Perrillo, "Metformin in the treatment of non-alcoholic steatohepatitis: a pilot open label trial," *Alimentary Pharmacology and Therapeutics*, vol. 20, no. 1, pp. 23–28, 2004.

[46] R. Kazemi, M. Aduli, M. Sotoudeh et al., "Metformin in nonalcoholic steatohepatitis: a randomized controlled trial," *Middle East Journal of Digestive Diseases*, vol. 4, no. 1, pp. 16–22, 2012.

[47] C. H. A. Eu, W. Y. A. Lim, S. H. Ton, and K. B. A. Kadir, "Glycyrrhizic acid improved lipoprotein lipase expression, insulin sensitivity, serum lipid and lipid deposition in high-fat diet-induced obese rats," *Lipids in Health and Disease*, vol. 9, article 81, 2010.

13

Risk Factors for Additional Surgery after Iatrogenic Perforations due to Endoscopic Submucosal Dissection

Gi Jun Kim, Sung Min Park, Joon Sung Kim, Jeong Seon Ji, Byung Wook Kim, and Hwang Choi

Division of Gastroenterology, Department of Internal Medicine, College of Medicine, The Catholic University of Korea, Seoul, Republic of Korea

Correspondence should be addressed to Joon Sung Kim; kijoons@catholic.ac.kr

Academic Editor: Tatsuya Toyokawa

Objectives. Endoscopic resection (ER) is commonly performed to treat gastric epithelial neoplasms and subepithelial tumors. The aim of this study was to predict the risk factors for surgery after ER-induced perforation. *Methods.* We retrospectively reviewed the data on patients who received gastric endoscopic submucosal dissection (ESD) or endoscopic mucosal resection (EMR) between January 2010 and March 2015. Patients who were confirmed to have perforation were classified into surgery and nonsurgery groups. We aimed to determine the risk factors for surgery in patients who developed iatrogenic gastric perforations. *Results.* A total of 1183 patients underwent ER. Perforation occurred in 69 (5.8%) patients, and 9 patients (0.8%) required surgery to manage the perforation. In univariate analysis, anterior location of the lesion, a subepithelial lesion, two or more postprocedure pain killers within 24 hrs, and increased heart rate within 24 hrs after the procedure were the factors related to surgery. In logistic regression analysis, the location of the lesion at the anterior wall and using two or more postprocedure pain killers within 24 hrs were risk factors for surgery. *Conclusion.* Most cases of perforations after ER can be managed conservatively. When a patient requires two or more postprocedure pain killers within 24 hrs and the lesion is located on the anterior wall, early surgery should be considered instead of conservative management.

1. Introduction

Endoscopic resection (ER), such as endoscopic submucosal dissection (ESD) and endoscopic mucosal resection (EMR), is widely used to treat gastric epithelial lesions and subepithelial lesions [1–5]. Compared to surgery, ER is less invasive [6–8] and is associated with better quality of life [9].

Among the various ER methods, ESD is preferred for the treatment of early gastric cancer without lymph node metastasis. An advantage of ESD is that it allows for *en bloc* and histologically complete resections [10, 11]. However, the disadvantage to ESD is that it is technically a more difficult procedure to perform and has a higher perforation rate than EMR [10, 11]. Iatrogenic perforations induced by gastric ESD and EMR have been reported to occur in approximately 4% and 1% of cases, respectively [10, 11]. Most perforations can be managed through endoscopic closure and conservative treatment, but surgery is required in rare cases [12–14].

A delay in deciding to perform surgery may cause fatal clinical outcomes in some patients. Therefore, it is important to determine whether additional surgery is required in patients with perforation after ER. Previous studies have reported several risk factors associated with gastric perforation caused by ER [15, 16]. However, no study has investigated the risk factors related to surgery in patients with iatrogenic gastric perforation by ER. The aim of this study was to predict the risk factors in patients who required surgery following ER-induced gastric perforation.

2. Materials and Methods

2.1. Patients. Patients underwent gastric EMR or ESD for gastric epithelial neoplasms or subepithelial lesions from January 2010 to March 2015, and the data were retrospectively reviewed. Patients diagnosed with ER-induced gastric perforations were included in this study. This study was approved by the Institutional Review Board of the Catholic University of Korea (OC16RISI0029).

2.2. Endoscopic Procedure. All endoscopic procedures were performed by five endoscopists (JSK, JSJ, BIL, BWK, and HC). ESD procedures were performed similar to the method described by Chung et al. [17]. EMR procedures were performed using two methods: EMR with circumferential precutting and EMR using a dual-channel endoscope (GIF-2T40; Olympus, Tokyo, Japan). EMR procedures were conducted in the same way as previously described [18].

2.3. Endoscopic and Histological Characteristics. The endoscopic characteristics of the lesions with perforation according to their location and size were retrospectively reviewed by two endoscopists (SMP and KJK). The vertical location of the lesion was classified into three regions (upper third including the fundus, cardia, and upper body; the middle third including the middle body, lower body, and angle; and the lower third including the antrum and pylorus). The circumferential location of the lesions was divided into four regions (lesser curvature, posterior wall, greater curvature, and anterior wall). The size of the lesion was defined as the longest length of the endoscopically resected specimen.

The resected specimens were mounted onto boards with pins and were fixed in 10% formalin. After fixation, the specimens were cut into 2 mm slices for histological diagnosis. The gastric epithelial lesions were classified according to the revised Vienna Classification [19]. The subepithelial lesions were diagnosed using immunohistochemical stains, including CD34, CD117, desmin, and S-100.

2.4. Characteristics of Procedure-Related Factors. En bloc resection was defined as the resection of the specimen in one piece. Complete resection was defined as the absence of remnant tumor tissue in any resected margin. Procedure time was measured using the time on the endoscopic image and was defined as the time between marking and finishing resection of the lesion.

2.5. Perforation. A patient was diagnosed with perforation when mesenteric fat or an intra-abdominal cavity was directly observed during the procedure (macroperforation) or when free air was observed on a plain chest X-ray or a computed tomography scan after the procedure without the endoscopist recognizing the gastric wall defect during the procedure (microperforation).

2.6. Management and Clinical Evaluation after the Procedure. Perforations confirmed or suspected during the endoscopic procedure were promptly closed using endoclips (HX-610-090L; Olympus, Tokyo, Japan) with or without detachable snares (MAJ 254 and MAJ 340; Olympus, Tokyo, Japan) (Figure 1). Some patients with perforation underwent percutaneous needle aspiration and received intravenous (IV) pain killers during or after the procedure to decrease their abdominal pain and were treated with antibiotics at the clinician's discretion. All patients with perforation underwent fasting until the peritoneal irritation sign and white blood cell (WBC) counts improved.

WBC counts, vital signs, physical exams, the degree of abdominal pain using a numerical rating scale, the amount of peritoneal free air, and the number of additional intravenous pain killers needed after the procedure were checked to evaluate the presence of peritonitis or sepsis. The maximum value for the white blood cell counts, heart rate, body temperature, the amount of free air, and the abdominal pain score within 24 hrs after the procedure were examined. The amount of peritoneal free air was measured using the length between the middle right diaphragm and the middle upper liver margin on a plain chest X-ray. The additional IV pain killers used after the procedure included meperidine and tramadol.

The patients underwent surgery when clinical symptoms and signs became worse depending on the judgment of the clinicians. Additional surgery was performed for EGCa that did not fulfill the extended criteria. The patients who underwent additional surgery for curative resection were classified into the nonsurgery group.

2.7. Statistical Analysis. Descriptive statistics were computed for all variables. Continuous data were compared using the Mann-Whitney U test. In univariate analysis, categorical data were compared using the χ^2 test or Fisher's exact test. Multivariate analysis was performed using logistic regression analysis with backward method for variables with $P < 0.05$ in univariate analyses to confirm the risk factors related to surgery caused by perforation. Variables with $P < 0.05$ in multivariate analyses were determined as the risk factors. All analyses were performed using SPSS for Windows (version 19; SPSS Inc., Chicago, IL, USA).

3. Results

3.1. Characteristics of the Patients with Gastric Lesions and Perforations. A total of 1183 patients received gastric ER. ESD and EMR were performed in 425 and 758 patients, respectively. Perforation occurred in 69 (5.8%) patients. Among these patients, perforations occurred in 60 (14.1%) patients in the ESD group and 9 (1.2%) patients in the EMR group.

In the 69 patients, the median age was 63 (48–85) years, and 44 of the 69 patients were male (63.8%). The most common vertical location and circumferential location of the perforation were in the middle third and the lesser curvature, respectively. The median size of the resected specimen was 4.0 (0.7–14.0) cm. The pathology of the lesion included adenomas in 36 cases, EGCa in 20 cases, gastrointestinal stromal tumors in seven cases, and other types of tumors in six cases. The median procedure time was 39 (6–215) min. Macroperforation and microperforation occurred in 45 (65.2%) patients and 24 (34.8%) patients, respectively. The basic characteristics of the 69 patients and their gastric lesions are summarized in Table 1.

3.2. Management and Clinical Symptoms within 24 hrs. Percutaneous needle aspiration within 24 hrs after perforation was performed in nine (13.0%) patients. The median use of postprocedure pain killers was one (1–7). The median size of free

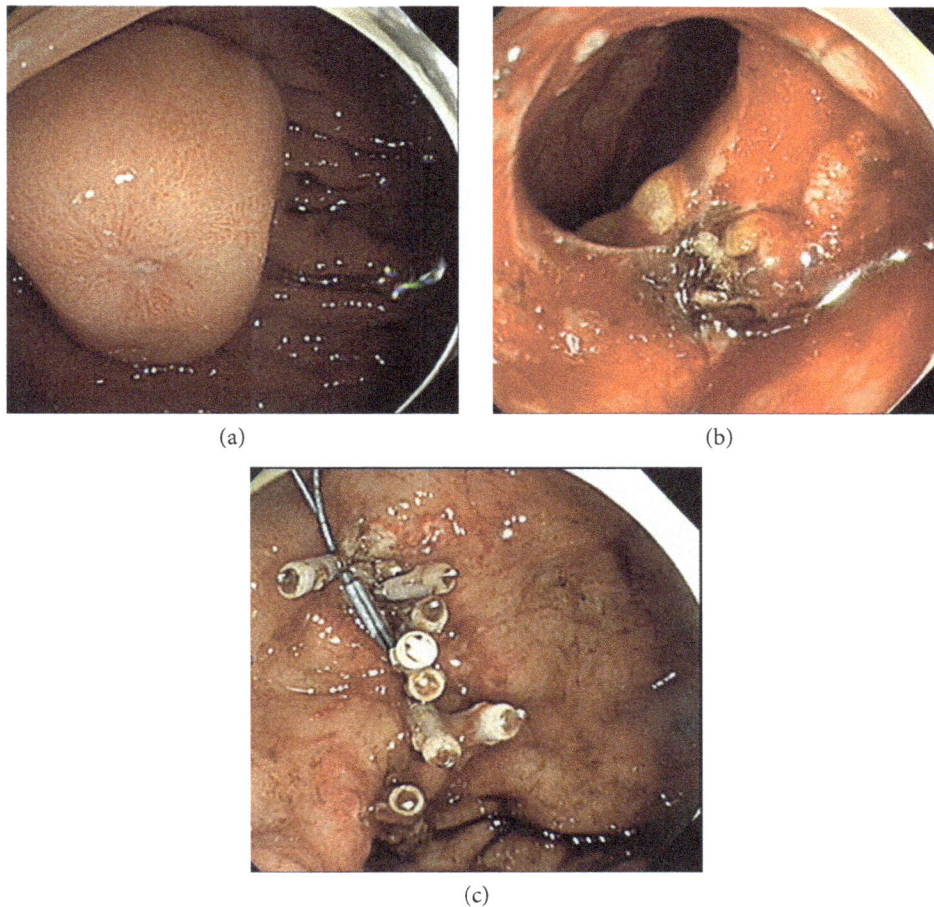

FIGURE 1: (a) A 2.8 cm GIST was observed on the anterior wall of the fundus. (b) An intra-abdominal space was detected through the perforation site during the procedure. (c) The perforation site was successfully closed using endoclips and a detachable snare.

air in the abdominal cavity was 2.6 (0.0–7.9) cm. The median count of white blood cells was 10,820/mm^3 (6190–21,540), and the median degree of body temperature was 36.3 (36.0–38.2) °C. The median heart rate was 78/min (56–112).

3.3. Surgery. 12 patients who received ESD underwent surgery following gastric perforation. In the EMR group, there were no patients who underwent surgery. Nine out of 12 underwent surgery because of peritonitis and sepsis caused by gastric perforation. The remaining three patients completely recovered with conservative management but received additional surgery due to noncurative resections. Therefore, these three patients were allocated into the non-surgery group (Figure 2). Among the nine patients, six, one, and two patients received surgery on the first, second, and fifth day after the procedure, respectively. Distal gastrectomy and laparoscopic wedge resections were performed in 2 and 7 patients, respectively (Table 2). All the nine patients have fully recovered after surgery and were discharged.

3.4. Risk Factors for Surgery Caused by ER-Induced Gastric Perforation. In univariate analyses, the following were identified as factors associated with surgery: location of

the lesion on the anterior wall ($P = 0.000$), a subepithelial lesion ($P = 0.021$), two or more postprocedure pain killers within 24 hrs ($P = 0.000$), and increased heart rate (≥ 100, $P = 0.026$) within 24 hrs after the procedure (Table 3). A logistic regression analysis for these four variables revealed that the location of the lesion on the anterior wall (odds ratio (OR) 20.56; 95% confidence interval (CI) 2.79–151.77, $P = 0.003$) and two or more postprocedure pain killers within 24 hrs (OR 15.13, 95% CI 2.03–112.72, $P = 0.008$) were the risk factors for surgery (Table 4).

4. Discussion

Gastric perforation is a serious complication associated with EMR and ESD. Although most perforations are managed through conservative treatment with endoscopic closure, surgery is needed in 2.5~3.3% of patients with perforation [12–14]. Previous studies reported that the upper area of the stomach, piecemeal resection, and long procedure times were risk factors associated with perforation after ESD [13–16, 20]. The upper area of the stomach has a thinner wall compared to other areas of the stomach and is more difficult to approach. Piecemeal resection may result from perforation that leads to

TABLE 1: Basic characteristics of the 69 patients with perforation.

	Total ($n = 69$)	Nonsurgery group ($n = 60$)	Surgery group ($n = 9$)	P value
Age, median (range) (years)	63 (48–85)	64 (48–85)	62 (50–76)	0.695
Male sex, n (%)	44 (63.8)	38 (63.3)	6 (66.7)	1.000
Location (vertical), n (%)				0.888
Upper third	16 (23.2)	14 (23.3)	2 (22.2)	
Middle third	38 (55.1)	32 (53.3)	6 (66.7)	
Lower third	15 (21.7)	14 (23.3)	1 (11.1)	
Location (circumferential), n (%)				0.000
Anterior wall	14 (18.8)	7 (11.7)	7 (77.8)	
Posterior wall	18 (26.1)	18 (30.0)	0 (0.0)	
Lesser curvature	24 (34.8)	24 (40.0)	0 (0.0)	
Greater curvature	13 (18.8)	11 (18.3)	2 (22.2)	
Resected size, median (range) (cm)	4.0 (0.7–14.0)	4.0 (1.2–10.0)	4.0 (0.7–14.0)	0.748
Histologic type, n (%)				0.008
Adenoma	36 (52.2)	34 (56.7)	2 (22.2)	
Early gastric cancer	20 (29.0)	18 (30.0)	2 (22.2)	
Gastrointestinal stromal tumor	7 (10.2)	5 (8.3)	2 (22.2)	
Leiomyoma	1 (1.4)	1 (1.7)	0 (0.0)	
Schwannoma	2 (2.9)	0 (0.0)	2 (22.2)	
No residual tumor	3 (4.3)	2 (3.3)	1 (11.1)	
Endoscopic procedure, n (%)				0.594
EMR	9 (13.0)	9 (15.0)	0 (0.0)	
ESD	60 (87.0)	51 (85.0)	9 (100)	
Procedure time, median (range) (min)	39 (6–215)	38 (6–215)	39 (8–109)	0.803
En bloc resection, n (%)	62 (89.9)	53 (88.3)	9 (100)	0.582
Complete resection, n (%)	53 (76.8)	48 (80.0)	5 (55.6)	0.197
Perforation, n (%)				0.147
Macroperforation	45 (65.2)	37 (61.7)	8 (88.9)	
Microperforation	24 (34.8)	23 (38.3)	1 (11.1)	
Endoclip use, n (%)	55 (79.7)	46 (76.7)	9 (100)	0.187
Percutaneous needle aspiration, n (%)	9 (13.0)	7 (11.7)	2 (22.2)	0.333
Size of the free air in the abdominal cavity, median (range) (cm)	2.6 (0.0–7.9)	2.5 (0.0–7.9)	4.1 (0.0–7.3)	0.838
Abdominal pain score (NRS), median (range)	4 (0–10)	2.0 (0–10)	6 (4–7)	0.002
Postprocedure pain killer use, median (range)	1 (0–7)	0 (0–5)	3 (1–7)	0.000
WBC count, median (range) (mm^3)	10,820 (6,190–21,540)	10,655 (6,190–19,140)	10,870 (9,450–21,540)	0.318
Body temperature, median (range) (°C)	36.3 (36.0–38.2)	36.3 (36.0–38.2)	36.7 (36.0–38.2)	0.149
Heart rate/min, median (range)	78 (56–112)	76 (56–112)	84 (68–110)	0.033

EMR: endoscopic mucosal resection; ESD: endoscopic submucosal dissection.

irritability in patients and difficulty in procedure. Long procedure times may be due to the large size of the lesion and may be dependent on the experience of the endoscopist. Previous studies focused on the risk factors associated with the development of perforation. Most perforations can be managed conservatively with endoscopic closure. However, surgery is required in rare cases. The risk factors associated with surgery after iatrogenic colon perforation have been reported [21]. However, no study has investigated the risk factors for surgery after ER-induced gastric perforation; thus, we performed this study.

In the present study, we found that two or more postprocedure pain killers within 24 hrs was a risk factor for surgery caused by gastric perforation. The greater use of postprocedure pain killers to control pain might imply an incomplete closure of the perforation site or the continuous leakage of gastric contents through the perforation site, which will lead to peritonitis or sepsis. Therefore, surgery should be considered in patients with uncontrolled pain who do not respond to analgesics.

Additionally, the location of the lesion on the anterior wall was a risk factor for surgery in this study. In this study,

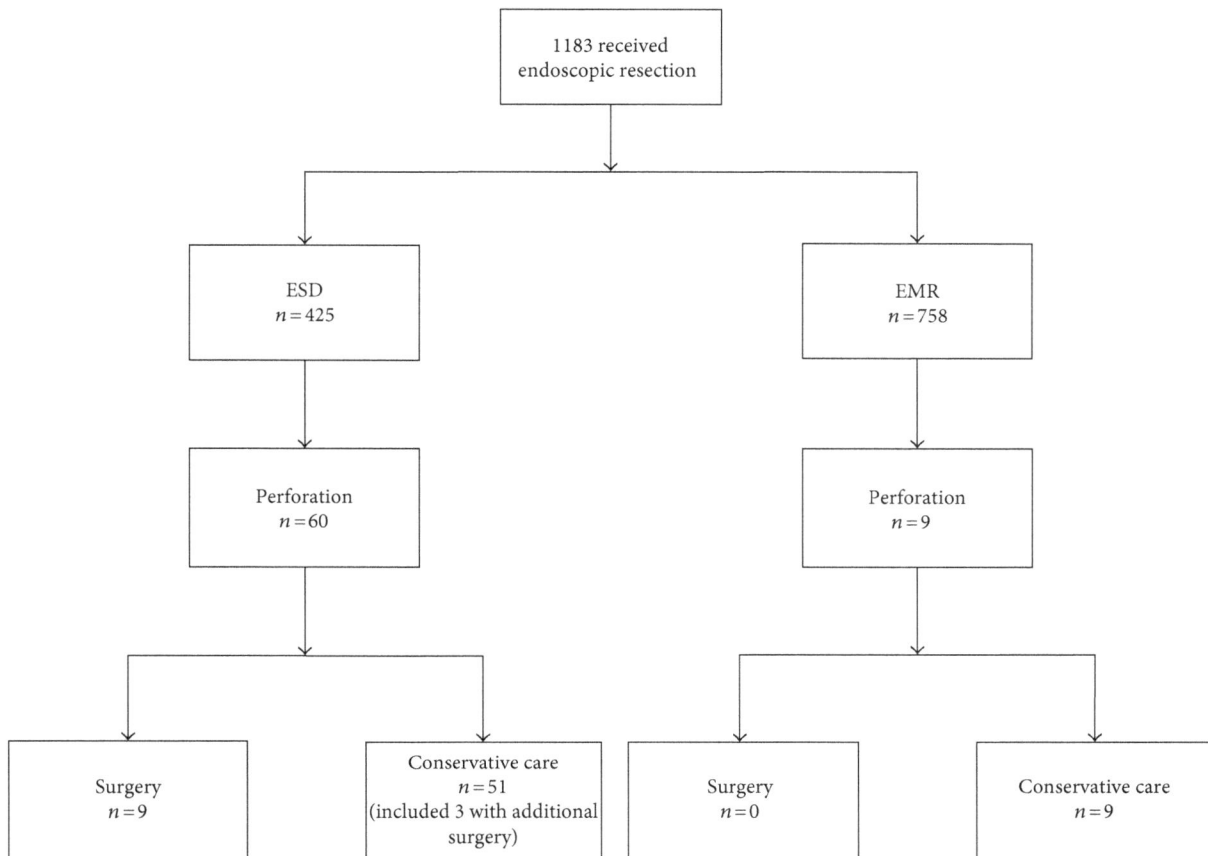

FIGURE 2: Patient selection and the clinical course of patients after gastric perforation caused by endoscopic resection. EMR, endoscopic mucosal resection; ESD, endoscopic submucosal dissection.

7 out of the 9 patients who underwent surgery had lesions located on the anterior wall; 6 out of the 7 patients had lesions in the upper or middle third of the stomach. Lesions on the anterior wall and in the upper and middle third appear to be in a difficult location to access and handle instruments. If a perforation occurs in that location, complete closure with endoscopic clips may be difficult. In addition, endoscopic procedures are normally performed in the lateral decubitus status, and gastric contents and blood clots may present in the upper area of the stomach due to gravity [22]. These materials can interrupt the visual field of the endoscopist and also interfere with endoscopic management when a perforation occurs. Additionally, these materials might leak through the perforation site during the procedure and induce peritonitis. Therefore, endoscopic closure should be performed earlier and more meticulously for lesions that are located on the anterior wall of the upper area of the stomach. If endoscopic closure is not performed satisfactorily, early surgery should be considered in patients with a perforation in this location.

According to a report by Cho et al. [21], the risk factors for early surgery after iatrogenic colonic perforation included large perforation (size ≥ 1 cm), leukocytosis (>10,000/mm^3), fever $\geq 37.0^\circ$C, severe abdominal pain (narcotic pain killer use ≥ 2), and a large amount of peritoneal free air (≥ 3 cm).

Among these risk factors, the only risk factor related to surgery after iatrogenic gastric perforation in the present study was two or more postprocedure pain killers within 24 hrs. The disparity in luminal contents may explain the difference in the risk factors for surgery after iatrogenic perforation of the colon and the stomach. Additionally, the present study included only perforations caused by ER, while the study by Cho et al. included perforations caused by diagnostic and therapeutic colonoscopy. The mechanism of perforation is different between diagnostic and therapeutic endoscopy [23, 24]. Most diagnostic perforations result from mechanical damage by the tip and shaft of the scope or a traction mechanism injury, while therapeutic perforation results from thermal injury. Therefore, diagnostic perforations are larger in size [25, 26] and need more surgical management than therapeutic perforation [24, 25]. This difference could lead to inconsistent results between the study by Cho et al. and the present study.

It is important for the attending physician to be able to determine when surgery is needed after gastric perforation caused by ER. Emergency surgery performed at night due to the deterioration of a patient's condition would be very stressful for both the surgeon and the patient. In order to avoid these worst-case scenarios, we believe, it is necessary to identify factors suggesting the need for surgery.

TABLE 2: Clinical characteristics, endoscopic findings, histology, surgical methods, and treatment results of patients with surgery.

Patient number	Sex	Age (years)	Tumor site (location/circumference)	Size[a] of the resected specimen (cm)	Histology	Time of surgery after ER (day)	Cause of surgery	Surgical method	Hospital stay (day)	Results of surgery
1	M	72	Middle third/anterior	4.0	EGCa	1	Peritonitis	LWR	28	Survival
2	M	62	Lower third/anterior	15.0	Adenoma	1	Peritonitis	TLDG c Billroth I anastomosis	9	Survival
3	M	60	Middle third/anterior	7.5	Adenoma	1	Peritonitis	LWR	6	Survival
4	F	76	Middle third/anterior	5.0	Adenoma	1	Peritonitis	LWR	17	Survival
5	M	54	Upper third/anterior	1.3	GIST	1	Peritonitis	LWR	8	Survival
6	M	62	Upper third/GC	5.5	EGCa	1	Peritonitis	DSG with Billroth II anastomosis	10	Survival
7	M	69	Upper third/anterior	1.0	GIST	5	Peritonitis	LWR	4	Survival
8	F	63	Middle third/GC	0.7	Schwannoma	5	Peritonitis	LWR	19	Survival
9	F	50	Middle third/anterior	3.0	Schwannoma	2	Peritonitis	LWR	8	Survival

[a]Tumor size was determined by the measurement of the ER specimen.
DSG: distal subtotal gastrectomy; EGCa: early gastric cancer; ER: endoscopic resection; GC: greater curvature; GIST: gastrointestinal stromal tumor; LWR: laparoscopic wedge resection; TLDG: totally laparoscopic distal gastrectomy.

TABLE 3: A univariate analysis of variables associated with surgery caused by gastric perforation after endoscopic resection.

Variable	Nonsurgery group ($n = 60$)	Surgery group ($n = 9$)	P value
Age ≥ 70 (years)	22 (36.7)	2 (22.2)	0.480
Male sex, n (%)	38 (63.3)	6 (66.7)	1.000
Location (vertical), upper third, n (%)	13 (21.7)	3 (33.3)	1.000
Location (circumferential), anterior, n (%)	7 (11.7)	7 (77.8)	0.000
Resected size ≥ 3 (cm), n (%)	49 (81.7)	6 (66.7)	0.373
Subepithelial lesion, n (%)	6 (10.0)	4 (44.4)	0.021
ESD, n (%)	51 (85.0)	9 (100)	0.594
En bloc resection, n (%)	53 (88.3)	9 (100)	0.582
Macroperforation, n (%)	37 (61.7)	8 (88.9)	0.147
Size of free air in the abdominal cavity ≥ 3 (cm), n (%)	35 (58.3)	3 (33.3)	0.281
Abdominal pain score (NRS) ≥ 7, n (%)	4 (6.7)	2 (22.2)	0.172
Postprocedure pain killer use ≥ 2, n (%)	9 (15.0)	7 (77.8)	0.000
WBC count > 12,000/mm^3, n (%)	14 (23.3)	3 (33.3)	0.679
Body temperature (>37.0°C), n (%)	9 (15.0)	3 (33.3)	0.183
Heart rate (≥ 100/min), n (%)	3 (5.0)	3 (33.3)	0.026

ESD: endoscopic submucosal dissection.

TABLE 4: Multivariate logistic regression analysis of risk factors for surgery caused by gastric perforation after endoscopic resection.

Variable	OR	95% CI	P value
Location (circumferential) Others versus anterior	20.56	2.79–151.77	0.003
Subepithelial lesion, n (%)	3.48	0.38–31.97	0.271
Postprocedure pain killer use ≥ 2, n (%)	15.13	2.03–112.72	0.008
Heart rate (≥ 100/min), n (%)	6.80	0.21–219.54	0.280

The present study has the following limitations: First, the present study was a retrospective study, which might lead to selection bias for the decision to perform surgery. Frequent use of pain killers may have influenced the endoscopists' decision to perform earlier surgery. In our experience, pain killers were not frequently needed when the perforation site is completely closed by clips. Thus, we believe that the need for two or more pain killers suggests inadequate closures and these patients may benefit from an earlier decision to surgery. Second, this was a single-center study with a small sample size. A multicenter study with a large sample size may be needed to apply the results of this study more generally. Finally, the perforation rate of ESD was higher than that of the previous reports and may have influenced the results.

5. Conclusion

In conclusion, the present study showed that the location of the lesion (on the anterior wall) and two or more postprocedure pain killers within 24 hrs were the risk factors for surgery caused by gastric perforation after ER. Therefore, early surgery for gastric perforation caused by ER should be considered in patients with these risk factors.

Competing Interests

The authors declare that there is no conflict of interests regarding the publication of this paper.

References

[1] Y. W. Min, B. H. Min, J. H. Lee, and J. J. Kim, "Endoscopic treatment for early gastric cancer," *World Journal of Gastroenterology*, vol. 20, no. 16, pp. 4566–4573, 2014.

[2] H. J. Chun, B. Keum, J. H. Kim, and S. Y. Seol, "Current status of endoscopic submucosal dissection for the management of early gastric cancer: a Korean perspective," *World Journal of Gastroenterology*, vol. 17, no. 21, pp. 2592–2596, 2011.

[3] M. Kato, T. Nishida, S. Tsutsui et al., "Endoscopic submucosal dissection as a treatment for gastric noninvasive neoplasia: a multicenter study by Osaka University ESD study group," *Journal of Gastroenterology*, vol. 46, no. 3, pp. 325–331, 2011.

[4] Z. He, C. Sun, Z. Zheng et al., "Endoscopic submucosal dissection of large gastrointestinal stromal tumors in the esophagus and stomach," *Journal of Gastroenterology and Hepatology*, vol. 28, no. 2, pp. 262–267, 2013.

[5] L. Wang, C. Q. Fan, W. Ren, X. Zhang, Y. H. Li, and X. Y. Zhao, "Endoscopic dissection of large endogenous myogenic tumors in the esophagus and stomach is safe and feasible: a

report of 42 cases," *Scandinavian Journal of Gastroenterology*, vol. 46, no. 5, pp. 627–633, 2011.

[6] Y. I. Kim, Y. W. Kim, I. J. Choi et al., "Long-term survival after endoscopic resection versus surgery in early gastric cancers," *Endoscopy*, vol. 47, no. 4, pp. 293–301, 2015.

[7] P. W. Chiu, A. Y. Teoh, K. F. To et al., "Endoscopic submucosal dissection (ESD) compared with gastrectomy for treatment of early gastric neoplasia: a retrospective cohort study," *Surgical Endoscopy*, vol. 26, no. 12, pp. 3584–3591, 2012.

[8] C. H. Park, H. Lee, D. W. Kim et al., "Clinical safety of endoscopic submucosal dissection compared with surgery in elderly patients with early gastric cancer: a propensity-matchedanalysis," *Gastrointestinal Endoscopy*, vol. 80, no. 4, pp. 599–609, 2014.

[9] J. H. Choi, E. S. Kim, Y. J. Lee et al., "Comparison of quality of life and worry of cancer recurrence between endoscopic and surgical treatment for early gastric cancer," *Gastrointestinal Endoscopy*, vol. 82, no. 2, pp. 299–307, 2015.

[10] Y. M. Park, E. Cho, H. Y. Kang, and J. M. Kim, "The effectiveness and safety of endoscopic submucosal dissection compared with endoscopic mucosal resection for early gastric cancer: a systematic review and metaanalysis," *Surgical Endoscopy*, vol. 25, no. 8, pp. 2666–2677, 2011.

[11] J. Lian, S. Chen, Y. Zhang, and F. Qiu, "A meta-analysis of endoscopic submucosal dissection and EMR for early gastric cancer," *Gastrointestinal Endoscopy*, vol. 76, no. 4, pp. 763–770, 2012.

[12] S. Minami, T. Gotoda, H. Ono, I. Oda, and H. Hamanaka, "Complete endoscopic closure of gastric perforation induced by endoscopic resection of early gastric cancer using endoclips can prevent surgery (with video)," *Gastrointestinal Endoscopy*, vol. 63, no. 4, pp. 596–601, 2006.

[13] K. Miyahara, R. Iwakiri, R. Shimoda et al., "Perforation and postoperative bleeding of endoscopic submucosal dissection in gastric tumors: analysis of 1190 lesions in low- and high-volume centers in Saga, Japan," *Digestion*, vol. 86, no. 3, pp. 273–280, 2012.

[14] M. Kim, S. W. Jeon, K. B. Cho et al., "Predictive risk factors of perforation in gastric endoscopic submucosal dissection for early gastric cancer: a large, multicenter study," *Surgical Endoscopy*, vol. 27, no. 4, pp. 1372–1378, 2013.

[15] K. Mannen, S. Tsunada, M. Hara et al., "Risk factors for complications of endoscopic submucosal dissection in gastric tumors: analysis of 478 lesions," *Journal of Gastroenterology*, vol. 45, no. 1, pp. 30–36, 2010.

[16] T. Ojima, K. Takifuji, M. Nakamura et al., "Complications of endoscopic submucosal dissection for gastric noninvasive neoplasia: an analysis of 647 lesions," *Surgical Laparoscopy, Endoscopy & Percutaneous Techniques*, vol. 24, no. 4, pp. 370–374, 2014.

[17] I. K. Chung, J. H. Lee, S. H. Lee et al., "Therapeutic outcomes in 1000 cases of endoscopic submucosal dissection for early gastric neoplasms: Korean ESD study group multicenter study," *Gastrointestinal Endoscopy*, vol. 69, no. 7, pp. 1228–1235, 2009.

[18] S. M. Park, J. S. Kim, J. S. Ji, H. Choi, B. I. Lee, and B. W. Kim, "Efficacy of endoscopic mucosal resections for the management of small gastric adenomas with low-grade dysplasia," *Scandinavian Journal of Gastroenterology*, vol. 50, no. 9, pp. 1175–1182, 2015.

[19] M. F. Dixon, "Gastrointestinal epithelial neoplasia: Vienna revisited," *Gut*, vol. 51, no. 1, pp. 130–131, 2002.

[20] T. Toyokawa, T. Inaba, S. Omote et al., "Risk factors for perforation and delayed bleeding associated with endoscopic submucosal dissection for early gastric neoplasms: analysis of 1123 lesions," *Journal of Gastroenterology and Hepatology*, vol. 27, no. 5, pp. 907–912, 2012.

[21] S. B. Cho, W. S. Lee, Y. E. Joo et al., "Therapeutic options for iatrogenic colon perforation: feasibility of endoscopic clip closure and predictors of the need for early surgery," *Surgical Endoscopy*, vol. 26, no. 2, pp. 473–479, 2012.

[22] H. Mori, H. Kobara, S. Fujihara et al., "Accurate hemostasis with a new endoscopic overtube for emergency endoscopy," *World Journal of Gastroenterology*, vol. 19, no. 17, pp. 2723–2726, 2013.

[23] J. Castellvi, F. Pi, A. Sueiras et al., "Colonoscopic perforation: useful parameters for early diagnosis and conservative treatment," *International Journal of Colorectal Disease*, vol. 26, no. 9, pp. 1183–1190, 2011.

[24] R. Magdeburg, M. Sold, S. Post, and G. Kaehler, "Differences in the endoscopic closure of colonic perforation due to diagnostic or therapeutic colonoscopy," *Scandinavian Journal of Gastroenterology*, vol. 48, no. 7, pp. 862–867, 2013.

[25] D. H. Yang, J. S. Byeon, K. H. Lee et al., "Is endoscopic closure with clips effective for both diagnostic and therapeutic colonoscopy-associated bowel perforation?" *Surgical Endoscopy*, vol. 24, no. 5, pp. 1177–1185, 2010.

[26] A. Y. Lo and H. L. Beaton, "Selective management of colonoscopic perforations," *Journal of the American College of Surgeons*, vol. 179, no. 3, pp. 333–337, 1994.

14

Extrahepatic Autoimmune Diseases in Patients with Autoimmune Liver Diseases: A Phenomenon Neglected by Gastroenterologists

Liping Guo,[1] Lu Zhou,[1] Na Zhang,[2] Baoru Deng,[1] and Bangmao Wang[1]

[1]*Department of Gastroenterology and Hepatology, Tianjin Medical University General Hospital, Tianjin 300052, China*
[2]*Department of Rheumatology, Tianjin Medical University General Hospital, Tianjin 300052, China*

Correspondence should be addressed to Lu Zhou; zhou_lu@126.com and Bangmao Wang; bmwang0926@outlook.com

Academic Editor: Paolo Gionchetti

Autoimmune liver diseases (AILDs) often coexist with other extrahepatic autoimmune diseases (EHAIDs). The spectrum of EHAIDs in patients with AILDs is similar, whereas the incidence is different. Notably, autoimmune thyroid disease and Sjogren's syndrome are the most common EHAIDs. Associated extrahepatic diseases may predate the appearance of AILDs or coincide with their onset. More frequently, they may appear during the course and even occur years after the diagnosis of AILDs. Importantly, associated EHAIDs may influence the natural course and prognosis of AILDs. To date, a definite pathophysiological pathway which contributes to the coexistence of AILDs and EHAIDs is still lacking. The current view of autoimmunity clustering involves a common susceptibility genetic background which applies to related pathologies. Herein, we review the current published researches regarding EHAIDs in patients with AILDs, particularly in relation to their clinical impact and pathophysiology. In managing patients with AILDs, gastroenterologists should be aware of the possibly associated EHAIDs to ensure a prompt diagnosis and better outcome.

1. Introduction

Autoimmune liver diseases (AILDs) fall into two broad categories, those with hepatic predominance such as autoimmune hepatitis (AIH) and those with predominance of cholestatic features such as primary biliary cirrhosis (PBC) and primary sclerosing cholangitis (PSC). The concurrence of clinical, biochemical, serological, and/or histological features suggesting AIH and PBC (or PSC) has been described as overlap syndrome (OS). Importantly, AILDs also coexist with other extrahepatic autoimmune diseases (EHAIDs) and conditions, thereby causing not only liver damage, but also extrahepatic injury. However, the relationship between AILDs and concomitant EHAIDs is strongly debated. Currently, two hypotheses exist: (i) it is thought that AILDs are part of multiple organ involvement in a systemic autoimmune disease, particularly in non-organ specific autoimmune diseases such as systemic lupus erythematosus (SLE), rheumatoid arthritis (RA), systemic sclerosis (SSc), and Sjogren's syndrome (SS);

(ii) it is thought that AILDs and concomitant extrahepatic autoimmune conditions are different disorders, linked by a common pathogenetic pathway, for example, the coexistence of AILDs and chronic lymphocytic thyroiditis, hyperthyroidism, myasthenia gravis, or pernicious anemia. Herein, we discuss EHAIDs in patients with AILDs, particularly in relation to their clinical impact and pathophysiology.

2. The Spectrum of EHIADs in Patients with AILDs

The spectrum of EHAIDs in patients with AILDs is similar in current reports, whereas the incidence is different (Table 1). Notably, autoimmune thyroid disease (AITD) and SS are the most common EHAIDs in patients with AILDs. Associated extrahepatic diseases may predate the appearance of AILDs or coincide with their onset. More frequently, they may appear during the course and even occur years after the

TABLE 1: Incidence of concomitant EHAIDs in AILDs.

	EHAIDs	Sjogren's syndrome	Autoimmune thyroid disease	Systemic lupus erythematosus	Rheumatoid arthritis	Systemic sclerosis or scleroderma	Inflammatory bowel disease	Dermatomyositis or polymyositis	Raynaud's phenomenon	Mixed connective tissue disease	Autoimmune thrombocytopenic purpura	Pernicious anemia	References
AIH	29.9–61.8%	1.4–34.5%	10.0–23.0%	0.7–18.8%	1.8–12.9%	1.2–3.5%	2.0–8.0%	3.6%	—	2.0–4.0%	1 case	—	[3–7]
PBC	36.5–67.4%	3.5–47.4%	14.4–23.8%	1.0–5.2%	1.8–17.0%	0.8–12.3%	2.0–7.5%	0.6–3.1%	18.0–24.0%	0.6–0.8%	1.0%	4.0%	[3, 8–11]
PBC-AIH OS	25.0–43.7%	8.5–20.8%	18.3%	2.8%	4.2%	1.4%	—	1 case	—	—	1 case	1.4%	[12–14]
PSC	60.0–80.0%	2 cases	7.6%	2 cases	5.6%	1 case	1.7–70.0%	—	—	—	—	—	[15–18]

EHAID: extrahepatic autoimmune disease; AILD: autoimmune liver disease; AIH: autoimmune hepatitis; PBC: primary biliary cirrhosis; PSC: primary sclerosing cholangitis; OS: overlap syndrome.

TABLE 2: Liver involvement in CTDs.

	Liver involvement	AIH	PBC	PSC	References
Systemic lupus erythematosus	3.0–79.0%	2.7–20.0%	2.7–15.0%	1 case	[1, 19–29]
Sjogren's syndrome	7.0–49.0%	6.0–47.0%	35.0–57.0%	11 cases	[22, 29–31]
Systemic sclerosis or scleroderma	1.1%	11 cases	51.2%	51.2%	[22, 29, 32–34]
Antiphospholipid syndrome	—	5 cases	1 case	1 case	[13, 35–37]
Dermatomyositis or polymyositis	—	7.1%	14.3%	—	[13, 38]

AIH: autoimmune hepatitis; PBC: primary biliary cirrhosis; PSC: primary sclerosing cholangitis.

diagnosis of AILDs. Watt et al. [1] reported that 84 of 160 (53%) PBC patients had at least one additional extrahepatic autoimmune condition, and 16 of 37 (43%) patients developed thyroid diseases prior to the detection of PBC, while 19 of 37 (51%) patients detected thyroid diseases at the same time or following the diagnosis of PBC; 10 of 12 (83%) patients developed sclerosis symptoms prior to the detection of PBC. Another report also showed that the onset time of AIH and dermatomyositis (DM) was uneven [2]. While explanations for the discrepancies in incidence and onset time are lacking, different geographical and genetic backgrounds in studies may be involved.

3. Nonspecific Liver Involvement or AILDs in the Course of EHIADs

Autoimmunity clustering frequently increases the difficulty of diagnosis. It is clinically important for gastroenterologists to early screen patients with AILDs for concomitant EHIADs and to make an accurate diagnosis according to their respective diagnostic criteria. Connective tissue diseases (CTDs) are systemic disorders that have an autoimmune basis and involve multiple organs or tissues, such as liver, kidney, and lung. Indeed, patients with CTDs often have concomitant liver abnormalities; about 3.0–79.0% of patients with SLE and 7.0–49.0% of patients with SS showed liver dysfunction (Table 2). When confronted with such patients, gastroenterologists need to classify these liver abnormalities as a primary liver disease with associated autoimmune, clinical, and laboratory features or a generalized liver involvement manifestation of CTDs. The classical example of this differential diagnosis dilemma is AIH and CTDs associated hepatitis, both of which have autoimmune symptoms. Antinuclear antibody (ANA) and immunoglobulin (Ig) G are not unique in AIH, which can be also positive in CTDs. On the other hand, patients with CTDs often show liver abnormalities as mentioned before. Therefore, it is big confusion to distinguish them just according to symptoms, physical signs, and autoantibodies. Liver biopsy may be helpful in such patients. Histopathological manifestations of CTDs associated hepatitis may vary from subclinical liver diseases with nonspecific changes to chronic active hepatitis, chronic persistent hepatitis, fibrosis, cirrhosis, nodular regenerative hyperplasia, and so on [17, 21].

Otherwise, external factors such as drugs can trigger susceptible patients with risk alleles of the major histocompatibility complex (MHC). Drug-induced autoimmune liver disease (DIAILD) refers to the latent autoimmunity with positive autoantibodies, including drug-induced liver injury (DILI), drug-induced-AIH (DI-AIH), and immunity mediated DILI (IM-DILI) [39]. It is important to remember that another main cause of biochemical liver abnormalities in patients with CTDs is drug-induced alterations. Almost all drugs in the armamentarium against SLE or other rheumatologic diseases may lead to liver toxicity, such as nonsteroidal anti-inflammatory drugs (NSAIDs). NSAID-associated liver injuries vary from slightly biochemical and histological abnormalities to severe liver fibrosis, cirrhosis, chronic liver failure, or even fulminant hepatic failure [22, 23]. A prospective study found that 28 of 260 (10.8%) patients with active SLE showed salicylate poisoning and biochemical liver abnormalities. In this study, 14 patients underwent liver biopsies, by which a nonspecific inflammatory reaction was confirmed. Additionally, immunosuppressive drugs such as antitumor necrosis factor- (TNF-) α were reported to induce liver injuries. The immune-mediated drug reaction in the liver must be monitored during using biologics [40]. Histological performances of AIH and DILI have certain similarities, including interface hepatitis, inflammatory cells infiltration in portal area, and centrilobular 3 zone necrosis [17, 41]. Suzuki et al. [42] compared 35 cases of DILI with 28 cases of AIH according to Ishak score, portal inflammatory cell types, penetration phenomenon, rosette, and cholestasis. The results showed that interface hepatitis, focal necrosis, and portal inflammation existed both in AIH and DILI; however, neutrophils infiltration in portal area and cholestasis were more common in DILI. In addition, Suzuki et al. [42] suggested that compared with AIH DILI had no obvious liver fibrosis. Other studies indicated that eosinophils infiltration was more common in DILI, but some findings showed that eosinophils infiltration was not conducive to distinguish DILI from AIH [31]. Therefore, in addition to medication history and clinical manifestations, liver biopsy is crucial to assist in distinguishing AILDs in the course of EHAIDs from CTDs associated or drug-induced liver injuries.

4. The Impact of Concomitant EHAIDs on the Natural Course and Prognosis of AILDs

Whether the concomitant EHAIDs affect the natural course and prognosis of AILDs is unclear as only a few related researches have been carried out. In a latest study from UK, Wong et al. [6] systematically assessed features and clinical impact of EHAID on AIH. Autoimmune skin diseases were more prevalent in AIH-2 than AIH-1 (21.9% versus 7.0%,

P = 0.009), which suggested that presence of EHAIDs might influence clinical phenotype of AIH at presentation. Personal history of EHAIDs was more commonly found in AIH patients with than without first-degree family history of EHAIDs [48/86 (55.8%) versus 169/446 (37.9%), P = 0.002]. AIH patients with EHAIDs were more often women (85.2% versus 76.1%, P = 0.008), had higher posttreatment IAIHG score (22 versus 20, P < 0.001), had less reactivity to smooth muscle antibodies (49.8% versus 65.0%, P < 0.001), were more likely to have mild fibrosis at diagnosis (20.9% versus 6.5%, P < 0.001), and less often had ascites (6.3% versus 13.6%, P = 0.008) and coagulopathy (1.18 versus 1.27, P = 0.013) at presentation. However, presence of EHAIDs did not significantly affect disease progression, prognosis, and survival in AIH.

Muratori et al. [43] investigated 608 Italian patients with AILDs (327 with AIH and 281 with PBC) for concomitant EHAIDs and assessed the incidence and clinical impact of associated EHAIDs on AILDs. AIH patients with EHAIDs showed significant female predominance (male/female: 63/163 versus 9/91). In addition, an EHAID was more often detected in patients with an onset of AIH devoid of any particular liver-related symptoms, and the concomitant EHAIDs did not modify the features of PBC patients.

Wang et al. [19] screened 322 Chinese PBC patients for the presence of CTDs and identified the differences in clinical features and laboratory findings between PBC patients with or without CTDs. Compared to patients with PBC alone, PBC-SLE patients had lower γ-glutamyl transpeptidase (γ-GGT) and immunoglobulin M (IgM) levels, suggesting that presence of SLE in PBC patients appeared to be associated with significantly less extensive liver damage and SLE might protect against progression of PBC by delaying cirrhosis and the need for liver transplantation; PBC-RA patients had higher serum immunoglobulin G (IgG) and alkaline phosphatase (ALP) levels, suggesting that presence of RA might be a harmful factor in the prognosis of PBC. The presence of SS, SSc, and polymyositis (PM) did not seem to have any impact on the clinical course and prognosis of PBC; however, their unique features emerged. PBC-SS patients were more likely to have fever and elevated erythrocyte sedimentation rate (ESR), a higher incidence of rheumatoid factor (RF) seropositivity, and interstitial lung disease (ILD), suggesting that patients with concomitant autoimmune disorders might have an aggravated inflammatory response; PBC-SSc patients had a higher incidence of ILD; PBC-PM patients had a higher white blood cell (WBC) count and incidence of myocardial involvement. In another study, adjusting for sex, age, log bilirubin, and ALP, the risk of transplantation or death from diagnosis was significantly lower in PBC-SSc (hazard ratio 0.116, P = 0.01) [44], suggesting that PBC patients with SSc had a better prognosis.

As mentioned before, the first two researches investigated the features and clinical impact of concomitant EHAIDs on AIH patients. Similar result was female predominance in AIH patients with concomitant EHAIDs. Besides analyses of some clinical features at AIH presentation and prognosis, Wong et al. [6] paid more attention to the personal and family EHAIDs history and impact of EHAIDs on AIH clinical phenotype.

The other three researches all analyzed the clinical features and prognosis of PBC patients with or without concomitant EHAIDs. Wang et al. [19] found that SLE or RA might be a beneficial or harmful factor in the prognosis of PBC, and SS, SSc, and PM seemed to have no impact on the clinical course and prognosis of PBC. However, the last paper suggested that concomitant SSc significantly lowered the risk of transplantation or death in PBC patients. Taken together, different EHAIDs may have different influences on the natural course and prognosis of AILDs. Certain EHAIDs may aggravate the systemic inflammatory response and liver damage, and others may alleviate the liver inflammatory response, consequently achieving a better prognosis. Meanwhile, it is worth paying more attention to the higher incidence of ILD in autoimmune clustering. Of course, differences between the researches may be due to entirely different population backgrounds. Furthermore, some multicenter researches with a large sample size and different population background are needed to explore and verify these findings.

5. Common Pathophysiological Pathways in AILDs and EHAIDs

Autoimmune diseases appear to result from a complex series of interactions between susceptibility genes, environment, and immune system. However, the researches on pathophysiological pathways of concomitant autoimmune diseases are still relatively limited. Recently, with the development of molecular genetics, human genome-wide association studies (GWAs) and risk-associated single nucleotide polymorphism (SNP) have revealed that these patterns of coexistence/overlap depend predominantly on genetic determinants [24–26, 32, 33, 35–38]. Most of these so-called susceptible gene loci are widely distributed in many autoimmune diseases and thus contribute strongly to their coexistence. The recently completed GWAs reported a significant connection between PBC and STAT4, which is also the prominent risk gene in AITD, type 1 diabetes, SLE, RA, SS, and inflammatory bowel disease (IBD) [24, 32, 36, 45]. Notably, the most commonly recorded connection between MHC and SSc was the HLA-B8, a DR3-containing haplotype. Interestingly, a high frequency of HLA-DR3 detected in PSC patients was also noted. Similarly, HLA-DRB1, HLA-DRB3, and HLA-DR4 have been suggested to contribute to the coexistence of PSC and IBD [46–49]. In addition, HLA-DR2, HLA-DR3, and IRF5 have been reported as the common susceptibility genes in both PBC and SS [25, 26], further indicating that a common genetic background contributes to the coexistence of AILDs and other extrahepatic autoimmune disorders.

The coexistence of SS and PBC is a major example of the so-called autoimmune clustering, and the underlying mechanism has been relatively well studied. Both of these autoimmune diseases are characterized by the progressive immune-mediated destruction of epithelial tissues, either in salivary and lacrimal glands or in the intrahepatic bile ducts. Antimitochondrial autoantibodies (AMAs) to the E2 subunit of the pyruvate dehydrogenase complex (PDC-E2) are serological hallmarks of PBC, which were detected in

95% of patients with PBC [50–52]. Surprisingly, the PBC autoantigen, PDC-E2, has been demonstrated to be present on the surface of salivary epithelial cells in the salivary glands of PBC patients with SS. Matsumoto et al. [53] found that SS and AILD had a similar immune and inflammatory response, especially $CD3^+$ T cells in related organizations, suggesting that the liver and salivary glands, lacrimal glands, or other secreting glands may have the same antigenicity. It is plausible to predict that on the basis of a similar susceptibility gene background environmental triggers (putatively infectious agents and xenobiotics) cause salivary or biliary epithelial cell apoptosis and immune tolerance breakdown to self-antigens which are not protected by PDC-E2, leading to the cellular immune response with predominant $CD4^+$ T cell infiltration and the mucosal immune response mediated by IgA [25, 26, 33, 38]. Therefore, common susceptibility gene backgrounds are involved in the pathophysiological pathways between PBC and SS.

Last but not least, autoimmune polyendocrine syndrome type 1 (APS-1) should be mentioned. It is a rare monogenetic recessive disorder caused by mutations in the autoimmune regulator (Aire) gene. Patients with APS-1 always developed SS, anemia, diabetes, alopecia, vitiligo, gastritis, and AIH, the last one affecting up to 20% of APS-1 patients [54], which provides a possible connection between AILD and some endocrine-associated autoimmune diseases. To summarize, common susceptibility genes, environmental triggers, and antigen cross-reaction cooperatively contribute to a possibly shared pathogenesis which is involved in the coexistence of AILDs and EHAIDs.

6. Conclusion

Commonly, more than one autoimmune condition can occur in same AILD patient. Herein, we discuss EHAIDs in patients with AILDs, particularly in relation to the clinical impact and pathophysiology of these diseases. The incidence of EHAIDs in AILDs and onset time of them can be different. These discrepancies might be explained by different geographical and genetic backgrounds between studies. Importantly, autoimmunity clustering frequently increases the difficulty of diagnosis. In particular, biochemical liver abnormalities in patients with CTDs are common, which may be the result of previous treatments with potentially hepatotoxic drugs or CTDs associated nonspecific liver involvement. Liver biopsy is crucial in distinguishing AILDs in the course of EHAIDs from CTDs associated or drug-induced liver injuries. In our review, it is worth mentioning that we first summarize and analyze a few researches regarding clinical features and impact of concomitant EHAIDs on AILDs. When overlapping with other extrahepatic autoimmune diseases, patients with AILDs manifest special clinical and laboratory features which may have an effect on the natural course and prognosis of AILDs. Certain EHAIDs may aggravate the systemic inflammatory response and liver damage, and others may alleviate the liver inflammatory response, consequently achieving a better prognosis. Furthermore, some multicenter researches with a large sample size and different population background are needed to explore and verify

these findings. Finally, we try to explore the pathophysiological pathway which contributes to the coexistence of AILDs and EHAIDs. Currently, it is widely recognized that a common susceptibility genetic background involves the autoimmunity clustering. Therefore, in managing patients with AILDs, gastroenterologists should be aware of concomitant EHAIDs to ensure a prompt diagnosis and better outcome. Future researches should pay more attention to the relationship between genomics and immune regulator factors and confirm a common and distinct pathway involved in the pathogeneses of autoimmunity clustering.

Competing Interests

The authors declare that they have no competing interests.

Authors' Contributions

Liping Guo wrote the paper; Lu Zhou, Na Zhang, Baoru Deng, and Bangmao Wang designed and reviewed the manuscript.

Acknowledgments

This work is supported by the National Natural Science Foundation of China (Grant no. 81200282 and no. 81470834).

References

[1] F. E. Watt, O. F. W. James, and D. E. J. Jones, "Patterns of autoimmunity in primary biliary cirrhosis patients and their families: a population-based cohort study," *QJM*, vol. 97, no. 7, pp. 397–406, 2004.

[2] C. Pamfil, E. Candrea, E. Berki, H. I. Popov, P. I. Radu, and S. Rednic, "Primary biliary cirrhosis—autoimmune hepatitis overlap syndrome associated with dermatomyositis, autoimmune thyroiditis and antiphospholipid syndrome," *Journal of Gastrointestinal and Liver Diseases*, vol. 24, no. 1, pp. 101–104, 2015.

[3] Y. Kurihara, T. Shishido, K. Oku et al., "Polymyositis associated with autoimmune hepatitis, primary biliary cirrhosis, and autoimmune thrombocytopenic purpura," *Modern Rheumatology*, vol. 21, no. 3, pp. 325–329, 2011.

[4] G. S. Hatzis, G. E. Fragoulis, A. Karatzaferis, I. Delladetsima, C. Barbatis, and H. M. Moutsopoulos, "Prevalence and longterm course of primary biliary cirrhosis in primary Sjögren's syndrome," *Journal of Rheumatology*, vol. 35, no. 10, pp. 2012–2016, 2008.

[5] R. Hua, H. Wu, X. W. Zhang, and Y. W. Sun, "Probable catastrophic antiphospholipid syndrome complicated with primary sclerosing cholangitis," *Journal of Digestive Diseases*, vol. 13, no. 11, pp. 601–603, 2012.

[6] G. W. Wong, T. Yeong, D. Lawrence et al., "Concurrent extrahepatic autoimmunity in autoimmune hepatitis: implications for diagnosis, clinical course and long-term outcomes," *Liver International*, 2016.

[7] G. W. Wong and M. A. Heneghan, "Association of extrahepatic manifestations with autoimmune hepatitis," *Digestive Diseases*, vol. 33, supplement 2, pp. 25–35, 2015.

[8] N. Bach and J. A. Odin, "Primary biliary cirrhosis: a Mount Sinai perspective," *The Mount Sinai Journal of Medicine*, vol. 70, no. 4, pp. 242–250, 2003.

[9] P. L. Bittencourt, A. Q. Farias, G. Porta et al., "Frequency of concurrent autoimmune disorders in patients with autoimmune hepatitis: effect of age, gender, and genetic background," *Journal of Clinical Gastroenterology*, vol. 42, no. 3, pp. 300–305, 2008.

[10] M. Kmieciak Le Corguillé, P. Rocher, C. Eugène et al., "Autoimmune hepatitis, acute pancreatitis, mixed connective tissue disease and Sjögren's syndrome. A case report," *Gastroenterologie Clinique et Biologique*, vol. 27, no. 8-9, pp. 840–841, 2003.

[11] M. J. Kaplan and R. W. Ike, "The liver is a common non-exocrine target in primary Sjögren's syndrome: a retrospective review," *BMC Gastroenterology*, vol. 2, article 21, 2002.

[12] S. Branger, N. Schleinitz, V. Veit et al., "Auto-immune hepatitis and antiphospholipids," *Revue de Medecine Interne*, vol. 28, no. 4, pp. 218–224, 2007.

[13] A. Floreani, I. Franceschet, N. Cazzagon et al., "Extrahepatic autoimmune conditions associated with primary biliary cirrhosis," *Clinical Reviews in Allergy and Immunology*, vol. 48, no. 2-3, pp. 192–197, 2015.

[14] J. K. Karp, E. K. Akpek, and R. A. Anders, "Autoimmune hepatitis in patients with primary Sjögren's syndrome: a series of two-hundred and two patients," *International Journal of Clinical and Experimental Pathology*, vol. 3, no. 6, pp. 582–586, 2010.

[15] T. Matsumoto, S. Kobayashi, H. Shimizu et al., "The liver in collagen diseases: pathologic study of 160 cases with particular reference to hepatic arteritis, primary biliary cirrhosis, autoimmune hepatitis and nodular regenerative hyperplasia of the liver," *Liver*, vol. 20, no. 5, pp. 366–373, 2000.

[16] C. Selmi, M. De Santis, and M. E. Gershwin, "Liver involvement in subjects with rheumatic disease," *Arthritis Research & Therapy*, vol. 13, no. 3, article 226, 2011.

[17] D. C. Rockey, S. H. Caldwell, Z. D. Goodman, R. C. Nelson, and A. D. Smith, "Liver biopsy," *Hepatology*, vol. 49, no. 3, pp. 1017–1044, 2009.

[18] E. A. Aleksandrova, E. Z. Burnevich, and E. A. Arion, "Systemic manifestations of primary sclerosing cholangitis," *Klinicheskaia Meditsina*, vol. 91, no. 4, pp. 38–42, 2013.

[19] L. Wang, F.-C. Zhang, H. Chen et al., "Connective tissue diseases in primary biliary cirrhosis: a population-based cohort study," *World Journal of Gastroenterology*, vol. 19, no. 31, pp. 5131–5137, 2013.

[20] S. Abraham, S. Begum, and D. Isenberg, "Hepatic manifestations of autoimmune rheumatic diseases," *Annals of the Rheumatic Diseases*, vol. 63, no. 2, pp. 123–129, 2004.

[21] W. I. Youssef and A. S. Tavill, "Connective tissue diseases and the liver," *Journal of Clinical Gastroenterology*, vol. 35, no. 4, pp. 345–349, 2002.

[22] M. Ramos-Casals, Roberto-Perez-Alvarez, C. Diaz-Lagares, M.-J. Cuadrado, and M. A. Khamashta, "Autoimmune diseases induced by biological agents: a double-edged sword?" *Autoimmunity Reviews*, vol. 9, no. 3, pp. 188–193, 2010.

[23] K. Visser, W. Katchamart, E. Loza et al., "Multinational evidence-based recommendations for the use of methotrexate in rheumatic disorders with a focus on rheumatoid arthritis: integrating systematic literature research and expert opinion of a broad international panel of rheumatologists in the 3E Initiative," *Annals of the Rheumatic Diseases*, vol. 68, no. 7, pp. 1086–1093, 2009.

[24] G. M. Hirschfield, X. Liu, C. Xu et al., "Primary biliary cirrhosis associated with *HLA*, *IL 12A*, and *IL12RB2* variants," *The New England Journal of Medicine*, vol. 360, pp. 2544–2555, 2009.

[25] C. Selmi, P. Invernizzi, M. Zuin, M. Podda, and M. E. Gershwin, "Genetics and geoepidemiology of primary biliary cirrhosis: following the footprints to disease etiology," *Seminars in Liver Disease*, vol. 25, no. 3, pp. 265–280, 2005.

[26] C. Selmi, M. J. Mayo, N. Bach et al., "Primary biliary cirrhosis in monozygotic and dizygotic twins: genetics, epigenetics, and environment," *Gastroenterology*, vol. 127, no. 2, pp. 485–492, 2004.

[27] Y. Liu, J. Yu, Z. Oaks et al., "Liver injury correlates with biomarkers of autoimmunity and disease activity and represents an organ system involvement in patients with systemic lupus erythematosus," *Clinical Immunology*, vol. 160, no. 2, pp. 319–327, 2015.

[28] M. H. El-Shabrawi and M. I. Farrag, "Hepatic manifestations in juvenile systemic lupus erythematosus," *Recent Patents on Inflammation and Allergy Drug Discovery*, vol. 8, no. 1, pp. 36–40, 2014.

[29] M. De Santis, C. Crotti, and C. Selmi, "Liver abnormalities in connective tissue diseases," *Best Practice and Research: Clinical Gastroenterology*, vol. 27, no. 4, pp. 543–551, 2013.

[30] Y. Akiyama, M. Tanaka, M. Takeishi, D. Adachi, A. Mimori, and T. Suzuki, "Clinical, serological and genetic study in patients with CREST syndrome," *Internal Medicine*, vol. 39, no. 6, pp. 451–456, 2000.

[31] H. Y. Ju, J. Y. Jang, S. W. Jeong et al., "The clinical features of drug-induced liver injury observed through liver biopsy: focus on relevancy to autoimmune hepatitis," *Clinical and Molecular Hepatology*, vol. 18, no. 2, pp. 213–218, 2012.

[32] A. Hewagama and B. Richardson, "The genetics and epigenetics of autoimmune diseases," *Journal of Autoimmunity*, vol. 33, no. 1, pp. 3–11, 2009.

[33] C. Selmi, P. L. Meroni, and M. E. Gershwin, "Primary biliary cirrhosis and Sjögren's syndrome: autoimmune epithelitis," *Journal of Autoimmunity*, vol. 39, no. 1-2, pp. 34–42, 2012.

[34] E. Savarino, M. Furnari, N. de Bortoli et al., "Gastrointestinal involvement in systemic sclerosis," *Presse Medicale*, vol. 43, no. 10, pp. 279–291, 2014.

[35] I. R. Mackay, "Clustering and commonalities among autoimmune diseases," *Journal of Autoimmunity*, vol. 33, no. 3-4, pp. 170–177, 2009.

[36] A. Martínez, J. Varadé, A. Márquez et al., "Association of the STAT4 gene with increased susceptibility for some immune-mediated diseases," *Arthritis & Rheumatism*, vol. 58, no. 9, pp. 2598–2602, 2008.

[37] T. S. Rodríguez-Reyna and D. Alarcón-Segovia, "Overlap syndromes in the context of shared autoimmunity," *Autoimmunity*, vol. 38, no. 3, pp. 219–223, 2005.

[38] C. Selmi and M. E. Gershwin, "The role of environmental factors in primary biliary cirrhosis," *Trends in Immunology*, vol. 30, no. 8, pp. 415–420, 2009.

[39] A. Castiella, E. Zapata, M. I. Lucena, and R. J. Andrade, "Drug-induced autoimmune liver disease: a diagnostic dilemma of an increasingly reported disease," *World Journal of Hepatology*, vol. 6, no. 4, pp. 160–168, 2014.

[40] S. Rodrigues, S. Lopes, F. Magro et al., "Autoimmune hepatitis and anti-tumor necrosis factor alpha therapy: a single center report of 8 cases," *World Journal of Gastroenterology*, vol. 21, no. 24, pp. 7584–7588, 2015.

[41] E. Björnsson, J. Talwalkar, S. Treeprasertsuk et al., "Drug-induced autoimmune hepatitis: clinical characteristics and prognosis," *Hepatology*, vol. 51, no. 6, pp. 2040–2048, 2010.

[42] A. Suzuki, E. M. Brunt, D. E. Kleiner et al., "The use of liver biopsy evaluation in discrimination of idiopathic autoimmune hepatitis versus drug-induced liver injury," *Hepatology*, vol. 54, no. 3, pp. 931–939, 2011.

[43] P. Muratori, A. Fabbri, C. Lalanne, M. Lenzi, and L. Muratori, "Autoimmune liver disease and concomitant extrahepatic autoimmune disease," *European Journal of Gastroenterology and Hepatology*, vol. 27, no. 10, pp. 1175–1179, 2015.

[44] C. Rigamonti, L. M. Shand, M. Feudjo et al., "Clinical features and prognosis of primary biliary cirrhosis associated with systemic sclerosis," *Gut*, vol. 55, no. 3, pp. 388–394, 2006.

[45] E. F. Remmers, R. M. Plenge, A. T. Lee et al., "STAT4 and the risk of rheumatoid arthritis and systemic lupus erythematosus," *The New England Journal of Medicine*, vol. 357, no. 10, pp. 977–986, 2007.

[46] R. Chapman, J. Fevery, A. Kalloo et al., "Diagnosis and management of primary sclerosing cholangitis," *Hepatology*, vol. 51, no. 2, pp. 660–678, 2010.

[47] S. N. Dastis, D. Latinne, C. Sempoux, and A. P. Geubel, "Ulcerative colitis associated with IgG4 cholangitis: Similar features in two HLA identical siblings," *Journal of Hepatology*, vol. 51, no. 3, pp. 601–605, 2009.

[48] Y. Goto, Y. Kurashima, and H. Kiyono, "The gut microbiota and inflammatory bowel disease," *Current Opinion in Rheumatology*, vol. 27, no. 4, pp. 388–396, 2015.

[49] M. A. Kriegel, "Self or non-self? The multifaceted role of the microbiota in immune-mediated diseases," *Clinical Immunology*, vol. 159, no. 2, pp. 119–121, 2015.

[50] G. M. Hirschfield, E. J. Heathcote, and M. E. Gershwin, "Pathogenesis of cholestatic liver disease and therapeutic approaches," *Gastroenterology*, vol. 139, no. 5, pp. 1481–1496, 2010.

[51] C. Selmi, I. R. Mackay, and M. E. Gershwin, "The autoimmunity of primary biliary cirrhosis and the clonal selection theory," *Immunology & Cell Biology*, vol. 89, no. 1, pp. 70–80, 2011.

[52] M. E. Gershwin and I. R. Mackay, "The causes of primary biliary cirrhosis: convenient and inconvenient truths," *Hepatology*, vol. 47, no. 2, pp. 737–745, 2008.

[53] T. Matsumoto, T. Morizane, Y. Aoki et al., "Autoimmune hepatitis in primary Sjögren's syndrome: pathological study of the livers and labial salivary glands in 17 patients with primary Sjögren's syndrome," *Pathology International*, vol. 55, no. 2, pp. 70–76, 2005.

[54] P. Obermayer-Straub, J. Perheentupa, S. Braun et al., "Hepatic autoantigens in patients with autoimmune polyendocrinopathy-candidiasis-ectodermal dystrophy," *Gastroenterology*, vol. 121, no. 3, pp. 668–677, 2001.

15

Low Prevalence of Clinically Significant Endoscopic Findings in Outpatients with Dyspepsia

Khaled Abdeljawad,[1] Antonios Wehbeh,[2] and Emad Qayed[1]

[1]Department of Medicine, Division of Digestive Diseases, Emory University School of Medicine, Atlanta, GA, USA
[2]Department of Medicine, Emory University School of Medicine, Atlanta, GA, USA

Correspondence should be addressed to Emad Qayed; eqayed@emory.edu

Academic Editor: Qasim Aziz

Background. The value of endoscopy in dyspeptic patients is questionable. *Aims.* To examine the prevalence of significant endoscopic findings (SEFs) and the utility of alarm features and age in predicting SEFs in outpatients with dyspepsia. *Methods.* A retrospective analysis of outpatient adults who had endoscopy for dyspepsia. Demographic variables, alarm features, and endoscopic findings were recorded. We defined SEFs as peptic ulcer disease, erosive esophagitis, malignancy, stricture, or findings requiring specific therapy. *Results.* Of 650 patients included in the analysis, 51% had a normal endoscopy. The most common endoscopic abnormality was nonerosive gastritis (29.7%) followed by nonerosive duodenitis (7.2%) and LA-class A esophagitis (5.4%). Only 10.2% had a SEF. Five patients (0.8%) had malignancy. SEFs were more likely present in patients with alarm features (12.6% versus 5.4%, $p = 0.004$). Age ≥ 55 and presence of any alarm feature were associated with SEFs (aOR 1.8 and 2.3, resp.). *Conclusion.* Dyspeptic patients have low prevalence of SEF. The presence of any alarm feature and age ≥ 55 are associated with higher risk of SEF. Endoscopy in young patients with no alarm features has a low yield; these patients can be considered for nonendoscopic approach for diagnosis and management.

1. Introduction

Dyspepsia is defined as chronic or recurrent pain or discomfort centered in the upper abdomen [1]. It involves a variety of symptoms such as epigastric pain or burning, early satiety, bloating, upper abdominal fullness, or nausea [2, 3]. Functional dyspepsia is defined by the Rome IV consensus as the presence of one or more of the following: bothersome postprandial fullness, bothersome early satiation, or bothersome epigastric pain or burning, with no evidence of structural disease to explain the symptoms. The criteria should be fulfilled for the last three months with symptom onset at least six months before diagnosis [4]. Dyspepsia is one of the most commonly encountered gastrointestinal complaints in the outpatient and inpatient settings. It is estimated that around 25–35% of the US population are affected by dyspepsia [3, 5, 6]. Dyspepsia has huge economic costs to patients and to the healthcare system. Patients with dyspepsia have lower work productivity and more sick leaves [7–10].

The approach for evaluating and managing patients with dyspepsia focuses on identifying high risk patients including those older than 55 years and those with one or more alarm features (bleeding, anemia, early satiety, unexplained weight loss, dysphagia, odynophagia, vomiting, family history of gastrointestinal cancer, previous esophagogastric malignancy, previous documented peptic ulcer, previous upper gastrointestinal surgery, lymphadenopathy, or an abdominal mass). It is recommended that these two groups of patients undergo Esophagogastroduodenoscopy (EGD) to exclude an organic pathology such as esophagogastric malignancy and peptic ulcer disease. Otherwise, patients can be managed by either the "test and treat" strategy for *H. pylori* or a trial of proton pump inhibitor (PPI) depending on the *H. pylori* prevalence [1, 11]. The yield of endoscopy in patients with dyspepsia is questionable and varies among studies; part of this variation is due to different definitions of dyspepsia used by different studies [6, 12]. A systematic review by Ford et al. examined studies that reported prevalence of endoscopic findings in outpatients with dyspepsia. A clinically significant finding was defined as erosive esophagitis, Barrett's esophagus, gastric or duodenal ulcer disease, and gastroesophageal malignancy. The pooled prevalence of significant endoscopic findings was 27.5% when using a broad definition of dyspepsia or 18% when including studies using the Rome criteria to define dyspepsia [13]. The most common clinically significant finding encountered was erosive esophagitis (20%) when using broad definition of dyspepsia or peptic ulcer disease (11%) when using the Rome criteria to define dyspepsia. Most of the included studies used a questionnaire to screen for eligible patients instead of medical staff evaluation, and in some studies all patients underwent endoscopy regardless of symptoms, age, or presence of alarm features [12, 14–18]. One study only included patients with positive *H. pylori* infection [19]. Those factors could have led to a higher prevalence of significant endoscopic findings. The utility of alarm features and age cutoff of 55 years in predicting the presence of significant endoscopic findings is unknown [20–22]. Furthermore, a large proportion of low risk patients with dyspepsia defined as younger than 55 and with no alarm features do not receive a trial of PPI or *H. pylori* testing prior to endoscopy [23]. In addition, it seems that many primary care physicians and even gastroenterologists do not define dyspepsia correctly and do not adhere to dyspepsia guidelines [24]. Due to the high prevalence of dyspepsia, a prompt endoscopy for every dyspeptic patient is not a practical approach, as this will lead to high costs and low yield of endoscopy [12, 25–27].

This study provides further clarification on the prevalence of significant endoscopic findings in outpatients with dyspepsia. It also evaluates the role of age and alarm features in clinical decision making regarding which patients should be referred to endoscopy. The primary aim of this study is to investigate whether age $\geq$ 55 and/or presence of any alarm feature predicts the presence of significant endoscopic findings (SEFs) in outpatients with dyspepsia at a large teaching hospital.

2. Methods

This is a retrospective study using the endoscopic procedure database at Grady Memorial Hospital in Atlanta, Georgia. This database prospectively collects information about all endoscopic procedures performed at the Gastroenterology unit, including procedure type, patient's medical record number, age, race, sex, procedure, indications, and findings. The study was approved by the Institutional Review Board. Inclusion criteria included all upper endoscopies performed in the outpatient setting for patients who were at least 18 year old and referred for dyspepsia between June 1, 2011, and July 1, 2015. Endoscopy referrals for patients with upper GI symptoms are made through the GI clinic, emergency department, primary care, and subspecialty physician offices. In our practice, most patients are seen in the GI clinic before their endoscopy. There are no specific referral criteria to the GI clinic. The decision to refer patients from the GI clinic to undergo upper endoscopy is at the discretion of the clinic physicians, based on age, severity of symptoms, and response to prior treatment. The medical record was carefully reviewed and the presence of dyspepsia symptoms (nausea, vomiting, epigastric pain/discomfort, postprandial fullness, belching, and early satiation) was recorded. Patients with heartburn and/or regurgitation were included only if they had accompanying dyspeptic symptoms. The medical record was also used to confirm endoscopic findings and collect further information about patients such as alcohol consumption, smoking status, and pertinent medications such as NSAIDs, PPI, H2-blockers, anticoagulants, ASA, and other antiplatelets. *H. pylori* infection status prior to endoscopy was recorded. At our institution, this is tested with the stool antigen test or serum antibody. Alarm features were recorded: (vomiting, weight loss, dysphagia, odynophagia, bleeding, anemia, early satiety, personal or family history of upper GI cancers, history of peptic ulcer disease, lymph node enlargement, or abdominal mass). Endoscopic findings were recorded in detail. We defined significant endoscopic findings as the presence of any of the following findings: gastric ulcer, duodenal ulcer, erosive esophagitis (LA grade B and higher), malignancy, stricture, or other findings that required specific therapy and were judged to have contributed to the patient's symptoms.

2.1. Statistical Analysis. Descriptive statistics were used to characterize patient demographic features. Continuous variables were summarized using mean and standard deviation, and categorical variables were summarized using number and percentage. We also categorized age as $\geq$55 and <55 years. We compared the presence of endoscopic findings in patients with and without alarm features and in patients within different age categories. The Chi-square test of independence was performed to examine the association of different endoscopic findings with the presence of alarm features. To examine the combined effect of age and presence of any alarm features on the presence of significant endoscopic findings, multivariate logistic regression was performed to examine the association of different factors (presence of any alarm feature, age $\geq$ 55, smoking, race, gender, PPI use, *H. pylori* status, NSAIDs, and alcohol) with the presence of significant endoscopic findings. Backward elimination was performed to remove nonsignificant covariates with a *p* value of >0.05.

3. Results

During the study period, 16,020 endoscopic procedures were performed, of which there were 4501 EGDs. Of those, 650 were performed for outpatients with dyspeptic symptoms and were included in the analysis. Table 1 shows the basic demographics of the study population. The average age was 48.4 years $\pm$ 12.6. Two-thirds of the patients were younger than 55 years; 473 (72.8%) were females; 423 (65.1%) were African Americans; 161 (24.8%) patients were smokers and 65 (9.5%) used alcohol heavily. Among all patients, 504 (77.5%) were using Nonsteroidal Anti-Inflammatory Drugs (NSAIDs) at the time of the procedure or preendoscopic clinic visit, and 456 (70.2%) patients were on a PPI. Aspirin was used by 114 (17.5%) patients. *H. pylori* status was unknown in 350 (53.8%) of the patients, positive and treated prior to

TABLE 1: Basics characteristics of outpatients with dyspepsia; Grady Memorial Hospital, Atlanta, Georgia, June 1, 2011–July 1, 2015.

Characteristic	n (650)	%
Age		
<55 years	433	66.6
≥55 years	217	33.4
Gender		
Female	473	72.8
Male	177	27.3
Race		
Black	423	65.1
Hispanic	112	17.2
White	57	8.8
Other	58	8.9
Smoking	161	24.8
Alcohol use		
None	456	70.2
Occasional	132	20.3
Heavy	62	9.5
Medications		
NSAIDs	504	77.5
PPI	456	70.2
H2-blocker	138	21.2
ASA	114	17.5
Other antiplatelets	7	1.1
Anticoagulant	5	0.8
H. pylori status prior to EGD		
Unknown	350	53.8
Positive and treated	140	21.5
Negative	126	19.4
Positive and not treated	34	5.2
Dyspepsia symptoms		
Epigastric pain	498	76.6
Nausea	280	43.1
Vomiting	170	26.2
Epigastric burning	138	21.2
Early satiety	79	12.2
Belching	34	5.2
Reflux symptoms		
Heartburns	172	26.5
Regurgitation	43	6.6
Alarm feature		
Vomiting	170	26.2
Weight loss	138	21.2
Anemia	103	15.8
Early satiety	79	12.2
Dysphagia	76	11.7
Previous peptic ulcer disease	41	6.3
Bleeding	38	5.8
Family history of GI cancer	29	4.5
Prior upper GI surgery	28	4.3
Previous GI cancer	12	1.8
Odynophagia	8	1.2
Lymphadenopathy or abdominal mass	4	0.6

NSAIDs: Nonsteroidal Anti-Inflammatory Drugs; PPI: proton pump inhibitor; ASA: aspirin; EGD: Esophagogastroduodenoscopy; GI: gastrointestinal.

endoscopy in 140 (21.5%) patients, negative in 126 (19.4%) patients, and positive and untreated prior to endoscopy in 34 (5.2%) of patients.

The most encountered dyspepsia symptom was epigastric pain (76.6%), followed by nausea (43.1%) and vomiting (26.2%). Among all patients, 65.7% had one or more alarm features. Vomiting was the most common alarm feature (26.2%), followed by weight loss (21.2%) and anemia (15.8%). Of note, 28 (4.3%) patients had prior upper GI surgery, such as Billroth I and II and Nissen fundoplication. There were no reported major complications or deaths related to endoscopy during the study period.

3.1. Endoscopic Findings. Table 2 shows the findings of endoscopy stratified by the presence or absence of alarm features. Among all patients, 321 (49.4%) had any endoscopic abnormality. This did not statistically differ between patients with alarm features versus no alarm features (48.7% versus 50.7%, resp., $p = 0.63$). Only 66 (10.2%) patients had significant endoscopic findings. This was more likely to be found in patients with alarm features compared to those without any alarm features (12.6% versus 5.4%, $p = 0.004$). The most common endoscopic abnormality was nonerosive gastritis (29.7%), followed by nonerosive duodenitis (7.2%) and Los Angeles class A esophagitis (5.4%). Peptic ulcer disease was found in 26 (4%) of patients. This was more likely to be found in patients with alarm features compared to those without any alarm features (5.4% versus 1.3%, $p = 0.01$). Malignancy was found in only 5 (0.8%) patients, all of whom had one or more alarm features. Two patients had gastric adenocarcinoma, one had GIST tumor, one had MALT lymphoma, and one had squamous cell carcinoma of the esophagus.

Other SEFs were found in 25 (3.8%) patients. There were no significant differences in the presence of other SEFs between patients with and without alarm features (4.7% versus 2.2%, resp., $p = 0.12$). Other nonsignificant endoscopic findings (benign polyps and nonobstructive Schatzki's ring) were found in 6% of patients, and they were similar in distribution between patients with and without alarm features (6.7% versus 5.2%, resp., $p = 0.41$).

3.2. Significant Endoscopic Findings according to Age. SEFs in patients with and without alarm features as stratified by age are shown in Table 3. Older patients had a higher likelihood of having significant endoscopic findings. The prevalence of endoscopic abnormalities in patients without alarm features younger than 55 years was low (7/156, 4.5%), with the lowest prevalence in those younger than 40 years (1/64, 1.6%). The presence or absence of alarm features was predictive of SEFs among the main age categories (<55, ≥55).

Multivariable logistic regression analysis showed that age ≥55, presence of any alarm feature, and smoking were significantly associated with the presence of SEFs (Table 4). Having more than one of these risk factors significantly increases the chance of SEFs. Race, gender, PPI use prior to endoscopy, *H. pylori* status, NSAIDs, and alcohol use were not associated with SEFs.

TABLE 2: Endoscopic findings in outpatients with dyspepsia, stratified by alarm features; Grady Memorial Hospital, Atlanta, Georgia, June 1, 2011–July 1, 2015.

Characteristic	All patients		No alarm features		Any alarm feature		p value
	n (650)	%	n (223)	34.3%	n (427)	65.7%	
Any endoscopic abnormality	321	49.4	113	50.7	208	48.7	0.63
Significant endoscopic abnormality	66	10.2	12	5.4	54	12.6	0.004
Any peptic ulcer disease	26	4	3	1.3	23	5.4	0.01
Gastric	17	2.6	3	1.3	14	3.3	0.14
Duodenal	11	1.7	0	0	11	2.6	0.02
Gastritis							
Erosive	43	6.6	15	6.7	28	6.6	0.93
Nonerosive	193	29.7	74	33.2	119	27.9	0.16
Duodenitis							
Erosive	5	0.8	1	0.4	4	0.9	0.5
Nonerosive	47	7.2	14	6.3	33	7.7	0.54
Malignancy	5	0.8	0	0	5	1.2	0.1
Esophagitis							
Los Angeles class A	35	5.4	11	4.9	24	5.6	0.71
Los Angeles classes B, C, and D	16	2.5	5	2.2	11	2.6	0.79
Other significant endoscopic findings	25	3.8	5	2.2	20	4.7	0.12
Anastomotic stricture	4		0		4		
Candida esophagitis	4		0		4		
Anastomotic ulcer	3		0		3		
Severe hemorrhagic gastritis	3		2		1		
Barrett's esophagus	3		1		2		
Esophageal benign stricture	2		0		2		
Esophageal varices	2		1		1		
Extrinsic compression	1		0		1		
Gastric bezoar	1		0		1		
Paraesophageal hernia	1		1		0		
Fobi-ring erosion	1		0		1		
Other nonsignificant endoscopic findings	37	6	15	6.7	22	5.2	0.41
Benign polyps	31		12		19		
Nonobstructive Schatzki's ring	6		3		3		

LA: Los Angeles.

4. Discussion

In this study, we found a low prevalence of significant endoscopic findings (10.2%) in outpatients with dyspepsia, and the majority of these were found in patients with alarm features. The prevalence of malignancy was extremely low (5 cases, 0.8%), and all 5 cases were present in patients with alarm features. This highlights the low yield of endoscopy in patients with dyspepsia and calls for a more conservative, nonendoscopic approach in management. This is especially true in patients without alarm features and younger than 55 years, where the prevalence of SEFs was 4.5%. While this could arguably be considered a significant percentage, none of these patients had malignancy. It is unlikely that treatment would significantly change in this small group of patients if they had undergone endoscopy, given that PPI and *H. pylori* testing are the mainstay of treatment. This study confirms the role of alarm features and age ≥ 55 in predicting the presence of SEFs. Patients with alarm features were more likely to have SEF compared to those with no alarm features (12.7 versus 5.4%, $p = 0.004$). Patients with both alarm features and age ≥55 had a 17% chance of having SEFs. Alarm feature and age ≥ 55 remained significant predictors of SEFs in multivariate analysis. In addition, we found that smoking is as useful in predicting SEFs as age ≥55 (aOR of 1.8 for both risk factors). Previous studies showed that smoking could increase the risk of peptic ulcerations [28–31]. Therefore, smoking could be considered an independent alarm feature and an important element in clinical decision making when stratifying patients with dyspepsia to undergo endoscopy. As expected, we found that combining several risk factors increased the chance of SEFs. For example, patients ≥ 55 years with any alarm feature had 4.2 (CI: 1.8–9.5) higher odds of having SEFs when compared to patients who were <55 years without alarm features (aOR 4.2).

In our study, we included patients with prior upper GI surgeries who are at risk of anastomotic complications such

TABLE 3: Significant endoscopic findings in patients with and without alarm features stratified by age; Grady Memorial Hospital, Atlanta, Georgia, June 1, 2011–July 1, 2015.

Age	No alarm features	With any alarm feature	p value
<55	7/156 (4.5%)	28/277 (10.1%)	0.04
<40	1/64 (1.6%)	8/104 (7.7%)	NS
40–54	6/92 (6.5%)	20/173 (11.6%)	NS
≥55	5/67 (7.5%)	26/150 (17.3%)	0.045
Total	12/223 (5.4%)	54/427 (12.6%)	0.004

NS: not significant.

TABLE 4: Multivariate analysis of association of risk factors with significant endoscopic findings; Grady Memorial Hospital, Atlanta, Georgia, June 1, 2011–July 1, 2015.

Risk factor(s)	aOR (95% CI)	p value
Any alarm feature	2.3 (1.2–4.4)	0.01
Age ≥ 55	1.8 (1.1–3)	0.02
Smoking	1.8 (1.1–3.1)	0.03
Any alarm feature and age ≥ 55	4.2 (1.8–9.5)	0.0007
Any alarm feature and smoking	4.1 (1.8–9.4)	0.0005
Any alarm feature, age ≥ 55, and smoking	7.5 (2.9–19)	<0.0001

aOR: adjusted odds ratio. Final model included any alarm feature, age ≥ 55, and smoking. Race, gender, PPI use prior to endoscopy, H. pylori status, NSAIDs, and alcohol use had a nonsignificant association with endoscopic findings and were removed from the final model.

as marginal ulcers and anastomotic strictures [32–35]. Prior GI surgery was considered an alarm feature. Of 28 patients with prior upper GI surgery, 9 (32%) had significant findings (four anastomotic strictures, 3 anastomotic ulcers, one Fobiring erosion, and one candida esophagitis). This group of patients is at high risk of complications and endoscopy is always warranted to investigate upper GI symptoms.

Despite the low yield of endoscopy in outpatients with dyspepsia, a negative endoscopy can improve patient satisfaction and relieve anxiety due to fear of serious illnesses [36, 37]. In our study, the most common SEF was peptic ulcer disease (4%). We found lower prevalence of erosive esophagitis due to including patients with GERD only if they had accompanying dyspepsia symptoms. Our study found a low prevalence of malignancy in patients with dyspepsia (0.8%) which is comparable to previous studies (<0.5%) [13]. The study revealed a relatively lower prevalence of SEFs compared to other studies due to multiple factors. Previous studies were statistically heterogeneous [12, 14–19, 38]. Patients in our study were evaluated in the outpatient settings, given an appointment for their endoscopy, which usually takes several weeks to complete. In the meanwhile, they might be given a trial of PPI or asked to discontinue possible culprit medications, such as NSAIDs. This could have allowed the healing of some lesions and prevented their detection at the time of endoscopy. However, this is reflective of daily practice and should not be considered a weakness in this study.

Our study has several limitations. It had a retrospective design, was performed in a single center, and lacked cost analysis. In a randomized clinical trial, Laheij et al. randomized patients with dyspepsia referred to endoscopy to either prompt endoscopy followed by directed medical treatment versus empirical treatment with PPI followed by testing and treating H. pylori in the case of relapse [30]. They found that the empirical drug treatment resulted in less diagnostic endoscopies, lower costs, and equal effectiveness in the first year of follow-up. We did not collect data on celiac disease serologies in our patients because we do not routinely screen patients with dyspepsia for celiac disease in our practice. The prevalence of celiac disease in patients with dyspepsia varies between 0.5 and 2% [39]. This is expected to be much lower in our hospital where the majority of patients are African Americans (65%). Therefore, we do not think there were missed cases of celiac disease in our patient population.

Our study has several strengths. Despite our retrospective design, we were able to extract all information about patient demographics, symptoms and signs, and endoscopic findings from the medical record. Furthermore, we attempted to examine the utility of endoscopy in patients with dyspepsia in a more pragmatic setting rather than a randomized clinical trial. We did not find prior treatment with PPI or H. pylori status to be predictive of endoscopic findings, probably due to the low prevalence of peptic ulcer disease (4%). We also focused our study on outpatients with dyspepsia, as inpatients tend to have more severe symptoms and comorbidities, and therefore the approach to their management should be separate from outpatients. Finally, we chose to define "significant endoscopic findings" as one composite outcome that includes findings pertinent to the patients' management and related to their symptoms. We did not consider simple erosive or nonerosive gastroduodenal inflammation as a significant finding given that it is unlikely to contribute to the patients' symptoms or alter their long-term management. Previous studies showed poor association of these findings with dyspeptic symptoms [40, 41]. Erosive esophagitis class B and higher was considered significant, as it would require long-term maintenance treatment with PPI.

In summary, the prevalence of significant endoscopic findings in outpatients with dyspepsia is low, particularly in patients younger than 55 years and without alarm features. Guidelines should highlight the low yield of endoscopy in this group of patients and recommend nonendoscopic workup or empiric therapy as alternatives to endoscopy. Those patients should also be reassured that their symptoms are unlikely related to an underlying significant pathology and should be encouraged to defer endoscopy. The presence of any alarm feature, age ≥ 55, and smoking are all independent predictors of significant endoscopic findings. An approach to outpatients with dyspepsia that considers an age cutoff ≥ 55 and presence of any alarm features as indications for endoscopy is a simple and straightforward management strategy. However, a scoring system that considers multiple additional risk factors (such as smoking) is likely to improve the yield of endoscopy in dyspepsia and allow for a more accurate stratification of patients to endoscopic workup versus nonendoscopic workup or empiric therapy. Further studies are required to clarify the role of each alarm feature in predicting significant endoscopic findings and compile a more concise list of predictive risk factors to be used as a scoring system that guides clinical decision making.

Abbreviations

SEF: Significant endoscopic findings
GERD: Gastroesophageal reflux disease
H. pylori: *Helicobacter pylori*
PPI: Proton pump inhibitor
EGD: Esophagogastroduodenoscopy
NSAIDs: Nonsteroidal Anti-Inflammatory Drugs
ASA: Aspirin
GI: Gastrointestinal
LA: Los Angeles
GIST: Gastrointestinal stromal tumors
MALT: Mucosa associated lymphoid tissue
CI: Confidence interval
aOR: Adjusted odds ratio.

Competing Interests

The authors have no conflict of interests to declare.

References

[1] N. J. Talley and N. Vakil, "Guidelines for the management of dyspepsia," *American Journal of Gastroenterology*, vol. 100, no. 10, pp. 2324–2337, 2005.

[2] J. Tack and N. J. Talley, "Functional dyspepsia—symptoms, definitions and validity of the Rome III criteria," *Nature Reviews Gastroenterology and Hepatology*, vol. 10, no. 3, pp. 134–141, 2013.

[3] J. Tack, N. J. Talley, M. Camilleri et al., "Functional Gastroduodenal Disorders," *Gastroenterology*, vol. 130, no. 5, pp. 1466–1479, 2006.

[4] D. A. Drossman and W. L. Hasler, "Rome IV—functional GI disorders: disorders of gut-brain interaction," *Gastroenterology*, vol. 150, no. 6, pp. 1257–1261, 2016.

[5] E. Castillo, M. Camilleri, G. Locke III et al., "A community-based, controlled study of the epidemiology and pathophysiology of dyspepsia," *Clinical Gastroenterology and Hepatology*, vol. 2, no. 11, pp. 985–996, 2004.

[6] A. C. Ford, A. Marwaha, R. Sood, and P. Moayyedi, "Global prevalence of, and risk factors for, uninvestigated dyspepsia: a meta-analysis," *Gut*, vol. 64, no. 7, pp. 1049–1057, 2015.

[7] L. Agréus and L. Borgquist, "The cost of gastro-oesophageal reflux disease, dyspepsia and peptic ulcer disease in Sweden," *PharmacoEconomics*, vol. 20, no. 5, pp. 347–355, 2002.

[8] R. A. Brook, N. L. Kleinman, R. S. Choung, A. K. Melkonian, J. E. Smeeding, and N. J. Talley, "Functional dyspepsia impacts absenteeism and direct and indirect costs," *Clinical Gastroenterology and Hepatology*, vol. 8, no. 6, pp. 498–503, 2010.

[9] O. Nyren, H. O. Adami, S. Gustavsson, L. Lööf, and A. Nyberg, "Social and economic effects of non-ulcer dyspepsia," *Scandinavian Journal of Gastroenterology. Supplement*, vol. 109, pp. 41–47, 1985.

[10] G. B. Sander, L. E. Mazzoleni, C. F. D. M. Francesconi et al., "Influence of organic and functional dyspepsia on work productivity: the HEROES-DIP study," *Value in Health*, vol. 14, no. 5, pp. S126–S129, 2011.

[11] A. Shaukat, A. Wang, R. D. Acosta et al., "The role of endoscopy in dyspepsia," *Gastrointestinal Endoscopy*, vol. 82, no. 2, pp. 227–232, 2015.

[12] R. M. Zagari, G. R. Law, L. Fuccio, P. Pozzato, D. Forman, and F. Bazzoli, "Dyspeptic symptoms and endoscopic findings in the community: the loiano-monghidoro study," *American Journal of Gastroenterology*, vol. 105, no. 3, pp. 565–571, 2010.

[13] A. C. Ford, A. Marwaha, A. Lim, and P. Moayyedi, "What is the prevalence of clinically significant endoscopic findings in subjects with dyspepsia? Systematic review and meta-analysis," *Clinical Gastroenterology and Hepatology*, vol. 8, no. 10, pp. 830.e2–837.e2, 2010.

[14] P. Aro, J. Ronkainen, T. Storskrubb et al., "Valid symptom reporting at upper endoscopy in a random sample of the Swedish adult general population: the Kalixanda study," *Scandinavian Journal of Gastroenterology*, vol. 39, no. 12, pp. 1280–1288, 2004.

[15] B. Bernersen, R. Johnsen, B. Straume, P. G. Burhol, T. G. Jenssen, and P. A. Stakkevold, "Towards a true prevalence of peptic ulcer: The Sorreisa Gastrointestinal Disorder Study," *Gut*, vol. 31, no. 9, pp. 989–992, 1990.

[16] P. H. Katelaris, G. H. K. Tippett, P. Norbu, D. G. Lowe, R. Brennan, and M. J. G. Farthing, "Dyspepsia, Helicobacter pylori, and peptic ulcer in a randomly selected population in India," *Gut*, vol. 33, no. 11, pp. 1462–1466, 1992.

[17] C.-L. Lu, H.-C. Lang, F.-Y. Chang et al., "Prevalence and health/social impacts of functional dyspepsia in Taiwan: A study based on the Rome Criteria Questionnaire Survey Assisted by Endoscopic Exclusion Among A Physical Check-up Population," *Scandinavian Journal of Gastroenterology*, vol. 40, no. 4, pp. 402–411, 2005.

[18] Y. Shaib and H. B. El-Serag, "The prevalence and risk factors of functional dyspepsia in a multiethnic population in the United States," *American Journal of Gastroenterology*, vol. 99, no. 11, pp. 2210–2216, 2004.

[19] T. Azuma, Y. Ito, H. Suto et al., "The effect of Helicobacter pylori eradication therapy on dyspepsia symptoms in industrial workers in Japan," *Alimentary Pharmacology and Therapeutics*, vol. 15, no. 6, pp. 805–811, 2001.

[20] G. A. J. Fransen, M. J. R. Janssen, J. W. M. Muris, R. J. F. Laheij, and J. B. M. J. Jansen, "Meta-analysis: the diagnostic value of alarm symptoms for upper gastrointestinal malignancy," *Alimentary Pharmacology and Therapeutics*, vol. 20, no. 10, pp. 1045–1052, 2004.

[21] P. Moayyedi, N. J. Talley, M. B. Fennerty, and N. Vakil, "Can the clinical history distinguish between organic and functional dyspepsia?" *Journal of the American Medical Association*, vol. 295, no. 13, pp. 1566–1576, 2006.

[22] N. Vakil, P. Moayyedi, M. B. Fennerty, and N. J. Talley, "Limited value of alarm features in the diagnosis of upper gastrointestinal malignancy: systematic review and meta-analysis," *Gastroenterology*, vol. 131, no. 2, pp. 390–401, 2006.

[23] J. P. Fiorenza, A. M. Tinianow, and W. W. Chan, "The initial management and endoscopic outcomes of dyspepsia in a low-risk patient population," *Digestive Diseases and Sciences*, vol. 61, no. 10, pp. 2942–2948, 2016.

[24] B. M. R. Spiegel, M. Farid, M. G. H. Van Oijen, L. Laine, C. W. Howden, and E. Esrailian, "Adherence to best practice guidelines in dyspepsia: a survey comparing dyspepsia experts, community gastroenterologists and primary-care providers," *Alimentary Pharmacology and Therapeutics*, vol. 29, no. 8, pp. 871–881, 2009.

[25] W. D. Chey and P. Moayyedi, "Review article: uninvestigated dyspepsia and non-ulcer dyspepsia-the use of endoscopy and the roles of *Helicobacter pylori* eradication and antisecretory therapy," *Alimentary Pharmacology & Therapeutics*, vol. 19, supplement 1, pp. 1–8, 2004.

[26] H. B. El-Serag and N. J. Talley, "Systematic review: the prevalence and clinical course of functional dyspepsia," *Alimentary Pharmacology and Therapeutics*, vol. 19, no. 6, pp. 643–654, 2004.

[27] A. B. R. Thomson, A. N. Barkun, D. Armstrong et al., "The prevalence of clinically significant endoscopic findings in primary care patients with uninvestigated dyspepsia: the Canadian Adult Dyspepsia Empiric Treatment-Prompt Endoscopy (CADET-PE) study," *Alimentary Pharmacology and Therapeutics*, vol. 17, no. 12, pp. 1481–1491, 2003.

[28] S. J. Konturek, W. Bielański, M. Płonka et al., "Helicobacter pylori, non-steroidal anti-inflammatory drugs and smoking in risk pattern of gastroduodenal ulcers," *Scandinavian Journal of Gastroenterology*, vol. 38, no. 9, pp. 923–930, 2003.

[29] J. H. Kurata and A. N. Nogawa, "Meta-analysis of risk factors for peptic ulcer: nonsteroidal antiinflammatory drugs, Helicobacter pylori, and smoking," *Journal of Clinical Gastroenterology*, vol. 24, no. 1, pp. 2–17, 1997.

[30] R. J. F. Laheij, J. L. Severens, E. H. Van De Lisdonk, A. L. M. Verbeek, and J. B. M. J. Jansen, "Randomized controlled trial of omeprazole or endoscopy in patients with persistent dyspepsia: a cost-effectiveness analysis," *Alimentary Pharmacology and Therapeutics*, vol. 12, no. 12, pp. 1249–1256, 1998.

[31] S. Rosenstock, T. Jørgensen, O. Bonnevie, and L. Andersen, "Risk factors for peptic ulcer disease: a population based prospective cohort study comprising 2416 Danish adults," *Gut*, vol. 52, no. 2, pp. 186–193, 2003.

[32] J. S. Bolton and W. C. Conway, "Postgastrectomy syndromes," *Surgical Clinics of North America*, vol. 91, no. 5, pp. 1105–1122, 2011.

[33] ASGE Bariatric Endoscopy Task Force, S. Sullivan, N. Kumar et al., "ASGE position statement on endoscopic bariatric therapies in clinical practice," *Gastrointestinal Endoscopy*, vol. 82, no. 5, pp. 767–772, 2015.

[34] B. E. Schneider, L. Villegas, G. L. Blackburn et al., "Laparoscopic gastric bypass surgery: outcomes," *Journal of Laparoendoscopic & Advanced Surgical Techniques and Videoscopy*, vol. 13, no. 4, pp. 247–255, 2003.

[35] C. A. Woodfield and M. S. Levine, "The postoperative stomach," *European Journal of Radiology*, vol. 53, no. 3, pp. 341–352, 2005.

[36] A. Quadri and N. Vakil, "Health-related anxiety and the effect of open-access endoscopy in US patients with dyspepsia," *Alimentary Pharmacology and Therapeutics*, vol. 17, no. 6, pp. 835–840, 2003.

[37] L. Rabeneck, K. Wristers, J. Souchek, and E. Ambriz, "Impact of upper endoscopy on satisfaction in patients with previously uninvestigated dyspepsia," *Gastrointestinal Endoscopy*, vol. 57, no. 3, pp. 295–299, 2003.

[38] Y. Zhao, D. Zou, R. Wang et al., "Dyspepsia and irritable bowel syndrome in China: a population-based endoscopy study of prevalence and impact," *Alimentary Pharmacology and Therapeutics*, vol. 32, no. 4, pp. 562–572, 2010.

[39] L. Petrarca, "Dyspepsia and celiac disease: prevalence, diagnostic tools and therapy," *World Journal of Methodology*, vol. 4, no. 3, pp. 189–196, 2014.

[40] R. Johnsen, B. Bernersen, B. Straume, O. H. Førde, L. Bostad, and P. G. Burhol, "Prevalences of endoscopic and histological findings in subjects with and without dyspepsia," *British Medical Journal*, vol. 302, no. 6779, pp. 749–752, 1991.

[41] G. N. J. Tytgat, "Role of endoscopy and biopsy in the work up of dyspepsia," *Gut*, vol. 50, no. 4, pp. iv13–iv16, 2002.

16

Tumor Size Is a Critical Factor in Adjuvant Chemotherapy for T_{3-4a}N0M0 Gastric Cancer Patients after D2 Gastrectomy

Shi Chen,[1] **Li-Ying Ou-Yang,**[2] **Run-Cong Nie,**[3] **Yuan-Fang Li,**[3] **Jun Xiang,**[1] **Zhi-Wei Zhou,**[3] **Ying-Bo Chen,**[3] **and Jun-Sheng Peng**[1]

[1]*The 6th Affiliated Hospital, Sun Yat-sen University, No. 26, Yuancun Erheng Road, Tianhe District, 510655 Guangzhou, China*
[2]*Department of Intensive Care Unit, Sun Yat-sen University Cancer Center, 651 Dongfeng East Road, 510060 Guangzhou, China*
[3]*Department of Gastropancreatic Surgery, Sun Yat-sen University Cancer Center, 651 Dongfeng East Road, 510060 Guangzhou, China*

Correspondence should be addressed to Ying-Bo Chen; chenyb@sysucc.org.cn and Jun-Sheng Peng; pengjunsheng@tom.com

Academic Editor: Ralf-Dieter Hofheinz

Aim. To investigate whether tumor size is a reasonable indication for adjuvant chemotherapy for T_{3-4a}N0M0 gastric cancer patients after D2 gastrectomy. *Method.* We performed a retrospective study of 269 patients with a histological diagnosis of T_{3-4a}N0M0 stage gastric cancer who underwent D2 radical surgery at the Sun Yat-sen University Cancer Center or the Sixth Affiliated Hospital of Sun Yat-sen University between January 2006 and December 2010. The follow-up lasted until June of 2015. Chi-square tests and Kaplan-Meier methods were employed to compare the clinicopathological variables and prognoses. *Result.* For this group of patients, univariate analyses revealed that tumor size ($p < 0.001$), pathological T stage ($p < 0.001$), and tumor location ($p = 0.025$) were significant prognostic factors. Adjuvant chemotherapy did not exhibit prognostic benefits. For patients with tumors larger than 5 cm, univariate analysis revealed that tumor location ($p = 0.007$), Borrmann type ($p = 0.039$), postoperative chemotherapy ($p = 0.003$), and pathological T stage ($p < 0.001$) were significant prognostic factors. Multivariate analysis revealed that postoperative chemotherapy and pathological T stage were independent prognostic factors. *Conclusion.* Our results imply that tumor size should be a critical factor in the decision to utilize adjuvant chemotherapy for T_{3-4a}N0M0 gastric cancer patients after D2 gastrectomy. Additional randomized controlled trials are required before this conclusion can be considered definitive.

1. Background

Gastric cancers are the fourth most common malignancies worldwide, and they are the second most lethal [1–3]. Gastrectomy with D2 lymphadenectomy is recommended as a standard surgery for gastric cancer patients and results in improved overall survival [4–6]. Moreover, adjuvant chemotherapy has been proven to improve the overall survival of advanced gastric cancer patients after D2 gastrectomy [7, 8]. However, for N0 patients, particularly T3 and T4a patients, the use of adjuvant chemotherapy remains controversial. Although N0-group patients were not found to benefit from adjuvant chemotherapy in an ACTS trial, stage II gastric cancer patients without lymph node metastases were not separately analyzed, and there were only 112 patients in the N0 group [7]. Moreover, in the CLASSIC trial, the N0

group also exhibited no survival benefit following adjuvant chemotherapy [8]. Thus, the question of how to select N0 patients for adjuvant chemotherapy, particularly stage II patients, remains unresolved. The role of postoperative chemotherapy in T3-T4a gastric cancer patients is still controversial. In addition to TNM stage, other risk factors should be identified for this patient group to select for whom postoperative chemotherapy would be beneficial. Tumor size is also an important characteristic of gastric cancer, and we found that it was an informative factor for chemotherapy selection.

Tumor size is another factor that can be evaluated in gastric cancer patients, although it is not listed in the staging systems of the UICC or JGCA for gastric cancer [9, 10]. Obviously, larger tumors are more advanced. In the present study, we performed a retrospective analysis that focused on these N0-group gastric cancer patients, compared the prognoses

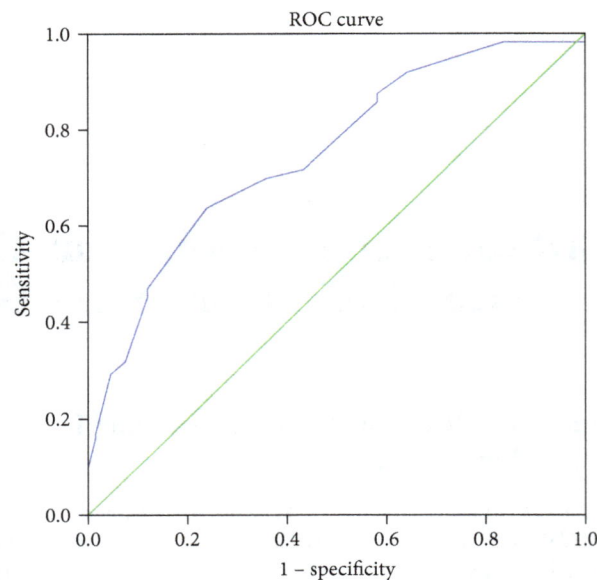

FIGURE 1: The AUC was 0.751, and the largest Youden index was 0.398, corresponding to a tumor size of 4.75 cm. However, we believed that, in the clinic, 5 cm is a more appropriate cut-off value for doctors seeking to decide whether the patient should receive postoperative chemotherapy.

TABLE 1: Clinical pathological data of the gastric cancer patients.

Clinical pathological data		Small gastric cancer patient group ($n = 148$ cases)		Large gastric cancer patient group ($n = 121$ cases)		p value
		Cases	%	Cases	%	
Age (years)	Median	58		62		
	Range	23–79		41–83		
Sex	Male	108	73.0	78	64.5	0.146
	Female	40	27.0	43	35.5	
Tumor location	Gastric cardia	55	37.2	75	62.0	
	Middle	21	14.2	14	11.6	<0.001
	Antrum	66	44.6	21	17.4	
	Total stomach	6	4.1	11	9.1	
CEA level	<5 μg/ml	135	93.1	93	76.9	<0.001
	≥5 μg/ml	10	6.9	28	23.1	
Borrmann type	I	2	1.4	2	1.7	
	II	69	46.6	50	41.3	0.145
	III	77	52.0	65	43.8	
	IV	0	0	4	6.2	
Histological grade	High differentiation	1	0.7	0	0	
	Median differentiation	37	25.0	46	38.0	0.103
	Low differentiation	87	58.8	57	47.1	
	Poor differentiation*	23	15.5	18	14.9	
T staging**	T3	130	87.8	97	80.2	0.093
	T4a	18	12.2	24	19.8	
LN harvested	15–29	121	81.8	106	87.6	0.237
	≥30	27	18.2	15	12.4	
Postoperative chemotherapy	Without	56	37.8	33	27.3	0.070
	With	92	62.2	88	72.7	

*Poorly differentiated cells: signet ring cell carcinoma, mucinous adenocarcinoma, undifferentiated carcinoma, etc. **The T and N staging for this group of patients is according to the AJCC 7th TNM staging system for gastric cancer.

according to different tumor size groups, and attempted to determine the prognostic value of tumor size in relation to adjuvant chemotherapy.

2. Materials and Methods

2.1. Ethics Statement. All of the patients provided written informed consent for their information to be stored in a hospital database. We obtained separate consent for the use of this information for research. Study approval was obtained from independent ethics committees at the Sixth Affiliated Hospital of Sun Yat-sen University and the Cancer Center of Sun Yat-sen University. This study was undertaken in accordance with the ethical standards of the World Medical Association Declaration of Helsinki.

2.2. Patient Inclusion and Exclusion Criteria. The inclusion criteria were as follows: (1) WHO performance status of 0 to 1; (2) histologically proven T3-4 adenocarcinoma of the stomach without evidence of lymph node metastasis; (3) no prior gastric surgery; (4) no previous radiotherapy or other treatments, including immunotherapy or traditional Chinese medicine; and (5) no synchronous or metachronous cancers.

2.3. Chemotherapy. Various chemotherapeutic regimens were considered in our research: 36 patients received Xeloda (1000 mg/m^2, D1–14, Q3W, cycles: 5.67 ± 1.15); 67 patients received the XELOX regimen (oxaliplatin: 130 mg/m^2 D1 + Xeloda 1000 mg/m^2, D1–14, Q3W, cycles: 5.53 ± 1.55); and 44 patients received the FOLFOX regimen (oxaliplatin: 85 mg/m^2 D1 + CF 400 mg/m^2 D1 + 5-Fu 2800 mg/m^2, D1-D2, Q2W, cycles: 8.52 ± 1.57). Of another 33 patients, 14 received the S-1 regimen (40–60 mg, bid, D1–14, Q3W, cycles: 5.71 ± 1.43); 13 received the CX regimen, (cisplatin: 60 mg/m^2 D1 + Xeloda 1000 mg/m^2, D1–14, Q3W, cycles: 4.92 ± 1.50); 5 received the SOX regimen (oxaliplatin: 85 mg/m^2 D1 + S-1 1000 mg/m^2, 40–60 mg, bid, D1–14, Q3W, cycles: 4.92 ± 1.50); and one received the DX regimen (docetaxel: 75 mg/m^2 D1 + Xeloda 1000 mg/m^2, D1–14, Q3W, cycles: 5).

2.4. Patient Characteristics. From January 2006 to December 2010, 269 consecutive patients with a histological diagnosis of T3-4N0 gastric cancer who underwent D2 radical surgery at the Sixth Affiliated Hospital of Sun Yat-sen University or the Sun Yat-sen University Cancer Center were included in this study. We divided the patients according to tumor size. We analyzed the ROC curve data and considered two balanced arms, selecting 5 cm as the cutoff value (Figure 1). Patients with gastric tumors of less than 5 cm were included in the small gastric cancer group, and patients with tumors greater than 5 cm were included in the large gastric cancer group. The clinicopathological factors are presented in Table 1.

2.5. Follow-Up. After treatment, the patients were monitored every month for the first year, every 3 months for the second year, and every 6 months thereafter, with regular follow-up assessments. Telephone calls and letters were used to follow up on the patients who were not able to attend regular follow-up assessments. Complete data were

TABLE 2: Univariate analysis of the overall survival in this group of gastric cancer patients.

Variables	n	Mean survival (months)	p value
Postoperative chemotherapy			0.543
With	180	58.01	
Without	89	56.08	
Tumor size			<0.001
<5 cm	148	63.25	
≥5 cm	121	47.95	
Tumor location			0.025
Upper	130	60.01	
Middle	35	46.20	
Lower	87	58.40	
Total	17	48.17	
Serum CEA level (ng/ml)			0.529
Normal	228	57.36	
Elevated	38	56.55	
Borrmann type			0.119
I	4	68.00	
II	119	59.58	
III	142	54.85	
IV	4	26.75	
Histological grade			0.300
High differentiation	1	72.00	
Median differentiation	83	61.71	
Low differentiation	144	61.05	
Poor differentiation	41	46.85	
T staging			<0.001
T3	227	59.61	
T4a	42	45.89	
LN harvested			0.160
15–29	227	58.31	
≥30	42	51.26	

collected for all 269 patients through December 2014. The following-up period ranged from 6 months to 90 months (median: 46 months).

2.6. Statistical Methods. A chi-square test was used to compare the categorical variables between the palliative operation group and the other groups. Student's *t*-tests were used to compare the continuous variables. Univariate survival analyses were performed using Kaplan-Meier methods. The survival curves were compared with the log-rank test. The statistical analyses were performed with SPSS software version 20.0 (SPSS Inc., Chicago, IL) for Windows. Statistical significance was defined as $p < 0.05$.

3. Result

3.1. Univariate Analyses of the Prognoses of Gastric Cancer Patients. According to the Kaplan-Meier analysis, tumor size

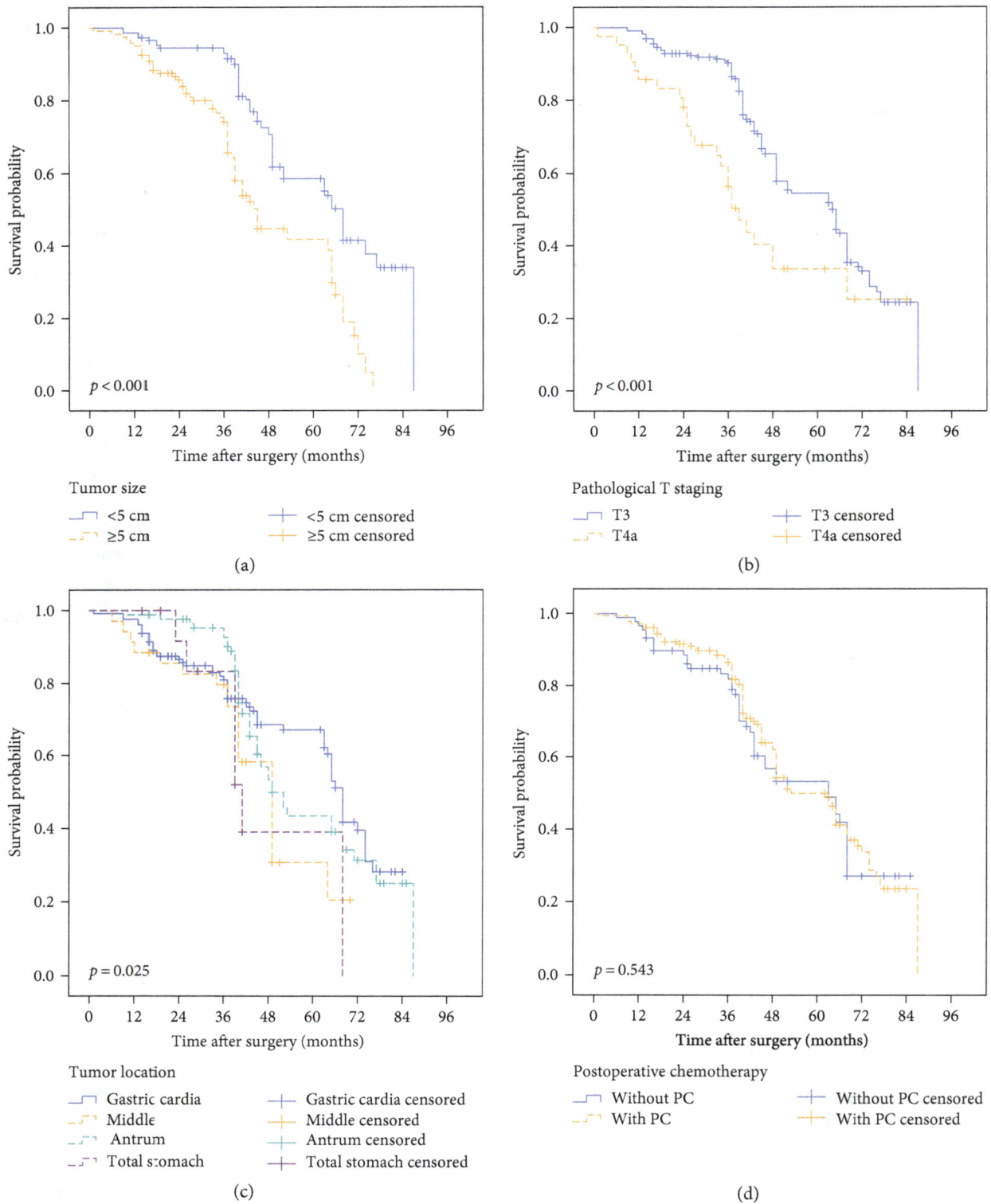

FIGURE 2: Univariate analysis of 267 T_{3-4a}N0M0 gastric cancer patients. (a) The mean survival times of patients with tumor sizes smaller than 5 cm and larger than 5 cm were 63.25 and 47.95 months, respectively ($p < 0.001$). (b) The mean survival times of the T3 and T4a patients in the study were 59.61 and 45.89 months, respectively ($p < 0.001$). (c) Tumor location was also a prognostic factor for this group of patients ($p = 0.025$). (d) Adjuvant chemotherapy did not have a prognostic benefit for this group of gastric cancer patients ($p = 0.543$).

TABLE 3: Multivariate analyses of overall survival in gastric cancer patients (Cox's regression model).

Variable	HR	95% CI	p value
OS in gastric cancer patients			
Tumor size	2.780	1.894–4.081	<0.001
CEA level	0.936	0.510–1.717	0.831
Tumor location	1.221	1.023–1.458	0.027
Pathological T staging	2.101	1.342–3.289	0.001

OS, overall survival; HR, hazard ratio; CI, confidence interval.

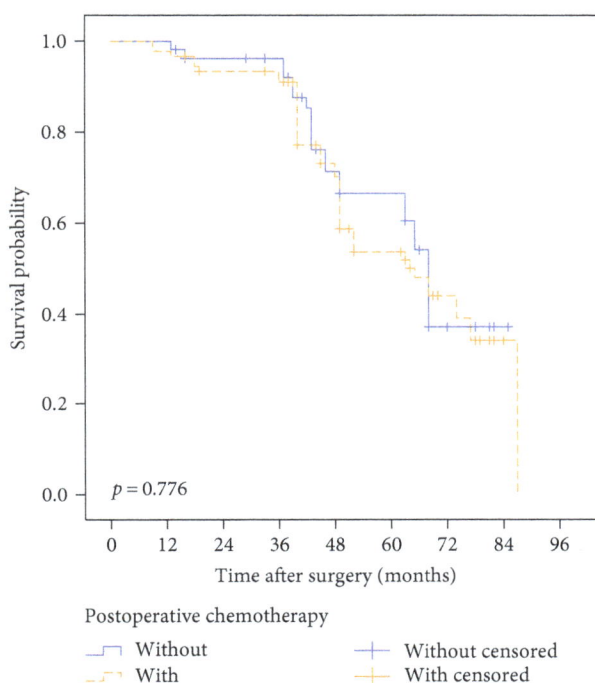

FIGURE 3: In the group of patients with tumor sizes of less than 5 cm, the median survival times of the chemotherapy and without chemotherapy groups were 64.43 months and 62.38 months, respectively ($p = 0.776$).

($p < 0.001$), pathological T stage ($p < 0.001$), and tumor location ($p = 0.025$) were risk factors (as shown in Table 2). However, no significant survival difference was found between the patients with postoperative chemotherapy and those without postoperative chemotherapy. The median survival times of the patients who received and did not receive postoperative chemotherapy were 58.0 months and 56.1 months, respectively ($p = 0.543$). The survival curves are illustrated in Figure 2.

3.2. Multivariate Analysis of the Prognoses of Gastric Cancer Patients.
Furthermore, we used the Cox regression model to analyze these risk factors in order to identify the independent risk factors. The results revealed that tumor size, tumor location, and pathological T stage were the only independent prognostic risk factors. All of these results are presented in Table 3.

3.3. Postoperative Chemotherapy Brings No Benefits for Stage II Gastric Cancer Patients with Tumors Less Than 5 cm in Size.
In the group of patients with tumor sizes of less than 5 cm, the postoperative chemotherapy did not show any benefit. As shown in Figure 3, the median survival times of the chemotherapy and without chemotherapy groups were 64.43 months and 62.38 months, respectively ($p = 0.776$).

3.4. Univariate Analyses of the Prognoses of Gastric Cancer Patients with Tumors Greater Than 5 cm in Size.
We first compared the clinicopathological factors between the postoperative chemotherapy and no postoperative chemotherapy groups of gastric cancer patients with tumors greater than 5 cm (Table 4). Kaplan-Meier analysis revealed that tumor location ($p = 0.007$), Borrmann type ($p = 0.039$), postoperative chemotherapy ($p = 0.003$), and pathological T

TABLE 4: Clinical pathological data of the gastric cancer patients whose tumor size is larger than 5 cm.

Clinical pathological data		Without postoperative chemotherapy group (n = 33 cases)		With postoperative chemotherapy group (n = 88 cases)		p value
		Cases	%	Cases	%	
Age (years)	Median	58		62		
	Range	23–79		41–83		
Sex	Male	20	60.6	58	65.9	0.368
	Female	13	39.4	30	34.1	
Tumor location	Gastric cardia	20	60.6	55	62.5	
	Middle	5	15.2	9	10.2	0.639
	Antrum	4	12.1	17	19.3	
	Total stomach	4	12.1	7	8.0	
CEA level	<5 μg/ml	27	81.8	66	75.0	0.296
	≥5 μg/ml	6	18.2	22	25.0	
Borrmann type	I	1	3.0	1	1.1	
	II	12	36.4	38	43.2	0.819
	III	19	57.6	46	52.3	
	IV	1	3.0	3	3.4	
Histological grade	High differentiation	0	0.0	0	0	
	Median differentiation	8	24.2	38	43.2	0.077
	Low differentiation	21	63.6	36	40.9	
	Poor differentiation*	4	12.1	14	15.9	
T staging**	T3	25	75.8	72	81.8	0.307
	T4a	8	24.2	16	18.2	
LN harvested	15–29	32	97.0	74	84.1	0.045
	≥30	1	3.0	14	15.9	

*Poorly differentiated cells: signet ring cell carcinoma, mucinous adenocarcinoma, undifferentiated carcinoma, etc. **The T and N staging for this group of patients is according to the AJCC 7th TNM staging system for gastric cancer.

stage ($p < 0.001$) were prognostic risk factors (Table 5). The survival curves are illustrated in Figure 4.

3.5. Multivariate Analysis of the Prognoses of Gastric Cancer Patients with Tumors Greater Than 5 cm in Size. Furthermore, we used the Cox regression model to analyze these risk factors in order to identify the independent risk factors for gastric cancer patients. Multivariate analysis revealed that Borrmann type, postoperative chemotherapy, and pathological T stage were independent prognostic factors for these patients (Table 6).

4. Discussion

Pathological stage can be used for gastric cancer patients to predict the risk of recurrence and prognosis. Stage I gastric cancer patients have a very low risk of recurrence [11] and are thus not indicated for postoperative chemotherapy. In contrast, stage IV gastric cancer patients can only accept palliative therapy, surgery, chemotherapy, and other treatments [12]. Until now, there has been great variability among the outcomes of patients with stage II/III GC; some patients are prone to suffer from locoregional or distant recurrence even after complete curative resection, whereas others achieve long-term survival [13]. Particularly for stage II gastric cancer patients, the controversy regarding the use of adjuvant chemotherapy following D2 gastrectomy persisted until the completion of the ACTS-GC and CLASSIC trials. The five-year outcomes of the ACTS-GC trial (S-1 versus surgery only) and the CLASSIC trial both indicated that stage II gastric cancer patients can benefit from postoperative chemotherapy [14, 15]. However, in these two clinical trials, the stage II gastric cancer patients included the T2N1M0 and T1N2M0 groups. Moreover, in the CLASSIC trial, the hazard ratio for adjuvant chemotherapy for N0 patients was 0.79 (CI: 0.39–1.60); thus, adjuvant chemotherapy was not advantageous in terms of prognostic improvement. Therefore, whether adjuvant chemotherapy is beneficial for lymph node-negative stage II gastric cancer patients remains unknown.

Because of the controversy regarding the role of postoperative chemotherapy in stage II gastric cancer patients, at our institution, we allowed patients and their relatives to decide whether the patients would receive postoperative chemotherapy. Some patients refused postoperative chemotherapy

TABLE 5: Univariate analysis of the overall survival in this group of gastric cancer patients.

Variables	n	Mean survival (months)	p value
Postoperative chemotherapy			0.003
With	88	51.23	
Without	33	38.93	
Tumor location			0.007
Upper	75	51.68	
Middle	14	34.24	
Lower	21	47.61	
Total	11	36.12	
Serum CEA level (ng/ml)			0.105
Normal	93	46.19	
Elevated	28	45.55	
Borrmann type			0.039
I	2	66.48	
II	50	53.52	
III	65	43.49	
IV	4	26.75	
Histological grade			0.217
High differentiation	0	—	
Median differentiation	46	53.26	
Low differentiation	57	43.27	
Poor differentiation	18	44.77	
T staging			<0.001
T3	97	53.39	
T4a	24	26.74	
LN harvested			0.479
15–29	106	47.49	
≥30	15	49.29	

because of the fear of chemotherapy-related adverse events, and others refused for economic reasons.

In the present study, we demonstrated that adjuvant chemotherapy does not benefit the survival of stage II gastric cancer patients without lymph node metastasis. The median survivals of the patients who did and did not receive adjuvant chemotherapy were 58.0 months and 56.1 months, respectively.

Precision therapy is thought to be the direction of future treatment strategies. Before molecular pathological techniques can be widely used to treat gastric cancer, it is important to determine how stage II gastric cancer patients can be properly selected to receive adjuvant chemotherapy to improve survival.

Although tumor size is not included in the current TNM staging system of the 7th AJCC, this factor still plays an important role in the prediction of the prognoses of gastric cancers due to the ease of its measurement. In Adachi's report, tumor size was strongly correlated with tumor progression parameters, such as the depth of invasion, the degree of lymph node metastasis, and the stage of the disease [16]. Wang et al. suggested that tumor size can efficiently and

reliably reflect lymph node status [17]. In the present trial, we found that tumor size was an independent prognostic factor for our group of $T_{3-4a}N0M0$ gastric cancer patients. Moreover, among these $T_{3-4a}N0M0$ gastric cancer patients with tumors greater than 5 cm, adjuvant chemotherapy was an independent prognostic factor. This finding indicates that adjuvant chemotherapy can benefit gastric cancer patients with tumors greater than 5 cm. In our study, we found that, among gastric cancer patients with tumor sizes larger than 5 cm, postoperative chemotherapy improved the prognosis. We therefore propose that postoperative chemotherapy should be performed in this group of patients.

The accurate cancer staging of each patient in clinical practice is crucial for helping clinicians select treatment plans. Although our sample was small, our results imply that tumor size may be useful for guiding adjuvant treatments for $T_{3-4a}N0M0$ gastric cancer patients. However, this study was a retrospective study and thus has limitations, such as confounding factors. Additional experiments and clinical trials are necessary to validate tumor size as a critical factor in determining whether adjuvant chemotherapy should be utilized for $T_{3-4a}N0M0$ patients following D2 gastrectomy.

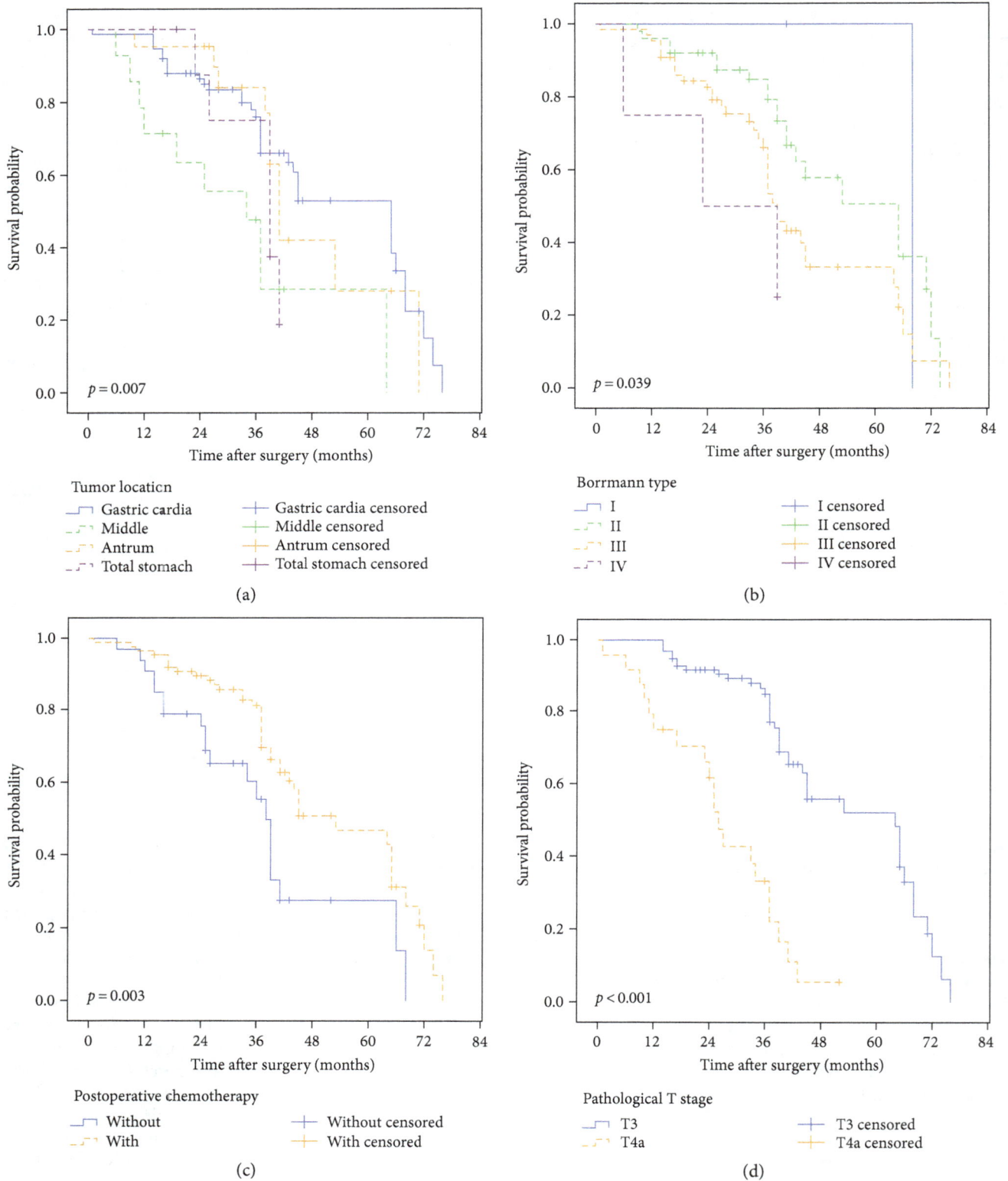

FIGURE 4: Univariate analysis of the prognosis of gastric cancer patients with tumor sizes larger than 5 cm. (a) The tumor location ($p = 0.007$), (b) Borrmann type ($p = 0.039$), (c) postoperative chemotherapy ($p = 0.003$), and (d) pathological T staging ($p < 0.001$) were the prognostic factors for these gastric cancer patients.

TABLE 6: Multivariate analyses of overall survival in gastric cancer patients whose tumor size was larger than 5 cm (Cox's regression model).

Variable	HR	95% CI	p value
OS in gastric cancer patients whose tumor size was larger than 5 cm			
Borrmann type	1.644	1.039–2.600	0.034
Tumor location	1.116	0.858–1.451	0.414
Pathological T staging	4.761	2.836–9.487	<0.001
Postoperative chemotherapy	0.489	0.281–0.851	0.011

OS, overall survival; HR, hazard ratio; CI, confidence interval.

Competing Interests

The authors declare that they have no competing interest.

Authors' Contributions

Shi Chen, Li-Ying Ou-Yang, and Run-Cong Nie contributed equally to this work.

Acknowledgments

This study was supported by the Specialized Research Fund for the Doctoral Program of Higher Education (20110171110075) and Guangdong Medical Research Foundation (no. A2015124).

References

[1] A. Jemal, R. Siegel, E. Ward, T. Murray, J. Xu, and M. J. Thun, "Cancer statistics, 2007," CA: a Cancer Journal for Clinicians, vol. 57, no. 1, pp. 43–66, 2007.

[2] F. Kamangar, G. M. Dores, and W. F. Anderson, "Patterns of cancer incidence, mortality, and prevalence across five continents: defining priorities to reduce cancer disparities in different geographic regions of the world," Journal of Clinical Oncology, vol. 24, no. 14, pp. 2137–2150, 2006.

[3] Y. Yamaoka, M. Kato, and M. Asaka, "Geographic differences in gastric cancer incidence can be explained by differences between Helicobacter pylori strains," Internal Medicine, vol. 47, no. 12, pp. 1077–1083, 2008.

[4] I. Songun, H. Putter, E. M. Kranenbarg, M. Sasako, and C. J. van de Velde, "Surgical treatment of gastric cancer: 15-year follow-up results of the randomised nationwide Dutch D1D2 trial," The Lancet Oncology, vol. 11, no. 5, pp. 439–449, 2010.

[5] A. Sierra, F. M. Regueira, J. L. Hernandez-Lizoain, F. Pardo, M. A. Martinez-Gonzalez, and J. A-Cienfuegos, "Role of the extended lymphadenectomy in gastric cancer surgery: experience in a single institution," Annals of Surgical Oncology, vol. 10, no. 3, pp. 219–226, 2003.

[6] C. W. Wu, C. A. Hsiung, S. S. Lo et al., "Nodal dissection for patients with gastric cancer: a randomised controlled trial," The Lancet Oncology, vol. 7, no. 4, pp. 309–315, 2006.

[7] S. Sakuramoto, M. Sasako, T. Yamaguchi et al., "Adjuvant chemotherapy for gastric cancer with S-1, an oral fluoropyrimidine," The New England Journal of Medicine, vol. 357, no. 18, pp. 1810–1820, 2007.

[8] Y. J. Bang, Y. W. Kim, H. K. Yang et al., "Adjuvant capecitabine and oxaliplatin for gastric cancer after D2 gastrectomy (CLASSIC): a phase 3 open-label, randomised controlled trial," The Lancet, vol. 379, no. 9813, pp. 315–321, 2012.

[9] T. Hayashi, T. Yoshikawa, K. Bonam et al., "The superiority of the seventh edition of the TNM classification depends on the overall survival of the patient cohort: comparative analysis of the sixth and seventh TNM editions in patients with gastric cancer from Japan and the United Kingdom," Cancer, vol. 119, no. 7, pp. 1330–1337, 2013.

[10] T. Waddell, M. Verheij, W. Allum et al., "Gastric cancer: ESMO-ESSO-ESTRO clinical practice guidelines for diagnosis, treatment and follow-up," European Journal of Surgical Oncology, vol. 40, no. 5, pp. 584–591, 2014.

[11] B. J. Dicken, D. L. Bigam, C. Cass, J. R. Mackey, A. A. Joy, and S. M. Hamilton, "Gastric adenocarcinoma: review and considerations for future directions," Annals of Surgery, vol. 241, no. 1, pp. 27–39, 2005.

[12] Y. J. Bang, E. Van Cutsem, A. Feyereislova et al., "Trastuzumab in combination with chemotherapy versus chemotherapy alone for treatment of HER2-positive advanced gastric or gastro-oesophageal junction cancer (ToGA): a phase 3, open-label, randomised controlled trial," The Lancet, vol. 376, no. 9742, pp. 687–697, 2010.

[13] H. H. Hartgrink, E. P. Jansen, N. C. van Grieken, and C. J. van de Velde, "Gastric cancer," The Lancet, vol. 374, no. 9688, pp. 477–490, 2009.

[14] M. Sasako, S. Sakuramoto, H. Katai et al., "Five-year outcomes of a randomized phase III trial comparing adjuvant chemotherapy with S-1 versus surgery alone in stage II or III gastric cancer," Journal of Clinical Oncology, vol. 29, no. 33, pp. 4387–4393, 2011.

[15] S. H. Noh, S. R. Park, H. K. Yang et al., "Adjuvant capecitabine plus oxaliplatin for gastric cancer after D2 gastrectomy (CLASSIC): 5 year follow-up of an open-label, randomised phase 3 trial," The Lancet Oncology, vol. 15, no. 12, pp. 1389–1396, 2014.

[16] Y. Adachi, T. Oshiro, M. Mori, Y. Maehara, and K. Sugimachi, "Tumor size as a simple prognostic indicator for gastric carcinoma," Annals of Surgical Oncology, vol. 4, no. 2, pp. 137–140, 1997.

[17] X. Wang, F. Wan, J. Pan, G. Z. Yu, Y. Chen, and J. J. Wang, "Tumor size: a non-neglectable independent prognostic factor for gastric cancer," Journal of Surgical Oncology, vol. 97, no. 3, pp. 236–240, 2008.

17

Procedure Time for Gastric Endoscopic Submucosal Dissection according to Location, considering Both Mucosal Circumferential Incision and Submucosal Dissection

Hironori Konuma,[1] Kenshi Matsumoto,[2] Hiroya Ueyama,[2] Hiroyuki Komori,[2] Yoichi Akazawa,[2] Misuzu Ueyama,[2] Yuta Nakagawa,[2] Takashi Morimoto,[1] Tsutomu Takeda,[2] Kohei Matsumoto,[2] Daisuke Asaoka,[2] Mariko Hojo,[2] Akihito Nagahara,[3] Takashi Yao,[4] Akihisa Miyazaki,[1] and Sumio Watanabe[2]

[1]Department of Gastroenterology, Juntendo Nerima Hospital, Tokyo, Japan
[2]Department of Gastroenterology, Juntendo University School of Medicine, Tokyo, Japan
[3]Department of Gastroenterology, Juntendo Sizuoka Hospital, Sizuoka, Japan
[4]Department of Human Pathology, Juntendo University School of Medicine, Tokyo, Japan

Correspondence should be addressed to Kenshi Matsumoto; kmatumo@juntendo.ac.jp

Academic Editor: Tatsuya Toyokawa

Background. Previous assessments of technical difficulty and procedure time for endoscopic submucosal dissection (ESD) of gastric neoplasms did not take into account several critical determinants of these parameters. However, two key phases of ESD determine the total procedure time: the mucosal circumference incision speed (CIS) and submucosal dissection speed (SDS). *Methods*. We included 302 cases of *en bloc* and R0 resection of gastric neoplasms performed by 10 operators who had completed the training program at our hospital. Twelve locations were classified based on multiple criteria, such as condition of surrounding mucosa, lesion vascularity, presence of submucosal fat, ulcers, scars, fibrosis, and scope and device maneuverability. Lesions in different locations were classified into three groups based on the length of the procedure: fast, moderate, or late. *Results*. A significant difference was found in CIS and SDS for each location ($p < 0.01$), which demonstrates the validity of this classification system. In several locations, CIS and SDS were not consistent with each other. *Conclusion*. CIS and SDS did not correspond to each other even for lesions in the same location. Consideration of ESD procedure time for gastric neoplasms requires a more elaborate classification system than that previously reported.

1. Introduction

The endoscopic submucosal dissection (ESD) technique was introduced to facilitate *en bloc* resection of early gastrointestinal neoplasms, which allows for precise histological diagnosis and minimizes the chances of recurrence [1, 2]. The popularity of ESD has rapidly increased in Asia and the rest of the world. Guidelines for ESD have been developed recently in Europe and the USA [3, 4].

However, the procedural complexity of ESD, especially for gastric neoplasms, tends to vary with the lesion location and vascularity, presence of ulcers, scars, and fibrosis. These factors also determine the risk of intraoperative complications such as perforation and catastrophic hemorrhage, more so in inexperienced hands. Therefore, the success of ESD, to a large extent, depends upon an in-depth understanding of the specific attributes of the lesion.

Recently, several studies have examined the technical challenges in performing ESD with respect to lesion location and procedural time. Scarred and undifferentiated lesions as well as those located in the upper third of the stomach were reported to be typically challenging and required more time [5, 6]. However, the classification of lesions based on location alone (namely, upper, middle, and lower) does

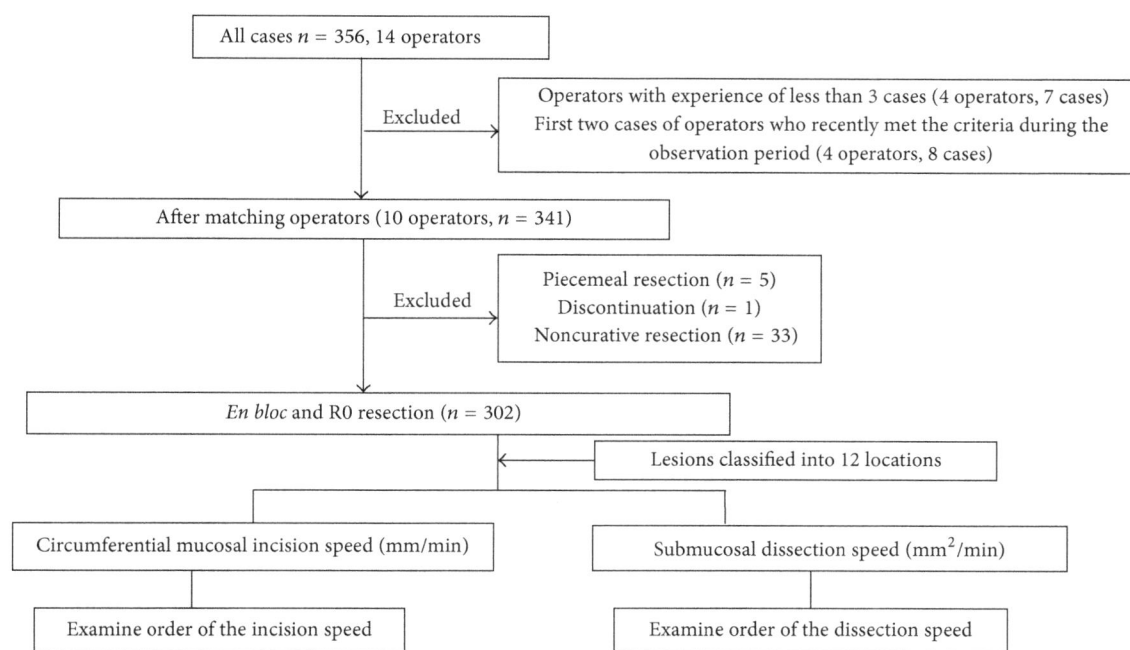

FIGURE 1: Study outline. Operators newly enrolled during the observation period and their first two cases.

not take into account the other determinants of procedural complexity while performing ESD [5, 7, 8]. For example, during circumferential incision at the greater curvature, the mucosa is thick and therefore harder to cut, and the bleeding is more than at other sites. Furthermore, ulcers, scars, and submucosal fibrosis (referred to as "hidden fibrosis" in this paper) tend to occur more commonly along the lesser curvature. Further, submucosal fibrosis is often detected only intraoperatively. Thus, in our opinion, the indicators for actual treatment difficulty or procedure time have been neglected in the classification methodology used in previous reports. Moreover, there are two critical phases that define the procedural complexity (and hence procedure time) for ESD: (1) the mucosal circumference incision phase (CIS) and (2) the submucosal dissection phase (SDS). We believe that these two aspects merit separate consideration.

In this study, all the situations in which procedure time was considered to be different are discussed and classified as new locations. Furthermore, the procedure time for each location is examined with regard to both the mucosal CIS and SDS.

2. Materials and Methods

2.1. Selection Criteria for ESD Operators. According to the training standards proposed by Tsuji et al. [9], ESD operators must have an experience of a minimum of 1,000 cases of upper gastrointestinal endoscopy, with 40 cases or more involving ESD assistance and 20 cases or more that required post-ESD prophylactic hemostasis at the ulcer site. Motivated by this training system to introduce ESD with greater safety, endoscopists at our institution observe and assist in ESD procedures for 1 year (approximately 150 cases). Subsequently,

they train on pig models for a minimum of 10 procedures. Endoscopists who have reached the level at which they no longer accidentally puncture are allowed to practice on humans. Furthermore, to minimize any difference in skills between operators, the inclusion criteria for enrollment in the present study consisted of operators who had performed the procedure on at least three humans with variations in procedure time in up to two procedures. For operators that were newly enrolled during the observation period, only those who met these criteria were included (Figure 1).

2.2. Target Lesions. Differentiated type, undifferentiated type, and mixed type (differentiated and undifferentiated) with an undifferentiated component of <20 mm were used according to the expanded criteria of ESD [7, 10, 11].

Adenomas that were considered precancerous included the following: (1) lesions >20 mm in diameter, (2) those with a depression, (3) those with rapid growth in a short time, and (4) those showing high-grade atypia on biopsy [12–14]. Furthermore, neuroendocrine cell tumors considered endoscopically curable and large benign polyps that are difficult to treat via endoscopic mucosal resection (EMR) due to risk of bleeding were also included in the present study, if treated with ESD.

2.3. Clinical Study of ESD. All cases of undifferentiated mixed type gastric cancer between April 1, 2009, and July 31, 2014, in which ESD was indicated as per the Japanese guidelines were reviewed [7, 11]. A total of 341 gastric ESD patients with 356 lesions were identified. Among these, operators and their patients who did not meet the selection criteria were excluded. Further, the first two cases of operators who recently met the criteria during the observation period were

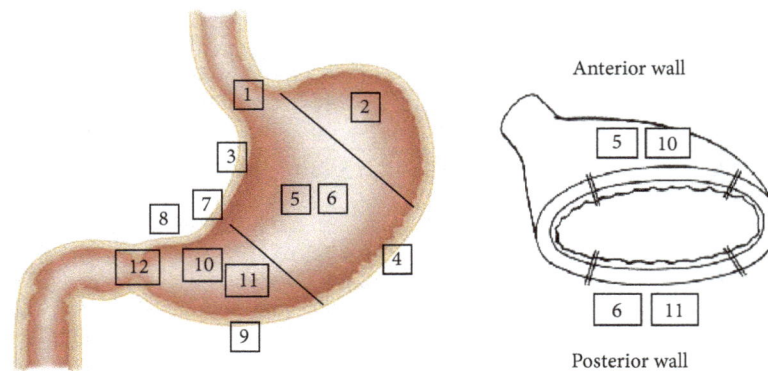

FIGURE 2: Twelve locations divided according to the consideration of a variable situation. 1: the lesion across the esophagogastric junction (AEGJ); 2: fornix; 3: lesser curvature of the body; 4: greater curvature of the body; 5: anterior wall of the body; 6: posterior wall of the body; 7: lesion across the angle; 8: lesser curvature of the antrum; 9: greater curvature of the antrum; 10: anterior wall of the antrum; 11: posterior wall of the antrum; 12: lesion across a pylorus ring (APR).

also excluded. Finally, piecemeal resection, discontinuation, and noncurative resection cases were also excluded to include only curative *en bloc* and R0 resection cases in the study (Figure 1).

2.4. Treatment Area Classification, Resected Lesion Circumference, and Area Calculation Method.

Prior to the observation period, six operators who met the criteria discussed each of the listed items for which the procedural complexity was expected to differ. These included the mucosa (pyloric, fundic, and cardiac areas), state of the submucosa (vascularity, ulcers, scars, and hidden fibrosis observed for the first time at dissection), and maneuverability of the endoscope and device when different from the type of scope used normally. On the basis of this discussion, a total of 12 locations were identified (Figure 2). Representative cases of these variations are shown in Table 3.

The 12 locations were as follows: 1: lesion at the esophagogastric junction (AEGJ); 2: fornix; 3: lesser curvature of the body; 4: greater curvature of the body; 5: anterior wall of the body; 6: posterior wall of the body; 7: lesion across the angle; 8: lesser curvature of the antrum; 9: greater curvature of the antrum; 10: anterior wall of the antrum; 11: posterior wall of the antrum; and 12: lesion across the pylorus ring (APR) (Figure 2). And we examined the proof of the validity of this taxonomy statistically.

Resected specimens were obtained by placing markings for the incision line 10 mm outside the lesion; then resection was performed outside this line for undifferentiated and mixed type lesions. For all other cases, markings for the incision line were placed 5 mm outside the lesion margin, and the incision was made outside this line. As the resected specimens were oval, the area and circumference were calculated from the long and short axes. Furthermore, the CIS per unit length (mm/min) and SDS per unit area (mm^2/min) were calculated for each location. Lastly, these were divided into three groups according to the median resected length/min and the median unit area for each location from the CIS and SDS in order of

size. Next, these groups were further stratified according to procedure time (fast, moderate, and late groups).

2.5. ESD Procedure.

The main endoscope used was GIF Q260J (Olympus, Tokyo, Japan); in duodenum bulb, a reverse maneuver is not possible with the GIF-Q260J, so, in all lesions of duodenum bulb, we used GIF-Q260 (Olympus, Tokyo, Japan). When a closed approach was difficult, the endoscope was changed to GIF 2TQ260M (Olympus, Tokyo, Japan). For the injection solution, a mixture of normal saline with 1% indigo carmine dye was used. In the event of poor uptake, an adequate amount of sodium hyaluronate with high viscosity was used. For basic techniques, we performed a precut in the region of the mucosa using a dual knife (KD-650, Olympus, Tokyo, Japan). Then, a mucosal circumferential incision was made using the dual knife or insulation-tipped (IT) knife 2 (KD-611L, Olympus, Tokyo, Japan). Submucosal dissection was performed using the IT knife 2 and/or a dual knife (especially if a dual knife was used for the scar tissue). In the event of active bleeding or if prominent blood vessels were present, hemostasis was ensured using a coagrasper (FD-410LR, Olympus, Tokyo, Japan). A high-frequency surgical unit for cutting and coagulation (Erbotom VIO300D, ERBE, Tubingen, Germany) was employed.

2.6. Definition.

Curative resection was defined as per the expanded criteria of ESD [7] in the case of an R0 and *en bloc* resection. Ulcers and scars that were observed on preprocedural endoscopy were represented as an "ulcer or scar." Fibrosis first observed in the submucosal layer at the time of treatment was recorded as "hidden fibrosis." Instances where hemostasis was required more frequently than usual or when preincisional coagulation was required due to presence of several submucosal blood vessels were defined as "much time to hemostasis." Tumor morphology was expressed according to the Paris classification [15], and pathological findings were documented as per the Vienna classification [16].

This study was conducted in accordance with the Declaration of Helsinki and was approved by the Institutional Review Boards at Juntendo University Hospital.

2.7. Statistical Analysis. Interquartile range (IQR) was calculated to determine variations in incisional circumference length (per unit length) for each location and the dissected area. With regard to operator skill differences for each location, large deviations were marked with an "*x*."

Outliers were defined as "cases exceeding 1.5 times the interquartile range above the third quartile." Data pertaining to categorical variables are presented as constituent ratios. Between-group differences in case of normally distributed variables were assessed using one-way Analysis of Variance; nonnormally distributed variables were assessed using Kruskal-Wallis or Steel-Dwass tests, as appropriate. Fisher's exact test or χ^2 test was used for all the other analyses. Odds ratios, absolute differences, 95% Confidence Intervals (CI), and *p* values are reported. Statistical significance was defined as $p < 0.05$. All statistical analyses were performed using SASS version 9.4 (SAS Institute, Cary, NC, USA).

3. Results

3.1. Results of the Validity of 12 Locations Classification. In this classification system, we found a significant difference between different groups for all CIS and SDS in each location, demonstrating the validity of this classification method ($p < 0.01$) (Table 4).

3.2. Study Outline. A total of 10 operators participated in the study: six operators who completed the training program prior to the observation period and had experience performing ESD on at least three patients, plus four newly added operators with ESD experience of at least three patients. On the basis of operator adaptations, 341 lesions remained for 10 operators. Furthermore, we excluded five cases that finally became piecemeal and snaring resection. In addition, we excluded one case in which the procedure was discontinued. Among the cases in which *en bloc* resection was performed, 33 noncurative resections (lesions invading the submucosa and positive lymphovascular invasion, positive margins, or expanded indication [7]) were excluded. Therefore, a total of 302 lesions treated by curative resection (*en bloc* and R0 resection) were included in the analysis (Figure 1).

3.3. Baseline Clinical Results. A total of 302 lesions were examined in the study; the male-to-female ratio was 2.5 : 1. Macroscopically, flat, and depressed types accounted for >95% of the total lesions. The median tumor diameter was 11 mm, and the median size of the resected specimen was 34 mm. The most common histological tumor type was differentiated adenocarcinoma (81.8%); mixed types containing a differentiated type and ≤20 mm undifferentiated types accounted for 4.0%; lesions of an undifferentiated type accounted only for 1.7% of the total number of lesions. Adenomas represented 11.9% of the cases. In addition, there was one case of a neuroendocrine tumor and one of a

Table 1: Baseline characteristics of gastric tumors.

Characteristics	Value	(%)
Sex (females : males)	80 : 222 (1 : 2.5)	
Age, years, median (range)	73 (40–92)	
Morphology		
Protruded (0-I)	11	(3.7)
Flat (0-II b, 0-II a)	143 (6, 137)	(47.4)
Depressed (0-II a + II c, 0-IIc)	147 (138, 9)	(48.8)
Submucosal tumor	1	(0.3)
Tumor size (mm), median (range)	11 (2–60)	
Specimen size (mm), median (range)	34 (14–110)	
Histology		
Adenoma	36	(11.9)
Differentiated type	247	(81.8)
Mix type (differentiated + undifferentiated type (<20 mm))	12	(4)
Undifferentiated type	5	(1.7)
Others*	2	(0.7)
Ulcer or scar	24	(7.9)
Hidden fibrosis	35	(11.6)
Much time to hemostasis	51	(16.9)
Perforation	7	(2.3)
Delayed bleeding	9	(3.0)

*Others: one case was neuroendocrine tumor and another was hyperplastic polyp.

Table 2: Classification of lesions by location ($n = 302$).

Location number	n	(%)
1: AEGJ	5	(1.7)
2: fornix	7	(2.3)
3: lesser curvature of the body	33	(10.9)
4: greater curvature of the body	21	(7.0)
5: anterior wall of the body	22	(7.3)
6: posterior wall of the body	46	(15.2)
7: across the angle	34	(11.3)
8: lesser curvature of the antrum	45	(14.9)
9: greater curvature of the antrum	17	(5.6)
10: anterior wall of the antrum	34	(11.3)
11: posterior wall of the antrum	34	(11.3)
12: APR	4	(1.3)

AEGJ: across the esophagogastric junction; APR: across the pyloric ring.

hyperplastic polyp. Ulcers or scars were confirmed in 7.9% of cases, and hidden fibrosis in 11.6%. Moreover, much time to hemostasis was observed in 16.9% of the cases. Complications involving perforation occurred in 2.3% and delayed bleeding in 3% of cases, comparable to results that have been reported elsewhere (Table 1) [1, 2, 17–19].

3.4. Results for Each Classified Location. The breakdown of the number of cases according to 12 classified locations is shown in Table 2. The lesions were most commonly found on the posterior wall of the gastric body ($n = 46$ [15.2%]), while those extending to the pyloric ring were least common

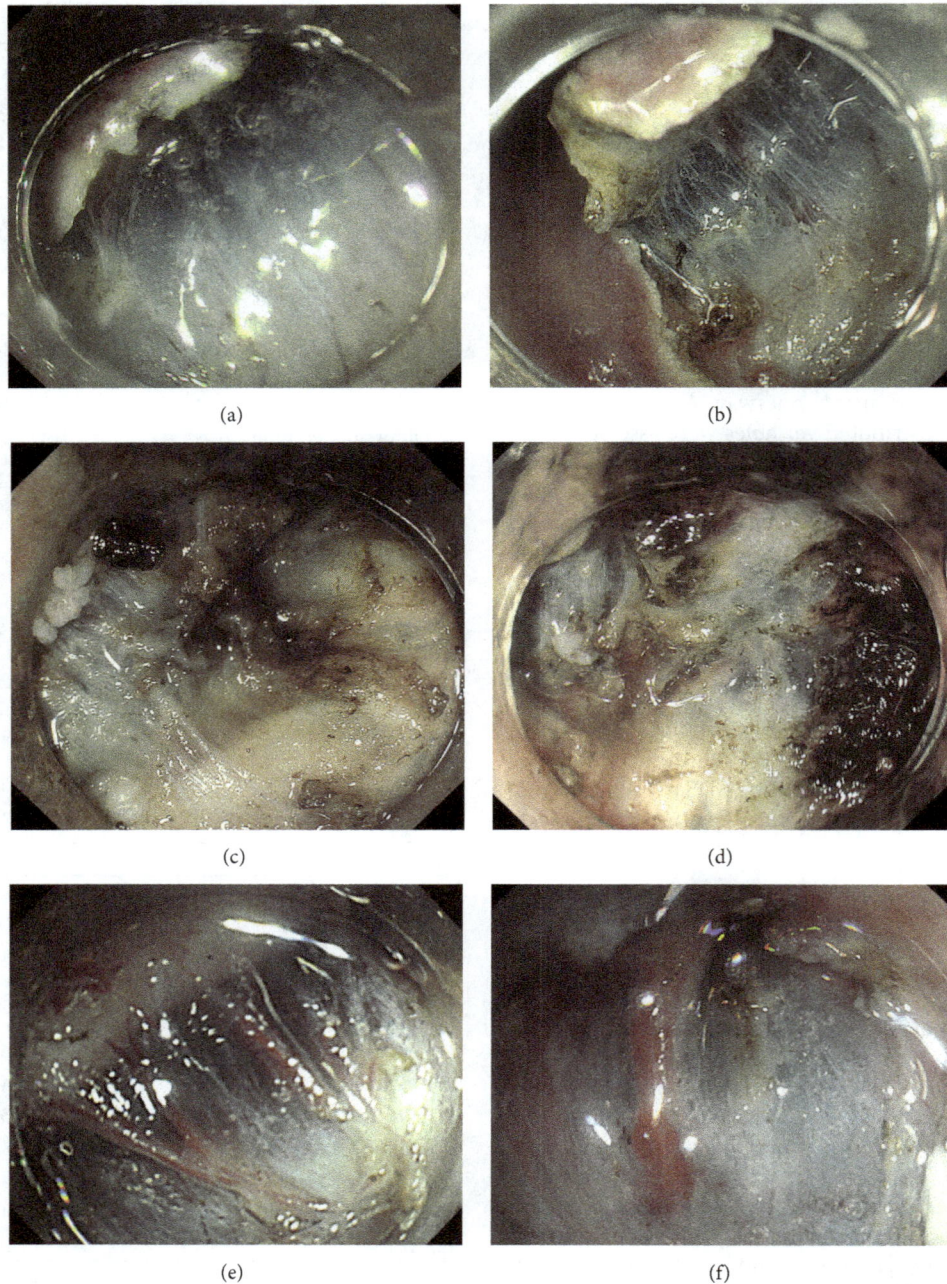

FIGURE 3: Variations of lesser curvature. (a, b) Easy case of submucosa. (c, d) "Hidden fibrosis." (e, f) Many perforating vessel case.

($n = 4$ [1.3%]). The clinicopathological characteristics by lesion location are listed in Table 3. No significant between-group difference was observed with respect to age ($p = 0.24$). Ulcers or scars exceeded 10% in four locations including the following: (1) AEGJ, location 1 (20%); (2) fornix, location 2 (14.3%); (3) angle, location 7 (11.8%); and (4) greater curvature of the antrum, location 9 (11.8%).

A high rate of hidden fibrosis was observed in fornix, location 2 (28.6%), and the lesser curvature of the body, location 3 (24.2%) (Figure 3). In addition, other locations in which fibrosis exceeded 10% were the posterior wall of the

body, location 6 (17.4%), and the lesions across the angle, location 7 (17.6%). It is important to note that a high rate of fibrosis of 24% was observed in the lesser curvature of the body (location 6), despite the fact that ulcers or scars were found in only 6.1% of these cases.

Much time to hemostasis was in the following, in descending order: (1) AEGJ (location 1), 60%; (2) fornix (location 2), 42.9%; (3) lesser curvature of the body (location 3), in 30.3%; (4) posterior wall of the body (location 6), 28.3%; (5) lesion across the angle (location 7), 26.5%; (6) anterior wall of the body (location 5), 22.7%; and (7) greater curvature

TABLE 3: Characteristics of the cases in the 12 locations.

Location	n	Mean age	Sex Females : males	Ulcer or scar (%)	Hidden fibrosis (%)	Much time to hemostasis (%)	Tumor size (mm), median	Circumference (mm), median	Resected area (mm^2), median
1	5	64.4	1 : 4	1/5 (20)	1/5 (20)	3/5 (60)	12	206.9	3187.1
2	7	72.1	2 : 5	1/7 (14.3)	2/7 (28.6)	3/7 (42.9)	10.5	182.3	2637.6
3	33	72.4	7 : 26	2/33 (6.1)	8/33 (24.2)	10/33 (30.3)	13.5	195.3	2901.4
4	21	69.5	3 : 18	2/21 (9.5)	2/21 (9.5)	3/21 (14.3)	16	201.8	3165.1
5	22	72.4	4 : 18	1/22 (4.5)	2/22 (9.1)	5/22 (22.7)	14	200	3132.2
6	46	70.1	12 : 34	4/46 (8.7)	8/46 (17.4)	13/46 (28.3)	14.5	182.2	2637.6
7	34	74.1	10 : 24	4/34 (11.8)	6/34 (17.6)	9/34 (26.5)	18	226.8	4042.8
8	45	72.6	14 : 31	4/45 (8.9)	4/45 (8.9)	2/45 (4.4)	18.5	219.2	3733.5
9	17	71.5	3 : 14	2/17 (11.8)	1/17 (5.9)	0/17 (0)	10.5	182.5	2625
10	34	72.2	12 : 22	1/34 (2.9)	0/34 (0)	1/34 (2.9)	12	183.6	2512
11	34	74.4	9 : 25	1/34 (2.9)	0/34 (0)	2/34 (5.9)	12	173.1	2373.8
12	4	76	3 : 1	1/4 (25)	1/4 (25)	0/4 (0)	14	211.1	3504.2
p value		0.24				<0.05	<0.01	<0.01	<0.01

1: the lesion across the esophagogastric junction (AEGJ); 2: fornix; 3: lesser curvature of the body; 4: greater curvature of the body; 5: anterior wall of the body; 6: posterior wall of the body; 7: the lesion across the angle; 8: lesser curvature of the antrum; 9: greater curvature of the antrum; 10: anterior wall of the antrum; 11: posterior wall of the antrum; 12: the lesion across the pylorus ring (APR).

TABLE 4: Mucosal circumference incision speed and submucosal dissection speed cut (speed per minute) in descending order.

Rank	Location	Mucosal circumference incision speed Median (mm/min) range	Interquartile range	Location	Submucosal dissection speed Median (mm²/min)	Interquartile range
1	9	19.3 (3.8–39.3)	18.3	10	214.6 (47.1–942)	174.5
2	10	18.0 (5.9–81.7)	10.9	9	204.1 (55.8–653.1)	309.3
3	11	15.6 (3.8–95.8)	13.7	11	175.1 (34.1–576.9)	201.2
4	8	13.9 (3.3–35.2)	11.3	8	118.2 (19.3–502.4)	114.1
5	4	12.8 (4.2–24.0)	8.6	3	116.7 (23.1–440.4)	159.4
6	3	12.4 (2.9–34.1)	10.7	5	116.0 (15.2–338.2)	92.7
7	5	11.5 (2.6–35.5)	10.4	4	96.4 (55.9–316.5)	61.2
8	2	10.0 (3.1–30.4)	12.5	6	93.5 (7.6–506.6)	80.1
9	7	9.2 (2.5–40.3)	8.15	7	92.5 (20.9–474.4)	125.9
10	6	8.2 (1.7–26.5)	6.6	1	91.1 (12.8–157)	97.7
11	1	7.6 (2.9–11.2)	6.4	2	66.6 (7.6–141.3)	49.2
12	12	4.5 (3.3–6.1)	2.2	12	43.5 (12.2–236.4)	170.9
p value		<0.01			<0.01	

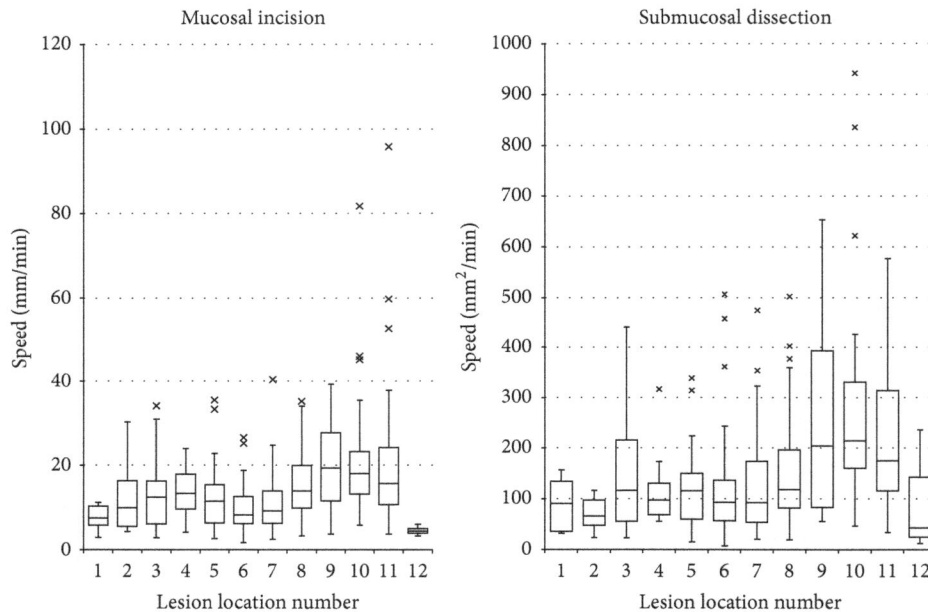

FIGURE 4: Interquartile range of the mucosal incision and submucosal dissection speed. This figure shows a graph of the mucosal incision and submucosal dissection speed of each of the 12 locations. By noting the interquartile range, the variation in the rate was clear.

of the body (location 4), in 14.3%, with a higher rate at the lesser curvature of the body (location 3) than at the greater curvature of the body (location 4).

Table 3 shows that a significant difference was observed in the tumor diameter between each location ($p < 0.05$). Furthermore, a significant difference was also observed for the circumference of the resected specimen or the area of the resected specimen between each location. Overall, the variations in the values were statistically significant ($p < 0.01$).

Table 4 shows the variations in the resection time in descending order of size of the median circumference incisional length per minute and median dissected area of the submucosal layer. The IQR for each location is graphically

presented in Figure 4. A significant variation in overall CIS and SDS was found by location ($p < 0.01$).

Regarding CIS, while the speed was faster for lesions of the antrum than for those at other locations, it was slowest for the antral area along the lesser curvature, location 8 (median: 13.9 mm/min). The overall incisional speed was slower for the gastric body than for the antral area and was the slowest for location 6, the posterior wall of the gastric body (median: 8.2 mm/min). The second slowest location (i.e., 11th position) was location 1, AEGJ (median: 7.6 mm/min), and the slowest location was location 12, APR (median: 4.5 mm/min).

In contrast, the greatest IQR was found for the antral area along the greater curvature, location 9. Although the

TABLE 5: Subgroup analyses by procedure time for mucosal incision and submucosal dissection on ESD.

	Mucosal incision				Submucosal dissection			
	Location	Rate, median (range)	Interquartile range	p value	Location	Rate, median (range)	Interquartile range	p value
Fast group	8, 9, 10, 11	15.6 (3.3–95.8)	12		8, 9, 10, 11	170.5 (19.3–942.0)	178.7	
Moderate group	2, 3, 4, 5	12.4 (2.6–35.5)	10.6	$p < 0.01$	3, 4, 5, 6	97.7 (7.6–506.6)	79.7	$p < 0.001$
Late group	1, 6, 7, 12	8.2 (12.2–474.4)	6.7	$p < 0.01$	1, 2, 7, 12	89.2 (12.2–474.4)	90.4	0.42

1: the lesion across the esophagogastric junction (AEGJ); 2: fornix; 3: lesser curvature of the body; 4: greater curvature of the body; 5: anterior wall of the body; 6: posterior wall of the body; 7: the lesion across the angle; 8: lesser curvature of the antrum; 9: greater curvature of the antrum; 10: anterior wall of the antrum; 11: posterior wall of the antrum; 12: the lesion across the pylorus ring (APR).

incisional speed was slow in the AEGJ and APR, the IQR was small, with little variation in speed.

With respect to SDS, as expected, the overall speed was fast for antral lesions; however, when dissecting areas around the antrum, the speed was slowest for location 8, the lesser curvature of the antrum (median: 118.2 mm^2/min). The antrum exhibited a large IQR, and, overall, the speed tended to vary greatly at the same sites of the antrum. The variation was particularly high in location 9, the greater curvature of the antrum. For the gastric body, the speed was the slowest for location 6, the posterior wall, similar to the case for CIS. However, the greatest variation in the dissection speed was observed for location 3, the lesser curvature (IQR: 159.40). The SDS for the AEGJ, APR, and fornix was lower than that for other locations.

The second slowest SDS (i.e., the 11th position) was the fornix, and the slowest was for the APR. The fornix was at the eighth place with respect to CIS but at the eleventh place for SDS. The greatest IQR for SDS was observed for location 9, the greater curvature of antrum (IQR = 309.3).

3.5. Grouping of CIS and SDS for Each Location. The results are shown in Table 5. The fornix had the fifth highest speed for CIS, placing it in the moderate group, whereas, for SDS, it was the second slowest overall, placing it in the late group. Furthermore, the time required for CIS at the posterior wall of the gastric body was the third overall, placing it in the late group. However, for SDS, the dissection speed was fifth overall, placing it in the moderate group, similar to other lesions of the body. For both APR and AEGJ, CIS and SDS were slow, placing them in the late group.

With regard to CIS, a significant difference was observed between the fast and moderate groups and between the moderate and late groups ($p < 0.01$). For SDS, no significant difference was observed between the moderate and late groups ($p = 0.42$). However, a remarkably high difference was observed between the fast and moderate groups ($p < 0.001$) (Table 5).

4. Discussion

With regard to the ESD difficulty by location, the longest reported procedure time has been reported for the upper third of the posterior wall [6, 19]. However, these previous studies did not take into account other factors that tend to vary with the location of the lesions; these include technical considerations (e.g., device angle and scope maneuverability) and lesion characteristics (e.g., vascularity, ulceration, scarring, fibrosis, characteristics of contiguous mucosa, and submucosa). Furthermore, the determinants of CIS and SDS are distinct, but procedural complexity in previous studies was only assessed with respect to overall procedure time.

In the present study, unlike conventional location classification methods, we incorporated several key variables that determine procedural complexity. Additionally, we also examined CI and SD as separate factors. Using this classification system, we found a significant difference between different groups for all CIS and SDS in each location, demonstrating the validity of this classification method ($p < 0.01$) (Table 4).

Undifferentiated lesions have been reported to be more difficult to assess [6]. This may be explained by the fact that the differentiated type is covered by a thin layer of atrophic mucosa, which makes it relatively easy to dissect the mucosa and submucosa. In contrast, the mucosa surrounding the undifferentiated type tumor is rarely atrophic. This may be attributed to the fact that the incisional diameter may have been much larger than the actual lesion because of rich mucosal vascularity. Moreover, in lesions with the presence of a large number of blood vessels and fat in submucosa, the incisional line was marked approximately 10 mm away from the lesion. As shown Table 3, at every location, there were significant differences in tumor size ($p < 0.5$). But actual resected specimen sizes are variable. For that reason, when the tumors were of an undifferentiated or mixed type, there was a need to make a larger excision. Endoscopically, when there is an ulcer or scar in order to allow the scope access to the under mucosa a larger than normal incision must be made, this may have resulted in the more significant difference in circumference (mm) and resected area (mm^2) ($p < 0.01$). If the procedure were to take place in area with a large amount of blood vessels with factors written above taking effect, the time needed to stop the hemorrhage and much time to hemostasis would prolong the procedure time. In the case of an ulcer or scar, the time needed to excise the scar in addition to the larger than normal incision would also result in a longer procedure time. Hidden fibrosis can only be known at the time of dissection; thus it can said that it has no correlation with the factors mentioned above.

Regarding the overall ESD, the incisional and dissection speed was faster in the case of antral lesions than those for other locations. However, the IQR tended to vary greatly during the actual dissection (Figure 4). We believe that this was due to the relative ease of dissection in this region; there were large differences in the performance of experienced and inexperienced operators despite our stringent operator selection criteria. However, for the procedures involving the antrum, both the incision and dissection speeds at the lesser curvature for CID and SDS were slower than those of other antral sites. We believe that this was because, in the lesser curvature of the antrum, the endoscopic device and lesion can readily become perpendicular to each other, and the lesion site may be relatively difficult to approach with the scope in this position. In locations other than the antrum, particularly the AEGJ and fornix, ESD tends to be challenging even for experienced operators, which may be responsible for the relatively low variability in the procedure time.

The SDS varied greatly in lesions in the lesser curvature of the body, relative to that in other locations of the body (IQR = 159.4). The gastric angle and lesser curvature of the body are sites in which ulcers and scars are common. However, in the lesser curvature of the body, hidden fibrosis is often incidentally discovered during endoscopic dissection, regardless of the lack of scars; of note, we also found fibrosis in 24.2% of the dissections in this area in the present study. Therefore, increased time is required for detachment when the submucosa is not sufficiently lifted by local injection. Furthermore, the lesser curvature of the body can be difficult to approach with a scope or device depending on the shape of the stomach. Moreover, some lesions were viewed perpendicularly, which may have been responsible for the high variability in the incisional speed among lesions located at the same gastric body site. Moreover, it was initially believed that the greater curvature had more blood vessels and hemostasis. However, in clinical practice, more cases of much time to hemostasis were observed for the lesser curvature lesions (30.3% versus 14.3% for the greater curvature lesions) (Table 3).

While increased perilesional vascularity in the case of ulcers, scars, and hidden fibrosis is believed to be another potential reason for the occurrence of many blood vessels, several perforating branches of blood vessels to submucosa in the lesser curvature are also contributory factors. However, a difference in the presence or absence of blood vessels and fibrosis in the lesser curvature greatly affects the procedure; therefore, it is not straightforward to predict the time required for dissection. Consequently, we suggest that expert operators with experience in difficult situations always be prepared to take turns at any time.

Differences in CIS and SDS between the fast, moderate, and late groups were found in the fornix (location 2) and in the posterior wall of the body (location 6). The fornix was classified in the moderate group for CIS, but the late group for SDS. This is because the scope and device end up perpendicular to the lesion and thus it is difficult to maneuver

horizontally as both the submucosa and muscularis were thin.

The posterior wall of the body was classified into the moderate group for SDS, but the late group for CIS. We believe that this was attributed to the fact that reverse maneuver was considered to be difficult for the circumferential incision, in addition to the fact that there were more large blood vessels and fat in the mucosa and submucosa than in the other sites. However, upon completion of the circumferential incision, not as many blood vessels or as much fat was observed in the submucosa as that at the time when the circumferential incision was performed, and, therefore, dissection was considered easier than the circumferential incision. Locations that became classified into the late group for both CIS and SDS included the following: location 1, AEGJ; location 7, across the angle; and location 12, APR.

Maneuverability for the AEGJ (location 1) is considered to be poor due to the following reasons: hemostatic treatment is difficult due to several palisade blood vessels traversing the submucosa; dissection is difficult due to inflammatory adhesions caused by gastroesophageal reflux disease or other conditions; the working space on the oral side of the lesion is narrow due to the requirement for the intraesophageal maneuver; and reverse maneuver on the anal side is difficult to move the scope closer to the lesion. The angle (location 7) has a sharp anatomical bend and, therefore, must be approached from various angles. It is also a common site for ulcers and scars, which cause adhesions and render the dissection more challenging. APR requires resection of the pylorus ring (location 12) and reverse maneuver in the narrow bulbous working space as well as precautions for prevention of duodenal perforation. Consequently, it was assumed to be the location in which numerous techniques were most required. For the reasons provided above, in APR, reverse maneuver was not possible with the GIF-Q260J typically used. In all cases, the scope had to be changed to GIF-Q260, which has the greatest flexibility in the tip structure. Furthermore, to ensure the working space for this location, it is important to use a scope without the tip hood mounted so as not to impede inversion.

Initially, we believed that the greater curvature belonged to the late group for both the CIS and SDS, on the basis of the mucosal thickness, blood vessels, and the amount of fat. However, in our analysis, it was found to belong to the moderate group.

Complications involving perforation occurred in 2.3% and delayed bleeding in 3% of cases, comparable to results that have been reported elsewhere (Table 1) [1, 2, 17–19]. However, our hospital is a specialized center for ESD; many cases including lesions with high difficulty and high complications have been treated at our hospital. Thus, we believe that such a condition is rather rare compared with that at other hospitals.

The limitations of this study include the fact that it was a single-center study, and there may be a bias according to the endoscopist who performed the ESD.

In the present study, a more detailed classification of the resection sites was used than those that have been previously described; this inevitably reduced the sample size for each lesion location. However, a larger sample size would have made it challenging to perform a detailed study. Apart from location, we did not analyze other determinants of ESD duration and speed. However, we were able to clarify submucosal fibrosis and confirmed, for the first time upon dissection in the lesser curvature of the body, locations at which hemostasis can be difficult (e.g., the greater curvature of the body).

It has been reported that the prolongation of ESD duration increases the rate of complications [20, 21], and, thus, it is also very important to choose the lesion treatment with a clear expectation of the time requirements for each stage (e.g., incision and dissection) in consideration of the skill level of the operator.

5. Conclusion

In the present study, we compared CIS and SDS in ESD of gastric lesions and reported the CIS and SDS for different locations for the first time. On the basis of our results, we predicted the CIS and SDS according to different locations and clarified the underlying factors that affect procedural complexity and speed.

Competing Interests

The authors declare that there are no competing interests or financial ties relevant to the publication of this paper.

Authors' Contributions

Hironori Konuma (endoscopist of this study) collected, analyzed, interpreted the data, and drafted the manuscript. Kenshi Matsumoto (corresponding author and endoscopist of this study) planned and executed the study, analyzed and interpreted the data, and revised the manuscript. Yoichi Akazawa, Hiroyuki Komori, Misuzu Ueyama, Yuta Nakagawa, Tsutomu Takeda, Takashi Morimoto, Kohei Matsumoto, and Hiroya Ueyama were endoscopists of this study. Daisuke Asaoka and Mariko Hojo collected the data. Takashi Yao (Professor) provided the pathological analysis. Akihito Nagahara (Professor) was an endoscopist of this study. Professors Akihisa Miyazaki and Sumio Watanabe revised the paper.

Acknowledgments

The authors would like to thank Shizuru Matsuoka, a statistical specialist, for providing appropriate statistical advice.

References

[1] T. Gotoda, H. Yamamoto, and R. M. Soetikno, "Endoscopic submucosal dissection of early gastric cancer," *Journal of Gastroenterology*, vol. 41, no. 10, pp. 929–942, 2006.

[2] M. Muto, S. Miyamoto, A. Hosokawa et al., "Endoscopic mucosal resection in the stomach using the insulated-tip needle-knife," *Endoscopy*, vol. 37, no. 2, pp. 178–182, 2005.

[3] S. V. Kantsevoy, D. G. Adler, J. D. Conway et al., "Endoscopic mucosal resection and endoscopic submucosal dissection," *Gastrointestinal Endoscopy*, vol. 68, no. 1, pp. 11–18, 2008.

[4] P. Pimentel-Nunes, M. Dinis-Ribeiro, T. Ponchon et al., "Endoscopic submucosal dissection: European Society of Gastrointestinal Endoscopy (ESGE) Guideline," *Endoscopy*, vol. 47, no. 9, pp. 829–854, 2015.

[5] A. Imagawa, H. Okada, Y. Kawahara et al., "Endoscopic submucosal dissection for early gastric cancer: results and degrees of technical difficulty as well as success," *Endoscopy*, vol. 38, no. 10, pp. 987–990, 2006.

[6] I.-K. Chung, J. H. Lee, S.-H. Lee et al., "Therapeutic outcomes in 1000 cases of endoscopic submucosal dissection for early gastric neoplasms: Korean ESD Study Group Multicenter Study," *Gastrointestinal Endoscopy*, vol. 69, no. 7, pp. 1228–1235, 2009.

[7] Japanese Gastric Cancer Association, "Japanese gastric cancer treatment guidelines 2010 (ver. 3)," *Gastric Cancer*, vol. 14, no. 2, pp. 113–123, 2011.

[8] O. Goto, M. Fujishiro, S. Kodashima, S. Ono, and M. Omata, "Is it possible to predict the procedural time of endoscopic submucosal dissection for early gastric cancer?" *Journal of Gastroenterology and Hepatology*, vol. 24, no. 3, pp. 379–383, 2009.

[9] Y. Tsuji, K. Ohata, M. Sekiguchi et al., "An effective training system for endoscopic submucosal dissection of gastric neoplasm," *Endoscopy*, vol. 43, no. 12, pp. 1033–1038, 2011.

[10] T. Gotoda, A. Yanagisawa, M. Sasako et al., "Incidence of lymph node metastasis from early gastric cancer: estimation with a large number of cases at two large centers," *Gastric Cancer*, vol. 3, no. 4, pp. 219–225, 2000.

[11] T. Hirasawa, T. Gotoda, S. Miyata et al., "Incidence of lymph node metastasis and the feasibility of endoscopic resection for undifferentiated-type early gastric cancer," *Gastric Cancer*, vol. 12, no. 3, pp. 148–152, 2009.

[12] K. Nakamura, H. Sakaguchi, and M. Enjoji, "Depressed adenoma of the stomach," *Cancer*, vol. 62, no. 10, pp. 2197–2202, 1988.

[13] G. Tamura, K. Sakata, S. Nishizuka et al., "Allelotype of adenoma and differentiated adenocarcinoma of the stomach," *Journal of Pathology*, vol. 180, no. 4, pp. 371–377, 1996.

[14] G. Tamura, "Molecular pathogenesis of adenoma and differentiated adenocarcinoma of the stomach," *Pathology International*, vol. 46, no. 11, pp. 834–841, 1996.

[15] R. J. Schlemper, I. Hirata, and M. F. Dixon, "The macroscopic classification of early neoplasia of the digestive tract," *Endoscopy*, vol. 34, no. 2, pp. 163–168, 2002.

[16] R. J. Schlemper, R. H. Riddell, Y. Kato et al., "The Vienna classification of gastrointestinal epithelial neoplasia," *Gut*, vol. 47, no. 2, pp. 251–255, 2000.

[17] H. J. Chun, B. Keum, J. H. Kim, and S. Y. Seol, "Current status of endoscopic submucosal dissection for the management of early gastric cancer: a Korean perspective," *World Journal of Gastroenterology*, vol. 17, no. 21, pp. 2592–2596, 2011.

[18] J. H. Lee, S. J. Hong, J. Y. Jang, S. E. Kim, and S. Y. Seol, "Outcome after endoscopic submucosal dissection for early gastric cancer in Korea," *World Journal of Gastroenterology*, vol. 17, no. 31, pp. 3591–3595, 2011.

[19] J. Y. Ahn, K. D. Choi, J. Y. Choi et al., "Procedure time of endoscopic submucosal dissection according to the size and location of early gastric cancers: analysis of 916 dissections performed by 4 experts," *Gastrointestinal Endoscopy*, vol. 73, no. 5, pp. 911–916, 2011.

[20] J. Y. Yoon, C. N. Shim, S. H. Chung et al., "Impact of tumor location on clinical outcomes of gastric endoscopic submucosal dissection," *World Journal of Gastroenterology*, no. 26, pp. 8631–8637, 2014.

[21] J. H. Yoo, S. J. Shin, K. M. Lee et al., "Risk factors for perforations associated with endoscopic submucosal dissection in gastric lesions: emphasis on perforation type," *Surgical Endoscopy and Other Interventional Techniques*, vol. 26, no. 9, pp. 2456–2464, 2012.

18

Solid-Pseudopapillary Tumor of the Pancreas: A Single Center Experience

Valentina Beltrame,[1] **Gioia Pozza,**[1] **Enrico Dalla Bona,**[1] **Alberto Fantin,**[2] **Michele Valmasoni,**[1] **and Cosimo Sperti**[1]

[1]*Department of Surgery, Oncology and Gastroenterology, 3rd Surgical Clinic, University of Padua, Via Giustiniani 2, 35128 Padua, Italy*
[2]*Gastroenterology Unit, University of Padua, Via Giustiniani 2, 35128 Padua, Italy*

Correspondence should be addressed to Cosimo Sperti; csperti@libero.it

Academic Editor: Atsushi Irisawa

Aim of this study was to review the institutional experience of solid-pseudopapillary tumors of the pancreas with particular attention to the problems of preoperative diagnosis and treatment. From 1997 to 2013, SPT was diagnosed in 18 patients among 451 pancreatic cystic neoplasms (3.7%). All patients underwent preoperative abdominal ultrasound, computed assisted tomography, and tumor markers (CEA and CA 19-9) determinations. In some instances, magnetic resonance, positron emission tomography, and endoscopic ultrasound with aspiration cytology were performed. There were two males and 16 females. Serum CA 19-9 was slightly elevated in one case. Preoperative diagnosis was neuroendocrine tumor ($n = 2$), mucinous tumor ($n = 2$), and SPT ($n = 14$). Two patients underwent previous operation before referral to our department: one explorative laparotomy and one enucleation of SPT resulting in surgical margins involvement. All patients underwent pancreatic resection associated with portal vein resection ($n = 1$) or liver metastases ($n = 1$). One patient died of metastatic disease, 77 months after operation, and 17 are alive and free with a median survival time of 81.5 months (range 36–228 months). Most of SPT can be diagnosed by CT or MRI, and the role of other diagnostic tools is very limited. We lack sufficient information regarding clinicopathologic features predicting prognosis. Caution is needed when performing limited resection, and long and careful follow-up is required for all patients after surgery.

1. Introduction

Solid-pseudopapillary tumor (SPT) is a distinct variety among cystic neoplasms of the pancreas. Although rare, this type of tumor is increasingly seen in clinical practice because of widespread availability of imaging modalities and better awareness of the disease. In a review of English literature from 1933 to 2003, a total of 718 SPTs were collected, including pediatric cases [1]; in a recent review of Law et al. in 2014 [2], a total of 2744 patients with SPT were identified, of whom 2410 were observed from 2000 to 2012. Solid-pseudopapillary tumor is generally considered an indolent lesion with low malignant potential; it occurs most frequently in young women. Favorable prognosis after surgical resection has been invariably reported. However, some cases of locally infiltrating or metastatic variety, or recurrences after surgery, have been described in a significant percentage of 10–15% of patients [3]. Long-term survival is reported even for metastatic disease, but some patients will eventually die for disease's progression, suggesting a widely variable and not clearly elucidated biology of the tumor.

We report our experience of SPTs with particular attention to identify the problems in differential diagnosis, the clinicopathological features predicting behaviour, and the treatment and outcome after tumor's resection.

2. Patients and Methods

We retrospectively reviewed the patients who underwent surgical resection of SPT of the pancreas from the prospectively recorded database, between January 1997 and December 2013. We evaluated patients' demographic features, clinical presentation, imaging findings, surgical procedures, pathologic aspects, perioperative outcome, follow-up, and survival. All

TABLE 1: Clinicopathologic features of patients with pancreatic SPT.

Pts	Sex	Age	Site	Size	Treatment	Follow-up (months)
(1)	Female	54	Tail	4.0	DP	A,NED (228)
(2)	Female	13	Body	4.0	CP	A,NED (198)
(3)	Female	32	Tail	7.0	DP	A,NED (192)
(4)	Female	31	Tail	14.0	DP	A,NED (180)
(5)	Female	20	Tail	10.0	DP	A,NED (156)
(6)	Female	14	Tail	10.0	DP	A,NED (132)
(7)	Female	38	Body	3.0	DP	A,NED (96)
(8)	Male	59	Tail	11.0	DP	A,NED (94)
(9)	Female	40	Body	2.0	CP	A,NED (84)
(10)	Female	21	Head	8.0	PPPD	A,NED (79)
(11)	Female	13	Head	3.0	PPPD	A,NED (77)
(12)	Female	49	Head-body	10.0	TP + VR	DEAD (77)
(13)	Female	38	Tail	4.0	DPSP	A,NED (74)
(14)	Male	75	Tail	4.5	DP	A,NED (72)
(15)	Female	30	Tail	10.0	DP	A,NED (61)
(16)	Female	24	Body	7.0	DP	A,NED (50)
(17)	Female	14	Head	3.0	PPPD	A,NED (48)
(18)	Female	35	Tail	4.5	DP	A,NED (36)

DP = distal pancreatectomy; CP = central pancreatectomy; TP = total pancreatectomy; VR = venous resection; PPPD = pylorus-preserving pancreaticoduodenectomy; A = alive; NED = no evidence of disease; DPSP = distal pancreatectomy spleen-preserving.

patients preoperatively underwent serum carcinoembryonic antigen CEA and CA 19-9 examination, abdominal ultrasonography (US), and computed assisted tomography (CT). In some instances, magnetic resonance imaging (MRI), 18-FDG positron emission tomography (PET/CT), and endoscopic ultrasound (EUS) with fine-needle aspiration (FNA) were also performed. Pathologically, SPTs were classified as malignant if it showed extrapancreatic invasion, perineural or vascular invasion, pancreatic parenchyma invasion [4], or distant metastases. Follow-up included physical examination, serum tumor markers, and US and/or CT or MRI every 6 months for the first 5 years and then every year. PET/CT was performed when clinically suggested. The median follow-up period was 84 months (range 36–228 months).

3. Results

In the study period, 451 patients with cystic tumors of the pancreas were observed; among these, 18 (3.7%) were histologically proven to have SPT of the pancreas (Table 1). There were 16 females and 2 males, with a mean age of 34.2 years (range 13–75): both male patients were older compared to females. Patients presented abdominal pain or discomfort ($n = 9$) and palpable mass ($n = 6$); three patients were asymptomatic. The tumor averaged 7.0 cm in diameter (range 2–14 cm) and was located in the body and/or tail of the pancreas in 13 patients, in the head in 3 patients, and in the neck in two patients. Three patients had surgery in other hospitals before referral to our department: one patient had cystogastrostomy for an incorrect diagnosis of pancreatic pseudocyst; one had exploratory laparotomy and biopsy for a locally advanced pancreatic mass involving portal-mesenteric vein; and one young patient had enucleation of

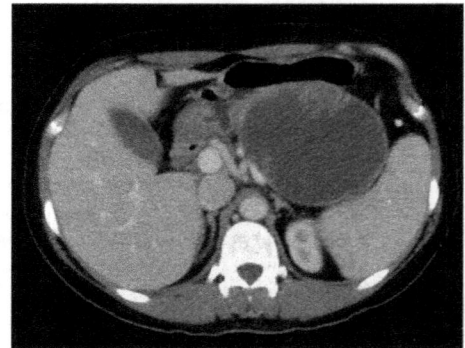

FIGURE 1: Computed tomography of the abdomen showing a large cystic mass with solid components in the body-tail of the pancreas (case number 13).

3 cm pancreatic head mass that showed surgical margins involvement at pathologic examination. Only one patient showed high serum CA 19-9 levels (92 U/mL; normal value < 37 U/mL). Preoperative radiological investigation included abdominal US and CT in all patients (Figure 1), MRI in 6 patients, and EUS + fine-needle aspiration in 5. Two patients had a correct cytologic diagnosis of SPT; 2 patients had a suggested diagnosis of neuroendocrine tumor (but with radiologic findings suggestive for SPT) and in one cytology was nondiagnostic. Ten patients underwent 18-FDG positron emission tomography (PET); in 7 patients there was a pathologic uptake of the radiotracer (mean SUV 8.8, range 2.6–24.0) (Figure 2). Two patients underwent 111-In-Octreoscan without pathologic uptake of the radiotracer. So, preoperative diagnosis was neuroendocrine tumor ($n = 2$),

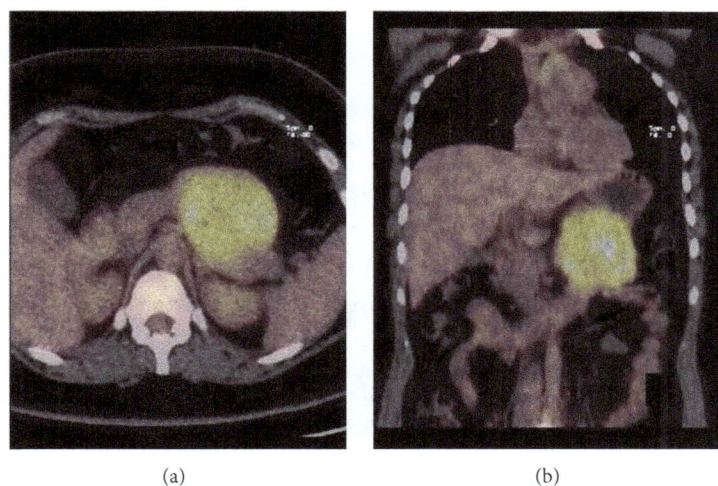

(a)   (b)

FIGURE 2: Positron emission tomography with CT acquisition (PET/CT) of the abdomen: axial (a) and coronal image (b) showing a pathologic uptake of FDG in a well-circumscribed, round mass in the tail of the pancreas (case number 15).

mucinous tumor (n = 2), and SPT (n = 14). Twelve patients underwent distal pancreatectomy (4 with spleen preservation and 2 with laparoscopic approach), 3 pylorus-preserving pancreaticoduodenectomy, 2 central pancreatectomy and 1 total pancreatectomy. One patient had associated resection of involved portal vein segment with jugular vein reconstruction. The invasion of portal vein was confirmed at pathological examination but no adjuvant chemotherapy was scheduled since the patient refused any other treatment. Another patient had synchronous resection of two small hepatic metastases. The patient reoperated after enucleation of pancreatic head lesion and underwent pancreaticoduodenectomy; pathological examination showed residual SPT.

All 18 patients had R0 resection, and there were no surgical mortalities. Postoperative complications occurred in 5 patients (28%); according to the International Study Group on Pancreatic Fistula (ISGPF) [5], one patient had Grade A, and four patients had Grade B pancreatic fistula, the latter requiring drainage under radiologic guidance.

Pathologic examination showed cellular atypia in 3 patients (numbers 5, 10, and 17), vascular invasion in 4 (numbers 5, 10, 12, and 13), perineural invasion in 4 (nr 9, 10, 16, 17), capsular invasion in 4 (numbers 3, 5, 9, and 10), and lymph node and liver metastases only in one patient (number 10). All but one patient (number 8) showed Mib 1 ≤ 1 (Table 2). B-catenin was always expressed. (Figure 3). One patient (number 10) had postoperative adjuvant therapy (gemcitabine regimen).

One patient died 77 months after operation, 45 months after tumor recurrence (liver metastases); the remaining patients are alive and well, free of disease with a median survival time of 81.5 months (range 36–228 months) (Figure 4).

4. Discussion

Solid-pseudopapillary tumor is a very rare neoplasm of the pancreas, accounting for only 1-2% of all exocrine pancreatic tumors [3]; in our experience we observed 18 SPTs among

TABLE 2: Clinicopathological features of Benign and Malignant SPT.

	Benign (n = 10)	Malignant (n = 8)
Age		
<40	7	6
≥40	3	2
Sex		
F	8	8
M	2	0
Tumor size		
<5	6	3
≥5	4	5
Tumor localization		
Head-neck	1	3
Body-tail	9	5
R0 resection	10	8
Pancreatic parenchyma/capsular invasion	0	4
Vascular invasion	0	4
Perineural invasion	0	4
Cellular atypia	0	3
Metastases	0	1
Mib1		
<1%	9	8
≥1%	1	0
Ki-67		
<4%	10	8
≥4%	0	0

a total of 451 (3.7%) cystic tumors of the pancreas from 1997 to 2013. In the last decade, there has been a significant increase in the number of SPTs published in the English literature [2], confirming the increasing interest toward this unique neoplasm. Most of our patients were female, at young age

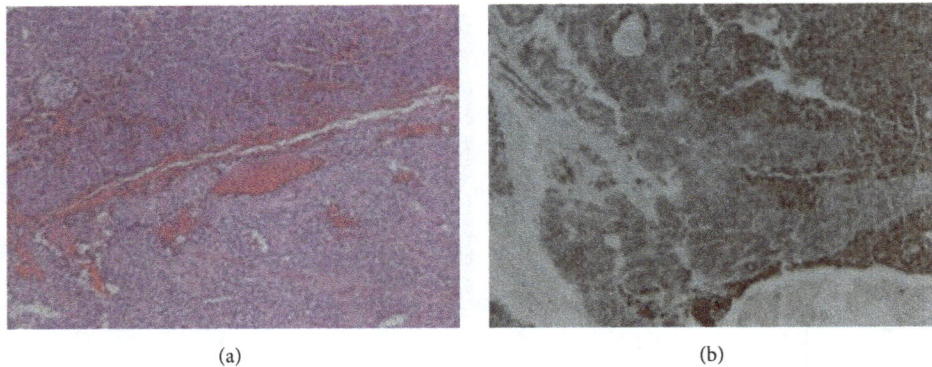

(a)   (b)

FIGURE 3: Hematoxylin and eosin stain (H&E, 100x) of SPT showing normal pancreas on the upper left side and neoplastic cells in the lower right side (a) and immunohistochemical β-catenin slide (100x) showing the different pattern of staining in normal pancreas (cytoplasmic) and in neoplastic pancreas (nuclear) (b).

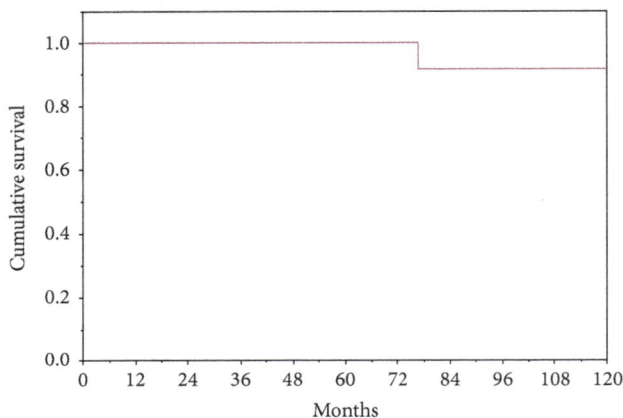

FIGURE 4: Kaplan-Meier survival curve of patients who underwent pancreatic resection of SPT.

(mean 34.2 years, range 13–75). Only two patients were males, older than females, both are alive and free of disease for 48 and 84 months, respectively. It has been reported that male patients have distinct patterns of onset and aggressiveness compared with female patients. Machado et al. [6] observed that SPTs in male patients were more aggressive than those in female patients, and they should be managed more radically. On the contrary, Cai et al. [7]. collected 16 male patients with SPTs, and observed that males were older than female patients and had a favorable outcome after surgery, with no recurrence or death of disease in the follow-up.

Clinical presentation of SPTs is not specific. The most frequent symptoms in our series were abdominal pain or discomfort, followed by abdominal mass; 2 patients were asymptomatic. These findings are well in accordance with previous reports [7–9]. Preoperative diagnosis of SPTs is generally made by CT or MRI imaging. Typically the tumor shows a large, well circumscribed, heterogeneous mass with varying solid and cystic components, generally demarcated by a peripheral capsule and occasional calcifications [10, 11]. These findings, together with other clinical findings, such as age and sex, may be sufficient for a correct diagnosis, as in

more half of our patients (Figure 1). Problems in differential diagnosis occur in the presence of small, solid lesions, or in large, unilocular cyst, or in male patients. Recently, EUS with FNA has been advocated as useful diagnostic tool also in SPTs. The diagnostic accuracy of EUS-FNA for SPT was found to be 75% in a multicentric experience of Jani et al. [12] in 2008. More recently, Law et al. [13] reported that the addition of EUS-FNA to a preoperative work-up of SPT significantly increased the diagnostic yield to 82.4%. In our experience, 5 patients underwent preoperative EUS-FNA: only 2 patients had a correct diagnosis of SPT. One patient had inconclusive results, and two had a suspected diagnosis of neuroendocrine tumor; this finding led us to perform octreotide scintigraphy and serum hormonal studies (both negative). However, CT and MR findings of these two patients were compatible with the diagnosis of SPT. In one patient EUS-FNA was complicated by mild acute pancreatitis. Recently, Virgilio et al. [14] reported a case of rupture of SPT following EUS-FNA. So the real utility of EUS in the diagnostic work-up of SPT is unclear and it appears indicated in very selected, doubtful cases.

Positron emission tomography with 18-FDG has an emerging role in the diagnosis and staging of pancreatic neoplasms, including cystic tumors [15]. The role of PET in these rare tumors is obviously not well defined. We perform preoperative PET in 10 patients: 7 showed a pathologic uptake in the tumor's area (Figure 2), while three patients did not. However, high accumulation of FDG in the tumor does not correlate with more aggressive behaviour, clinical characteristics, or histopathological features of malignancy, since all but one of these patients are alive without evidence of tumor's relapse. Dong et al. [16] studied 8 patients with SPTs who underwent preoperative PET; they found a relationship between standard uptake value (SUVmax) and histological malignancy of the tumor. However, all patients were alive without recurrence after surgery, although follow-up was very short.

Recently, Kang et al. [17] reported a large experience of 37 SPTs studied with 18-FDG PET; the pattern of FDG uptake in SPTs was not associated with histopathologic features suggestive of malignant potential. Moreover, SUVmax apparently increased according to the degree of Ki-67 expression, but without statistical significance. They concluded that the clinical usefulness of PET in SPTs needs to be further investigated. At the moment, it appears that 18-FDG PET does not have a substantial role in the diagnosis of SPTs.

In our series, only one patient presented with preoperative slight increase of serum CA 19-9, so the role of tumor markers in both the diagnosis and monitoring of the disease appears very limited.

SPT is generally considered as a tumor with low malignant potential. Although resection of the tumor provides a 5-year survival rate more than 95% [18], local recurrence or distant metastases can occur. Moreover a minority of patients show locally advanced or metastatic disease at their initial presentation. One patient presented with malignant locally advanced tumor, invading the portal vein. Total pancreatectomy with portal vein resection and reconstruction with jugular vein graft was performed, but the tumor recurred in the liver and the patient died 77 months after surgery. Locally infiltrative solid-pseudopapillary tumors of the pancreas occur infrequently; in 2008 we collected from English literature, a total of 20 patients with locally malignant SPT: 10 patients had portal vein or mesenteric vessels involvement (associated with liver metastases in two cases) and 10 had invasion of other organs (colon, spleen, kidney, adrenal gland, and omentum) [3].

A recent case series [19] of 131 consecutive resections for SPT has been published, showing only one case of metastatic disease at presentation and two cases of recurrence after resection of primary SPT. In all cases, capsular and/or pancreatic parenchyma invasion were found. No adjuvant or neoadjuvant chemotherapy has been administered. One patient eventually died because of disease progression 56 months after distal pancreatectomy. Cheng et al. [20] reported their experience of 8 patients with SPT infiltrating the portal-mesenteric vein, who underwent pancreatectomy associated with vascular resection. All but one patient were alive and free of disease after a median follow-up period of 67.5 months. One patient who underwent R1 resection died of liver recurrence 54 months after operation. So vascular invasion, although uncommon, does occur; vascular resection and reconstruction is warranted whenever possible, because long-term survival is not infrequent even in locally advanced disease.

Some reports found that a high Ki-67 mitotic index occurred more frequently in patients with malignant SPT and seems to be associated with a shorter survival [21–24]. Yang et al. [25] found that a Ki-67 $\geq$ 4% was significantly associated ($p < 0.001$) with recurrence. In our experience neither high Mib 1 nor Ki-67 $\geq$ 4% was associated with clinical or histopathological features of malignancy.

Recently, there is increasing interest in less aggressive surgical procedures for benign or border-line neoplasms of the pancreas, in order to preserve pancreatic function. So limited resection (i.e., enucleation, central pancreatectomy, spleen preservation, etc.) has been advocated also for SPTs [26]. However, one of our patients underwent pancreaticoduodenectomy for a previously enucleated SPT of the head of the pancreas that showed margin involvement at pathologic examination.

Recurrence after apparently radical resection of SPT is well reported: metastasis either at the time of presentation or, less commonly, some years after resection of the primary tumor develops in less than 15% of cases, and the liver is the most common site [18, 26].

One of our patients presented with synchronous liver metastases which were removed together with pancreaticoduodenectomy. Although there is no evidence of efficient chemotherapeutic drugs, adjuvant therapy with gemcitabine was performed, and the patient is alive, without recurrence, more than 6 years after surgery.

Resection of liver metastases is possible if the involvement of the liver is limited; survival after metastasis excision is good because of the indolent nature of the disease, and it appears that the 5-year survival is not significantly altered even in the presence of metastatic disease [18, 27]. Only occasional death from tumor, usually after many years, has been reported. Our experience confirms that, at present, there are no established clinical or histological criteria to predict the biological behaviour of SPT. While invasion of blood vessels, perineural infiltration, invasion of adjacent structures, and elevated mitotic rate are suggested to be associated with metastases and recurrence in some reports [25, 28, 29], they appear to be not related to prognosis in other experience [30], and the absence of these features does not preclude malignant behaviour [22], so long-term follow-up is warranted in all patients [31].

The utility of chemotherapy and radiotherapy for patients with SPT is substantially unknown, although there are some anecdotal reports of benefit [32–36]. Kang et al. [37] performed in vitro adenosine triphosphate based chemotherapy response assay in five resected SPT of the pancreas; cisplatin was shown to be the most effective single-chemotherapeutic agent. This finding has been reported in some previous experiences [38, 39] but not confirmed in others [40]. The limited number of reported cases explains the lack of standard treatment, and thus chemotherapeutic agents used are substantially experimental.

5. Conclusions

Solid-pseudopapillary tumor of the pancreas is an enigmatic tumor, mostly presenting with benign course or, less frequently, with aggressive behaviour or relapse after resection. Preoperative diagnosis is substantially made by CT or MRI in most cases. Because of its rarity, we lack sufficient information regarding clinicopathologic features predicting prognosis, and the role of radiochemotherapy in unresectable disease is clearly unknown. At moment, the biologic behaviour of SPT is unpredictable, so surgery remains the only chance of treatment even in locally or metastatic presentation. Long and careful follow-up is recommended after resection for all patients.

Competing Interests

The authors declare that they have no competing interests.

References

[1] T. Papavramidis and S. Papavramidis, "Solid pseudopapillary tumors of the pancreas: review of 718 patients reported in English literature," *Journal of the American College of Surgeons*, vol. 200, no. 6, pp. 965–972, 2005.

[2] J. K. Law, A. Ahmed, V. K. Singh et al., "A systematic review of solid-pseudopapillary neoplasms: are these rare lesions?" *Pancreas*, vol. 43, no. 3, pp. 331–337, 2014.

[3] C. Sperti, M. Berselli, C. Pasquali, D. Pastorelli, and S. Pedrazzoli, "Aggressive behaviour of solid-pseudopapillary tumor of the pancreas in adults: a case report and review of the literature," *World Journal of Gastroenterology*, vol. 14, no. 6, pp. 960–965, 2008.

[4] F. T. Bosman, F. Carneiro, and R. H. Hruban, *WHO Classification of Tumors of the Digestive System*, vol. 3, World Health Organization, Geneva, Switzerland, 4th edition, 2010.

[5] C. Bassi, C. Dervenis, G. Butturini et al., "Postoperative pancreatic fistula: an international Study Group (ISGPF) definition," *Surgery*, vol. 138, no. 1, pp. 8–13, 2005.

[6] M. C. C. Machado, M. A. C. Machado, T. Bacchella, J. Jukemura, J. L. Almeida, and J. E. M. Cunha, "Solid pseudopapillary neoplasm of the pancreas: distinct patterns of onset, diagnosis, and prognosis for male versus female patients," *Surgery*, vol. 143, no. 1, pp. 29–34, 2008.

[7] Y.-Q. Cai, S.-M. Xie, X. Ran, X. Wang, G. Mai, and X.-B. Liu, "Solid pseudopapillary tumor of the pancreas in male patients: report of 16 cases," *World Journal of Gastroenterology*, vol. 20, no. 22, pp. 6939–6945, 2014.

[8] P.-F. Yu, Z.-A. Hu, X.-B. Wang et al., "Solid pseudopapillary tumor of the pancreas: a review of 553 cases in Chinese literature," *World Journal of Gastroenterology*, vol. 16, no. 10, pp. 1209–1214, 2010.

[9] J. S. Estrella, L. Li, A. Rashid et al., "Solid pseudopapillary neoplasm of the pancreas: clinicopathologic and survival analyses of 64 cases from a single institution," *American Journal of Surgical Pathology*, vol. 38, no. 2, pp. 147–157, 2014.

[10] N. Vassos, A. Agaimy, P. Klein, W. Hohenberger, and R. S. Croner, "Solid-pseudopapillary neoplasm (SPN) of the pancreas: case series and literature review on an enigmatic entity," *International Journal of Clinical and Experimental Pathology*, vol. 6, no. 6, pp. 1051–1059, 2013.

[11] N. Guo, Q. B. Zhou, R. F. Chen et al., "Diagnosis and surgical treatment of solid pseudopapillary neoplasm of the pancreas: analysis of 24 cases," *Canadian Journal of Surgery*, vol. 54, no. 6, pp. 368–374, 2011.

[12] N. Jani, J. Dewitt, M. Eloubeidi et al., "Endoscopic ultrasound-guided fine-needle aspiration for diagnosis of solid pseudopapillary tumors of the pancreas: a multicenter experience," *Endoscopy*, vol. 40, no. 3, pp. 200–203, 2008.

[13] J. K. Law, A. Stoita, W. Weaver et al., "Endoscopic ultrasound-guided fine needle aspiration improves the pre-operative diagnostic yield of solid-pseudopapillary neoplasm of the pancreas: an international multicenter case series (with video)," *Surgical Endoscopy and Other Interventional Techniques*, vol. 28, no. 9, pp. 2592–2598, 2014.

[14] E. Virgilio, P. Mercantini, M. Ferri et al., "Is EUS-FNA of solid-pseudopapillary neoplasms of the pancreas as a preoperative procedure really necessary and free of acceptable risks?" *Pancreatology*, vol. 14, no. 6, pp. 536–538, 2014.

[15] C. Sperti, C. Pasquali, F. Chierichetti, G. Liessi, G. Ferlin, and S. Pedrazzoli, "Value of 18-fluorodeoxyglucose positron emission tomography in the management of patients with cystic tumors of the pancreas," *Annals of Surgery*, vol. 234, no. 5, pp. 675–680, 2001.

[16] A. Dong, Y. Wang, H. Dong, J. Zhang, C. Cheng, and C. Zuo, "FDG PET/CT findings of solid pseudopapillary tumor of the pancreas with CT and MRI correlation," *Clinical Nuclear Medicine*, vol. 38, no. 3, pp. e118–e124, 2013.

[17] C. M. Kang, A. Cho, H. Kim et al., "Clinical correlations with 18FDG PET scan patterns in solid pseudopapillary tumors of the pancreas: still a surgical enigma?" *Pancreatology*, vol. 14, no. 6, pp. 515–523, 2014.

[18] A. K. Madan, C. B. Weldon, W. P. Long, D. Johnson, and A. Raafat, "Solid and papillary epithelial neoplasm of the pancreas," *Journal of Surgical Oncology*, vol. 85, no. 4, pp. 193–198, 2004.

[19] G. Marchegiani, S. Andrianello, M. Massignani et al., "Solid pseudopapillary tumors of the pancreas: specific pathological features predict the likelihood of postoperative recurrence," *Journal of Surgical Oncology*, vol. 114, no. 5, pp. 597–601, 2016.

[20] K. Cheng, B. Shen, C. Peng, F. Yuan, and Q. Yin, "Synchronous portal-superior mesenteric vein or adjacent organ resection for solid pseudopapillary neoplasms of the pancreas: a single-institution experience," *The American Surgeon*, vol. 79, no. 5, pp. 534–539, 2013.

[21] L. H. Tang, H. Aydin, M. F. Brennan, and D. S. Klimstra, "Clinically aggressive solid pseudopapillary tumors of the pancreas: a report of two cases with components of undifferentiated carcinoma and a comparative clinicopathologic analysis of 34 conventional cases," *American Journal of Surgical Pathology*, vol. 29, no. 4, pp. 512–519, 2005.

[22] J. A. Adamthwaite, C. S. Verbeke, M. D. Stringer, P. J. Guillou, and K. V. Menon, "Solid pseudopapillary tumour of the pancreas: diverse presentation, outcome and histology," *Journal of the Pancreas*, vol. 7, no. 6, pp. 635–642, 2006.

[23] F. Yang, C. Jin, J. Long et al., "Solid pseudopapillary tumor of the pancreas: a case series of 26 consecutive patients," *The American Journal of Surgery*, vol. 198, no. 2, pp. 210–215, 2009.

[24] A. Yagcı, S. Yakan, A. Coskun et al., "Diagnosis and treatment of solid pseudopapillary tumor of the pancreas: experience of one single institution from Turkey," *World Journal of Surgical Oncology*, vol. 11, article 308, 2013.

[25] F. Yang, X. Yu, Y. Bao, Z. Du, C. Jin, and D. Fu, "Prognostic value of Ki-67 in solid pseudopapillary tumor of the pancreas: Huashan experience and systematic review of the literature," *Surgery*, vol. 159, no. 4, pp. 1023–1031, 2016.

[26] C. Zhang, F. Liu, H. Chang et al., "Less aggressive surgical procedure for treatment of solid pseudopapillary tumor: limited experience from a single institute," *PLoS ONE*, vol. 10, no. 11, Article ID e0143452, 2015.

[27] R. C. G. Martin, D. S. Klimstra, M. F. Brennan, and K. C. Conlon, "Solid-pseudopapillary tumor of the pancreas: a surgical enigma?" *Annals of Surgical Oncology*, vol. 9, no. 1, pp. 35–40, 2002.

[28] K. Nishihara, M. Nagoshi, M. Tsuneyoshi, K. Yamaguchi, and I. Hayashi, "Papillary cystic tumors of the pancreas: assessment of their malignant potential," *Cancer*, vol. 71, no. 1, pp. 82–92, 1993.

[29] H. Matsunou and F. Konishi, "Papillary-cystic neoplasm of the pancreas: a clinicopathologic study concerning the tumor aging and malignancy of nine cases," *Cancer*, vol. 65, no. 2, pp. 283–291, 1990.

[30] H. Zhang, W. Wang, S. Yu, Y. Xiao, and J. Chen, "The prognosis and clinical characteristics of advanced (malignant) solid pseudopapillary neoplasm of the pancreas," *Tumor Biology*, vol. 37, no. 4, pp. 5347–5353, 2016.

[31] J. K. Park, E. J. Cho, J. K. Ryu, Y.-T. Kim, and Y.-B. Yoon, "Natural history and malignant risk factors of solid pseudopapillary tumors of the pancreas," *Postgraduate Medicine*, vol. 125, no. 2, pp. 92–99, 2013.

[32] A. Maffuz, F. D. T. Bustamante, J. A. Silva, and S. Torres-Vargas, "Preoperative gemcitabine for unresectable, solid pseudopapillary tumour of the pancreas," *Lancet Oncology*, vol. 6, no. 3, pp. 185–186, 2005.

[33] J. A. Zauls, A. E. Dragun, and A. K. Sharma, "Intensity-modulated radiation therapy for unresectable solid pseudopapillary tumor of the pancreas," *American Journal of Clinical Oncology: Cancer Clinical Trials*, vol. 29, no. 6, pp. 639–640, 2006.

[34] Y. Takahashi, T. Fukusato, K. Aita et al., "Solid pseudopapillary tumor of the pancreas with metastases to the lung and liver," *Pathology International*, vol. 55, no. 12, pp. 792–796, 2005.

[35] P. Levy, J. Bougaran, and B. Gayet, "Pseudopapillary and solid tumor of the pancreas with diffuse peritoneal carcinomatosis: role of tumoral traumatism," *Gastroenterolgie Clinique et Biologique*, vol. 21, no. 10, pp. 789–791, 1997.

[36] J. F. Strauss, V. J. Hirsch, C. N. Rubey, and M. Pollock, "Resection of a solid and papillary epithelial neoplasm of the pancreas following treatment with cis-platinum and 5-fluorouracil: a case report," *Medical and Pediatric Oncology*, vol. 21, no. 5, pp. 365–367, 1993.

[37] C. M. Kang, H. Kim, Y. Cho et al., "In vitro adenosine triphosphate-based chemotherapy response assay (ATP-CRA) in solid pseudopapillary tumor of the pancreas," *Pancreas*, vol. 41, no. 3, pp. 498–500, 2012.

[38] J. O. Hah, W. K. Park, N. H. Lee, and J. H. Choi, "Preoperative chemotherapy and intraoperative radiofrequency ablation for unresectable solid pseudopapillary tumor of the pancreas," *Journal of Pediatric Hematology/Oncology*, vol. 29, no. 12, pp. 851–853, 2007.

[39] W. Rebhandl, F. X. Felberbauer, S. Puig et al., "Solid-pseudopapillary tumor of the pancreas (Frantz tumor) in children: report of four cases and review of the literature," *Journal of Surgical Oncology*, vol. 76, no. 4, pp. 289–296, 2001.

[40] H. Hofmann, R. Von Haken, J. Werner et al., "Unresectable isolated hepatic metastases from solid pseudopapillary neoplasm of the pancreas: a case report of chemosaturation with high-dose melphalan," *Pancreatology*, vol. 14, no. 6, pp. 546–549, 2014.

19

Endoscopic Approaches to the Treatment of Variceal Hemorrhage in Hemodialysis-Dependent Patients

Xiaoquan Huang,[1,2] Lili Ma,[1] Xiaoqing Zeng,[2] Jian Wang,[2] Jie Chen,[2] and Shiyao Chen[1,2]

[1]*Endoscopy Center and Endoscopy Research Institute, Zhongshan Hospital, Fudan University, Shanghai 200032, China*
[2]*Department of Gastroenterology, Zhongshan Hospital, Fudan University, Shanghai 200032, China*

Correspondence should be addressed to Shiyao Chen; chen.shiyao@zs-hospital.sh.cn

Academic Editor: Atsushi Irisawa

Background. Esophagogastric variceal hemorrhage leads to challenging situation in chronic kidney disease patients on maintenance hemodialysis. *Aims.* To determine the safety and efficacy of endoscopic approaches to patients with hemodialysis-dependent concomitant with esophagogastric varices. *Methods.* Medical records were reviewed from January 1, 2004, to December 31, 2015, in our hospital. Five consecutive hemodialysis-dependent patients with variceal hemorrhage who underwent endoscopic treatments were retrospectively studied. *Results.* The median age of the patients was 54 years (range 34–67 years) and the median follow-up period was 21.3 months (range 7–134 months). All the patients received a total of three times heparin-free hemodialysis 24 hours before and no more than 24 hours and 72 hours after endoscopic treatment. They successfully had endoscopic variceal ligation, endoscopic injection sclerotherapy, and/or N-butyl cyanoacrylate injection. The short-term efficacy is satisfying and long-term follow-up showed episodes of rebleeding. *Conclusions.* Endoscopic approaches are the alternative options in the treatment of upper gastroenterology variceal hemorrhage in hemodialysis-dependent patients without severe complications.

1. Introduction

The global prevalence and incidence of end-stage renal disease (ESRD) are increasing worldwide while the mortality among patients with ESRD observed large net reductions due to both dialysis and transplantation [1]. Cirrhotic patients with ESRD have increased complications and higher mortality rate [2]. The prevalence of cirrhosis was about 6.2% at the beginning of dialysis in a cohort study in Taiwan [3]. Esophagogastric variceal bleeding accounts for a mortality rate of approximately 15% in general population [4]. Evidence had proven endoscopic approaches are the most effective intervention for primary and secondary prevention of gastroesophageal variceal bleeding, recommended as the first-line option [5].

However, patients with marked impaired renal function undergoing hemodialysis and concomitant cirrhotic gastroesophageal varices remained intractable. Their fragile hemostasis states, caused by renal anemia, uremic platelet dysfunction, and use of anticoagulants [6, 7], lead to recurrent upper gastroenterology bleeding. Haskal and Radhakrishnan [8] had reported that transjugular intrahepatic portosystemic shunts (TIPS) were effective in controlling ascites and bleeding in dialysis-dependent patients but a high incidence of post-TIPS hepatic encephalopathy. Simultaneous liver-kidney transplantation (SLKT) is the best choice for them considering both survival and quality-adjusted life years [9, 10]. However, it takes time waiting for the donor and some patients died of massive variceal hemorrhage during the waiting period. Endoscopic treatment might be the alternative option to avoid massive variceal bleeding. The concerns of the endoscopic approach are the risk of bleeding and anesthesia management. To our knowledge, no literature reporting endoscopic treatment of varices in hemodialysis-dependent patients was found. In this study, we report our experiences in controlling esophagogastric variceal bleeding in hemodialysis-dependent patients.

2. Materials and Methods

2.1. Study Design. In this tertiary hospital-based retrospective case series study, a total of 2038 consecutive hospitalized patients with esophageal and/or gastric varices undergoing endoscopic therapy were screened. We included (1) patients who required maintenance hemodialysis; (2) patients confirmed to have liver cirrhosis by computed tomography; (3) patients confirmed to have varices by gastroscopy; and (4) patients who had endoscopic treatment for secondary prevention of variceal bleeding. We excluded patients who had endoscopic treatment before starting hemodialysis. We retrieved medical records including the emergency room and outpatient department from our hospital between January 1, 2004, and December 31, 2015. The end point was set at March 31, 2016. All the patients were followed up via phone calls and outpatient clinic visits. This retrospective report was approved by the institution's Ethics Committee and written informed consent was obtained from each patient. Median and range were shown to describe quantitative data.

2.2. Endoscopic Intervention. The devices and drugs used included the electronic endoscope GIF-XQ240/260 (Olympus, Tokyo, Japan), 6 multiband ligators (Cook Endoscopy, Winston-Salem, North Carolina, USA) or 7 multiband ligators (Boston Scientific, Natick, Massachusetts, USA), N-butyl-cyanoacrylate (Beijing Suncon Medical Adhesive, Beijing, China), lauromacrogol (Tianyu Pharmaceutical, China), lipiodol, and injection needle (Olympus NM-200 L-423, Tokyo, Japan).

Gastric varices were treated with N-butyl-cyanoacrylate using the sandwich method (lipiodol or 20% glucose or lauromacrogol-cyanoacrylate-lipiodol or 20% glucose or lauromacrogol). Each cyanoacrylate injection point was no more than 2.0 mL and an equal volume of lipiodol or 20% glucose or 2–8 mL lauromacrogol determined by the varix size according to our published study [11]. Multiple sites injection was an attempt to completely obturate the gastric varices in one session. To decrease the risk of a variceal tear, the needle sheath was held in the puncture site to prevent leakage of the cyanoacrylate and to ensure the varice has hardened before retracting the injector catheter.

Endoscopic variceal ligation (EVL) is the primary treatment selection for esophageal varices according to guideline and our experiences [12, 13]. Ligation was applied from 1 cm above the Z-line in a spirally ascending fashion, with no more than six or seven bands used per session. Endoscopic injection sclerosis (EIS) treatment is usually performed in patients who had multiple EVL sessions and as an attempt to eliminate the small esophageal varix. The initial injection started above the Z-line, and intravariceal or paravariceal injection of 10–30 mL per session of lauromacrogol was injected. Follow-up endoscopy was performed at an interval of no less than 2 months and treatment was repeated until complete obliteration was achieved.

2.3. Perioperative Management. All the patients required hemodialysis three times per week. Heparin-free dialysis was performed the day before the endoscopic procedure and postoperative heparin-free dialysis was performed no more than 24 hours after the procedures, and the third heparin-free dialysis was done more than 72 hours after the procedure. Patients did not receive any other anticoagulation drugs for a week. Later comes the routine usage of heparin dialysis. They were adequately treated with proton pump inhibitors (PPIs) after endoscopic treatment and no prophylactic antibiotics were used.

2.4. Anesthesia Management. The patient's general condition should be designated as American Society of Anesthesiologists (ASA) classification I, II, or III, and these patients underwent propofol sedation for endoscopy [14]. The initial dosage was 2 mg/kg, and 1 mg/kg was added by the anesthesiologist if body movement disturbed the procedure. Electrocardiogram, oxygen saturation, respiratory rate, and noninvasive blood pressure measurements were monitored during the endoscopic treatment.

2.5. Statistical Analysis. Statistical analysis was performed with SPSS 23.0 software (SPSS Inc., Chicago, Illinois, USA). Median and range were shown to describe continuous data.

3. Results

Five patients were enrolled in this study, and their demographic data were shown in Table 1. Of the five patients, there were three males and two females with the age of 54 years (range, 33–67 years) and the creatinine of 738 μmol/L (range, 542–1131 μmol/L) at the time of having the first endoscopic treatment. The etiologies of liver cirrhosis included hepatic B virus (HBV), hepatic C virus (HCV), and drug-induced-liver-injury (DILI) (aristolochic acid and unknown herb in traditional Chinese medicine). The primary diseases related to renal failure are chronic glomerulonephritis (80%) and aristolochic acid nephropathy (20%). Among these patients, one had hepatocellular carcinoma (HCC, patient 1) and another one had colorectal cancer (CRC, patient 4) before developing into gastroesophageal varices and starting maintenance hemodialysis. The liver function of these patients was mild impairment.

Among the five cases, the time interval between hemodialysis and first endoscopic treatment was 37.5 months (range 5.9–94.6 months). A total of 16 endoscopic procedures were performed including 11 EVLs, 2 EISs, and 3 N-butyl cyanoacrylate injections. The details of endoscopic treatment were shown in Table 2. All the procedures were secondary prophylaxis of bleeding. The changes before and after endoscopic treatment of gastric varices were shown in Figure 1. All the three cyanoacrylate injection procedures had immediate blood exudations and were controlled by rinsing with 8% ice norepinephrine solution. The esophageal varices were treated by ligations and sclerotherapy (Figures 2(a), 2(b), and 2(c)). No delay bleeding was observed when they were back to the ward. No complications such as infections, massive bleeding, or stroke were observed in these patients.

TABLE 1: Demographic data in five patients undergoing endoscopic treatment.

Patient number	Gender	Age	Etiology of cirrhosis	Primary renal disease	Creatinine (μmol/L)	eGFR (ml/min/1.73 m^2)	Time interval between hemodialysis start and first bleeding (months)	Varices type	Child-Pugh grade	Concomitant tumor
1	Male	34	HBV	Chronic glomerulonephritis	738	7.4	3.2	Only EV (G3)	B	HCC
2	Male	51	HCV	Chronic glomerulonephritis	878	5.6	34.9	Only GV (IGV)	B	/
3	Male	54	HBV	Chronic glomerulonephritis	1131	4.1	105.1	Only EV (G3)	B	/
4	Female	64	DILI*	Chronic glomerulonephritis	546	6.8	12.6	Both EV (G3) and GV (GOV-2)	A	CRC
5	Female	67	DILI†	Aristolochic acid nephropathy	542	7.4	81.9	Both EV (G3) and GV (GOV-1)	B	/

HBV, hepatitis B virus; HCV, hepatitis C virus; HCC, hepatocellular carcinoma; CRC, colorectal cancer; DILI, drug-induced liver injury. eGFR, estimate glomerular filtrate rate, using CKD-EPI (Chronic Kidney Disease Epidemiology Collaboration) equation. Esophageal varices, Grade 3 (EV, G3), were defined as large, coil-shaped EV occupying more than one-third of the lumen. Gastric varices (GV) were defined according to Sarin's classification as lesser curvature varices (gastroesophageal varices type 1, GOV-1), greater curvature varices (gastroesophageal varices type 1, GOV-1), greater curvature varices (GOV-2), or isolated gastric varices type (IGV). *Induced by unknown herb in traditional Chinese medicine. †Induced by aristolochic acid.

TABLE 2: Endoscopic treatment details of hemodialysis patients.

Patient number	Time interval between first bleeding and treatment (months)	Time interval* (months)	Treatment options *numbers	Total treatments	Rebleeding (within 3 months)	Rebleeding (after 3 months)	Follow-up (months)	Time interval between the end of treatment and death (months)	Outcome
1	2.7	5.9	EVL * 4 and EIS * 1	5	Yes	Yes	64.4	/	SLKT in 2013/alive
2	2.6	37.5	NBCA 1.5 ml and NBCA 0.5 ml	2	No	Yes	10.2	3.8	Die in May, 2014
3	1.7	94.6	EVL * 5 and EIS * 1	6	No	Yes	134.2	/	Alive
4	1.8	14.4	NBCA 4ml and EVL * 1	2	No	No	7.7	/	Alive
5	8.0	89.9	EVL * 1	1	No	No	21.3	21.7	Die in Aug, 2013

EVL, endoscopic variceal ligation; EIS, endoscopic injection sclerosis; NBCA, N-butyl-cyanoacrylate; SLKT, simultaneous liver-kidney transplantation.
*Time interval: the interval between hemodialysis start and first time receiving endoscopic treatment.

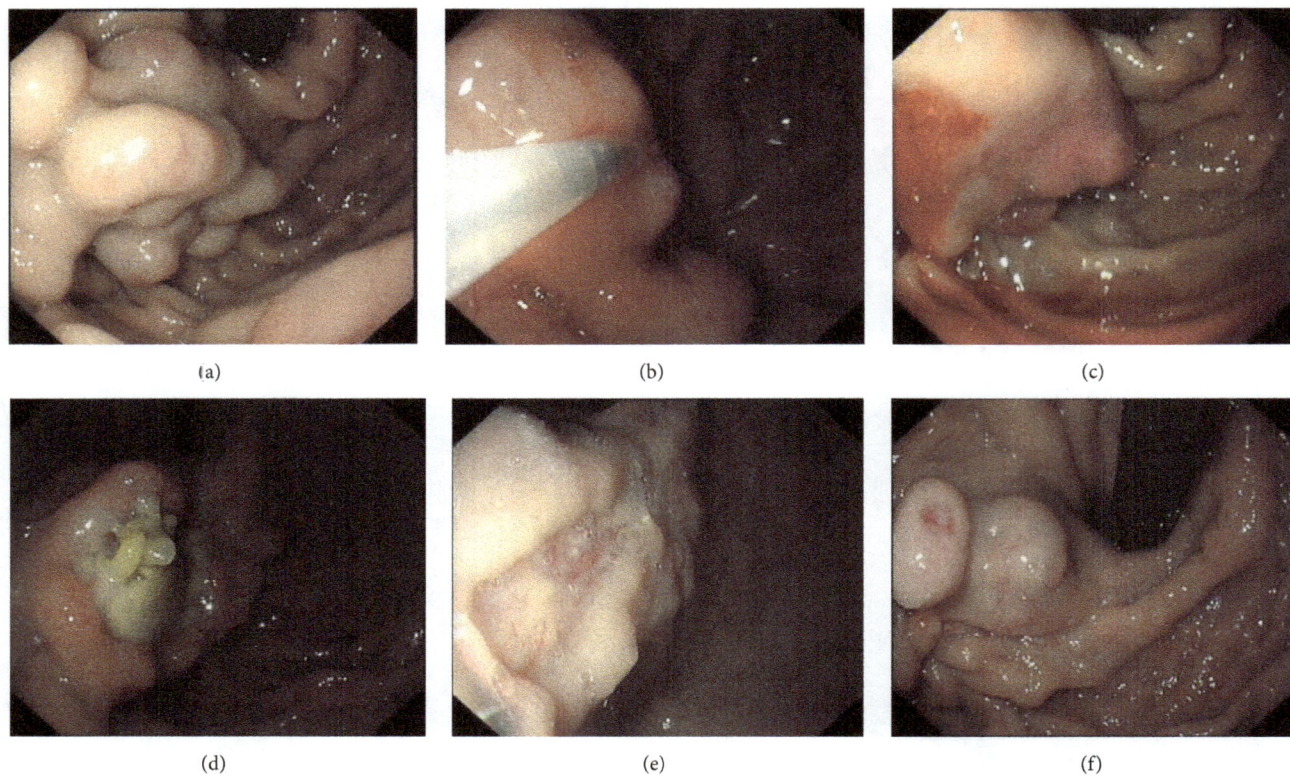

FIGURE 1: Gastric varices. (a) Isolate gastric varices vein (4 cm) before treatment. (b) Injecting 6 mL lauromacrogol + 1.5 mL N-butyl-cyanoacrylate + 4 mL lauromacrogol. (c) Mild blood exudation after injection; the injection site was rinsed with ice-cold norepinephrine. (d) Gastric ulceration in the injection site. (e) Scar of cyanoacrylate injection. (f) Recurrence of gastric varices in 10 months (patient 2).

Of the five patients, only one (20%) experienced rebleeding within 3 months after the endoscopic treatment and three (60%) suffered from nonlethal rebleeding episodes after 3 months. The median follow-up period was 21.3 months (range 7–134 months). Patient 1 received SLKT in 2013 and completely cured without severe complications (Figure 2(d)).

4. Discussion

An increasing number of patients with concurrent ESRD and varices make the management of variceal hemorrhage intractable. The concerns of endoscopic approaches are the risk of bleeding and anesthesia. Our experiences illustrate that endoscopic treatment is effective and relatively safe in these patients. All of our patients' esophageal varices were prominent in the distal esophagus, in contrast to the "downhill varices" in the proximal esophagus in hemodialysis patient with central venous catheters [15]. "Uphill" varices caused by cirrhotic portal hypertension are much easy to bleed. Endoscopic approaches are promising in the hemorrhage management [16].

While the impaired renal and hepatic functions increased the risk of sedation and propofol, an ultrashort acting hypnotic agent was given. Propofol is widely recommended in short endoscopic procedures and superior in terms of

patient's tolerance, maximum level of sedation achieved, and shorter recovery room times [17]. Only very little part of propofol clearance is through renal elimination. Its pharmacokinetics are minimally changed in patients with impaired liver and renal functions [18]. Patients sedated with propofol were confirmed to be safe and less invasive by a large amount of patients undergoing endoscopic treatments in our hospital. Closely monitoring the blood pressure and limitation of fluid infusion are required.

Because none of our patients had endoscopic procedures for the management of acute variceal hemorrhage, propofol sedation is possible in secondary prophylaxis for variceal hemorrhage. The sedation helps with the compliable of patients during treatments and reduces the possibility of bleeding and makes bleeding easy to control during injection. Extravascular injection of drugs is easy to cause gastric ulceration and precise intravascular injection can also reduce rebleeding risk [19]. In addition, the administration of propofol was by anesthesiologists, and we can immediately switch into intubation when necessary.

Little is known about the safety of long-term heparin-free hemodialysis; however, temporarily heparin-free hemodialysis without anticoagulation drug is beneficial to these patients for endoscopic procedures. Perioperative heparin-free dialysis reduced the risk of bleeding during endoscopic treatment and delay bleeding.

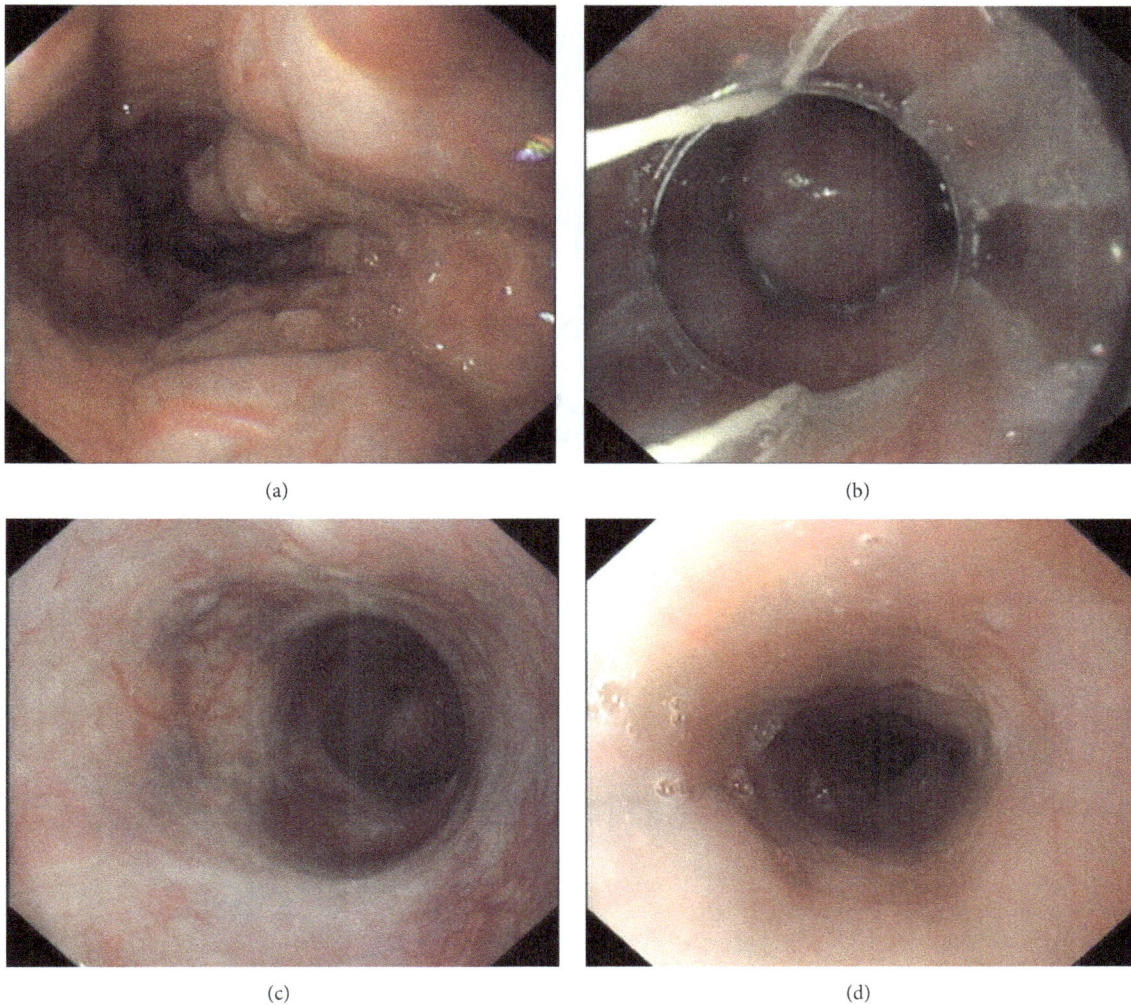

(a)

(b)

(c)

(d)

Figure 2: Esophageal varices. (a) Esophageal appearance before treatment. (b) Endoscopic variceal ligations. (c) Esophageal appearance after endoscopic variceal ligation procedures. (d) Brand new esophageal appearance after simultaneous liver-kidney transplantation (patient 1).

Long-term rebleeding episodes might be because of the high portal pressure in these patients. However, because of their poor general conditions, none of them had hepatic venous pressure gradient (HVPG) measurement. The actual pressure of these patients remained unknown. Further study will be required to evaluate the long-term outcomes in more patients.

In conclusion, for hemodialysis-dependent patients with esophagogastric varices, endoscopic approaches might be the alternative options to TIPS and SKLT, which reduce the risk of variceal hemorrhage without severe complications.

Disclosure

The funder had no role in the study design, data collection and analysis, decision to publish, or preparation of the manuscript.

Competing Interests

The authors declare that they have no competing interests.

Acknowledgments

The authors would like to thank all the staff in Department of Gastroenterology, Endoscopy Center and Endoscopy Research Institute, Department of Anesthesiology, and Department of Nephropathy of Zhongshan Hospital, Fudan University, for assistance. The study was supported by Innovation Fund of Shanghai Committee of Science and Technology (no. 15411950501).

References

[1] R. Saran, Y. Li, B. Robinson et al., "US renal data system 2015 annual data report: epidemiology of kidney disease in the

United States," *American Journal of Kidney Diseases*, vol. 67, no. 3, supplement 1, pp. A7–A8, 2016.

[2] T.-H. Hung, C.-C. Tsai, K.-C. Tseng et al., "High mortality of cirrhotic patients with end-stage renal disease," *Medicine*, vol. 95, no. 10, Article ID e3057, 2016.

[3] C.-C. Chien, J.-J. Wang, Y.-M. Sun et al., "Long-term survival and predictors for mortality among dialysis patients in an endemic area for chronic liver disease: A National Cohort Study in Taiwan," *BMC Nephrology*, vol. 13, no. 1, article 43, 2012.

[4] M. Bai, X. Qi, M. Yang, G. Han, and D. Fan, "Combined therapies versus monotherapies for the first variceal bleeding in patients with high-risk varices: a meta-analysis of randomized controlled trials," *Journal of Gastroenterology and Hepatology*, vol. 29, no. 3, pp. 442–452, 2014.

[5] R. de Franchis and B. V. Faculty, "Expanding consensus in portal hypertension: report of the Baveno VI Consensus Workshop: stratifying risk and individualizing care for portal hypertension," *Journal of Hepatology*, vol. 63, no. 3, pp. 743–752, 2015.

[6] P. Sood, G. Kumar, R. Nanchal et al., "Chronic kidney disease and end-stage renal disease predict higher risk of mortality in patients with primary upper gastrointestinal bleeding," *American Journal of Nephrology*, vol. 35, no. 3, pp. 216–224, 2012.

[7] G. Escolar, M. Díaz-Ricart, and A. Cases, "Uremic platelet dysfunction: past and present," *Current Hematology Reports*, vol. 4, no. 5, pp. 359–367, 2005.

[8] Z. J. Haskal and J. Radhakrishnan, "Transjugular intrahepatic portosystemic shunts in hemodialysis-dependent patients and patients with advanced renal insufficiency: safety, caution, and encephalopathy," *Journal of Vascular and Interventional Radiology*, vol. 19, no. 4, pp. 516–520, 2008.

[9] M. M. Doyle, V. Subramanian, N. Vachharajani et al., "Results of simultaneous liver and kidney transplantation: a single-center review," *Journal of the American College of Surgeons*, vol. 223, no. 1, pp. 193–201, 2016.

[10] B. Kiberd, C. Skedgel, I. Alwayn, and K. Peltekian, "Simultaneous liver kidney transplantation: a medical decision analysis," *Transplantation*, vol. 91, no. 1, pp. 121–127, 2011.

[11] X. Zeng, L. Ma, Y. Tzeng et al., "Endoscopic cyanoacrylate injection with or without lauromacrogol for gastric varices: a randomized pilot study," *Journal of Gastroenterology and Hepatology*, 2016.

[12] J. Chen, X.-Q. Zeng, L.-L. Ma et al., "Randomized controlled trial comparing endoscopic ligation with or without sclerotherapy for secondary prophylaxis of variceal bleeding," *European Journal of Gastroenterology & Hepatology*, vol. 28, no. 1, pp. 95–100, 2016.

[13] J. Chen, X. Q. Zeng, L. L. Ma et al., "Long-term efficacy of endoscopic ligation plus cyanoacrylate injection with or without sclerotherapy for variceal bleeding," *Journal of Digestive Diseases*, vol. 17, no. 4, pp. 252–259, 2016.

[14] B. K. Enestvedt, G. M. Eisen, J. Holub, and D. A. Lieberman, "Is the American Society of Anesthesiologists classification useful in risk stratification for endoscopic procedures?" *Gastrointestinal Endoscopy*, vol. 77, no. 3, pp. 464–471, 2013.

[15] L. Gessel and J. Alcorn, "Variants of varices: is it all 'downhill' from here?" *Digestive Diseases and Sciences*, vol. 60, no. 2, pp. 316–319, 2015.

[16] C. Froilán, L. Adán, J. M. Suárez et al., "Therapeutic approach to "downhill" varices bleeding," *Gastrointestinal Endoscopy*, vol. 68, no. 5, pp. 1010–1012, 2008.

[17] D. O. Faigel, T. H. Baron, J. L. Goldstein et al., "Guidelines for the use of deep sedation and anesthesia for GI endoscopy," *Gastrointestinal Endoscopy*, vol. 56, no. 5, pp. 613–617, 2002.

[18] J. Kanto and E. Gepts, "Pharmacokinetic implications for the clinical use of propofol," *Clinical Pharmacokinetics*, vol. 17, no. 5, pp. 308–326, 1989.

[19] L. Cheng, Z. Wang, C. Li, W. Lin, A. E. Yeo, and B. Jin, "Low incidence of complications from endoscopic gastric variceal obturation with butyl cyanoacrylate," *Clinical Gastroenterology and Hepatology*, vol. 8, no. 9, pp. 760–766, 2010.

20

The Emerging Role of miRNAs and Their Clinical Implication in Biliary Tract Cancer

Nina Nayara Ferreira Martins,[1] **Kelly Cristina da Silva Oliveira,**[1] **Amanda Braga Bona,**[2]
Marília de Arruda Cardoso Smith,[3] **Geraldo Ishak,**[1] **Paulo Pimentel Assumpção,**[1]
Rommel Rodríguez Burbano,[2] **and Danielle Queiroz Calcagno**[1]

[1]*Núcleo de Pesquisas em Oncologia, Universidade Federal do Pará, Belém, PA, Brazil*
[2]*Laboratório de Citogenética Humana, Instituto de Ciências Biológicas, Universidade Federal do Pará, Belém, PA, Brazil*
[3]*Universidade Federal de São Paulo, São Paulo, SP, Brazil*

Correspondence should be addressed to Danielle Queiroz Calcagno; danicalcagno@gmail.com

Academic Editor: Mario Scartozzi

Biliary tract cancers are aggressive malignancies that include gallbladder cancer and tumors of intra- and extrahepatic ducts and have a poor prognosis. Surgical resection remains the main curative therapy. Nevertheless, numerous patients experience recurrence even after radical surgery. This scenario drives the research to identify biliary tract cancer biomarkers despite the limited progress that has been made. Recently, a large number of studies have demonstrated that deregulated expression of microRNAs is closely associated with cancer development and progression. In this review, we highlight the role and importance of microRNAs in biliary tract cancers with an emphasis on utilizing circulating microRNAs as potential biomarkers. Additionally, we report several single-nucleotide polymorphisms in *microRNA* genes that are associated with the susceptibility of biliary tract tumors.

1. Background

Despite their relatively rare incidence, biliary tract cancers (BTCs) are an aggressive tumor group with poor prognosis and are characterized by early lymph node and systemic metastases [1]. These tumors include gallbladder cancer (GBC) and cholangiocarcinoma (CCA), which is divided into intrahepatic cholangiocarcinoma (iCCA) and extrahepatic cholangiocarcinoma (eCCA). Currently, surgical resection remains the only curative treatment for BTCs, and neoadjuvant chemoradiotherapy is not a standard option for patients with these malignancies. Moreover, many cases present with recurrence even after radical surgery, and patients with recurrent or metastatic BTCs usually have a poor outcome [2]. Therefore, there is a need for additional investigations to determine potential biomarkers of BTCs for early diagnosis, determining patient prognosis and the development of targeted therapy.

Recent studies have described microRNAs (miRNAs) as potential biomarkers in different cancer types [3–6]. However, miRNA expression and their implications in the diagnosis of, prognosis of, and therapeutic applications towards BTCs remain elusive.

miRNAs are small noncoding RNAs (18–25 nucleotides) that play important roles in the regulation of a large number of essential biological functions that are critical to the development of different cancer types, including cell proliferation, differentiation, apoptosis, migration, and invasion [7].

miRNA biogenesis initiates in the nucleus, where miRNA genes are usually transcribed by RNA polymerase II, resulting in a primary transcript of miRNA (pri-miRNAs) [8]. During the initial processing of pri-miRNAs, the Drosha-DGCR8 complex cleaves the pri-miRNA, releasing a hairpin structure named pre-miRNA (~70 nucleotides). Pre-miRNAs are transferred to the cytoplasm and converted into an miRNA duplex by Exportin-5 and the Dicer-TRBP complex, respectively. Then, a helicase separates the double-stranded miRNA to produce one stable single-stranded miRNA, while the other strand is processed for autolytic degradation. The stable mature miRNA strand is loaded into the RNA-induced silencing complex (RISC) to mechanistically target the 3′ untranslated regions (3′UTRs) of protein coding mRNAs, thereby acting as posttranscriptional regulators by two mechanisms: mRNA degradation (when the sequences are perfect complements) and inhibition of translational initiation (when there is partial complementarily) [9]. Thus, miRNAs act as negative regulators of posttranscriptional gene expression of target mRNAs.

It has been well established that miRNAs could regulate approximately 60% of human genes, including many oncogenes and tumor suppressor genes; this phenomenon strengthens the importance of these noncoding RNAs as relevant regulators in cancer [10].

In this review, we focus on the roles and importance of miRNAs in BTCs and highlight the potential of circulating miRNAs as diagnostic and prognostic biomarkers. Therefore, we reported several single-nucleotide polymorphisms (SNPs) in *miRNA* genes associated with BTC susceptibility.

2. Roles and Clinical Significance of miRNAs in BTCs

A large number of deregulated miRNAs have been categorized as oncomiRs (oncogene miRNAs) and/or tsmiRs (tumor suppressor miRNAs) in cancer depending on the effect of the target mRNA.

In BTCs, several studies on miRNA expression have identified many upregulated oncomiRs and downregulated tsmiRs as well as their potential targets (Table 1).

One of the best-described miRNAs in BTCs is hsa-miR-21, which is usually identified as an oncomiR since its overexpression has been associated with invasion and metastasis [11–19, 21–25, 27, 30, 41, 47–50]. Liu et al. [13] observed that overexpression of hsa-miR-21 significantly promotes cell migration, invasion, and xenograft growth after transfection of hsa-miR-21 into CCA cell lines (QBC939 and RBE). Moreover, these authors showed decreased E-cadherin expression and increased N-cadherin and vimentin expression after hsa-miR-21 overexpression. Thus, hsa-miR-21 could induce the epithelial-mesenchymal transition (EMT) in CCA. In this process, epithelial cells lose their cell polarity and cell adhesion—probably due to the decrease of E-cadherin expression—which allows cells to migrate and invade surrounding tissues; this the loss of E-cadherin expression plays a key role in tumor invasion and metastasis.

Similarly, aberrant expression of miRNAs also induces EMT and enhances the metastatic potential of GBC cells [24, 51]. Bao et al. [51] reported that hsa-miR-101 overexpression inhibits the proliferation, migration, and invasion of GBC cells, induces the increased expression of E-cadherin and β-catenin, and causes decreased expression of vimentin. Furthermore, these authors observed that hsa-miR-101 downregulation was correlated with tumor size, invasion, lymph node metastasis, TNM stage, and poor survival in GBC

patients. These results indicate that hsa-miR-101 plays a tsmiR role and attenuates EMT and metastasis in GBC.

Accumulating evidence has indicated that hsa-miR-146b-5p presents critical tumor suppressor properties [52, 53]. Its expression was significantly downregulated in GBC tissue compared with adjacent nonneoplastic tissues. In addition, the overexpression of hsa-miR-146b-5p in the SGC-996 GBC cell line inhibited cell growth by enhancing apoptosis and arresting the cells at G1 phase. However, the enforced expression of *EGFR*, a cell surface protein that binds to epidermal growth factor (which inducing cell proliferation), reversed the ability of hsa-miR-146b-5p to inhibit proliferation. Moreover, hsa-miR-146b-5p expression levels were significantly correlated with tumor size and cancer progression [46].

Recent studies have described hsa-miR-135a-5p as having a tsmiR role [54–56]. In GBC, Zhou et al. [44] found that hsa-miR-135a-5p levels were significantly downregulated in tumors compared to adjacent nontumor gallbladder tissues and were correlated with neoplasms of histological grades III and IV. Additionally, this study identified *VLDLR* as a direct and functional target gene of hsa-miR-135a-5p in GBC tissues. Furthermore, the transfection with a hsa-miR-135a-5p mimetic inhibited the proliferative and colony-forming abilities of GBC cells by arresting the cells in G1/S phase. These data suggest that hsa-miR-135a-5p may inhibit the proliferation of GBC cells.

3. Circulating miRNAs as Potential BTCs Biomarkers

Several studies have reported that detectable miRNAs in bodily fluids (e.g., plasma, serum, urine, and saliva) are more stable in comparison with other circulating nucleic acids [57]. Therefore, circulating miRNAs may be noninvasive and specific diagnostic and/or prognostic molecular biomarkers for human diseases, including cancer [4, 7, 58, 59]. In BTCs, many circulating miRNAs seem to be reproducible and reliable potential biomarkers as well as possible therapeutic targets [60]. Table 2 summarizes the circulating miRNAs with potential diagnostic, prognostic, and predictive biomarker applications in BTCs.

In CCA patients, Cheng et al. [64] observed different expression levels of circulating hsa-miR-106a not only between CCAs and healthy controls but also among CCAs and benign bile duct diseases (e.g., primary bile duct stone and congenital biliary duct cysts). Furthermore, they identified decreased hsa-miR-106a levels in patients with lymph node metastasis compared with those without metastasis, indicating the possible role of hsa-miR-106a in the occurrence of lymph node metastasis.

Interestingly, Voigtländer et al. [65] found a distinct circulating miRNA profile in the bile and serum samples from CCA patients and patients with primary sclerosing cholangitis (PSC), a noncancerous disease. Furthermore, bile samples from patients with concomitant PSC and CCA (PSC/CCA) were also included in this study. Their results showed higher expression levels of hsa-miR-126, hsa-miR-26a, hsa-miR-30b, hsa-miR-122, and hsa-miR-1281 in PSC patients than those

TABLE 1: Deregulated miRNAs in BTCs.

miRNA	Tumor	Expression	Target	Roles in BTCs	Reference
hsa-miR-21	CCA	↑	PTEN	Invasion Migration Chemoresistance	[11–14]
		↓	TPM1	DNA methylation Histone deacetylation	[15]
		↓	15-PGDH HPGD	Inflammation	[16]
		↑	PDCD4	Lymph node metastasis Migration	[17–20]
		↑	RECK	Migration Metastasis	[21, 22]
		↑	TIMP3	Apoptosis	[18]
		↑	—	pTNM Prognosis	[23]
hsa-miR-20[a]	GBC	↑	SMAD7	Invasion Metastasis Migration Prognosis	[24]
hsa-miR-34a	CCA	↓	C-MYC	Progression	[25]
	GBC	↓	PNUTS	Proliferation Prognosis	[26]
hsa-miR-335	GBC	↓	BMI1	Invasion Lymph node metastasis pTNM Prognosis	[27, 28]
hsa-miR-148a	CCA	↓	DNMT1	Prognosis	[29]
hsa-miR-31	CCA	↑	RASA1	Apoptosis Proliferation	[30]
hsa-miR-200b/c	CCA	↓	SUZ12	Chemoresistance Invasion Migration	[28]
hsa-miR-210	CCA	↑	MNT	Progression	[25]
Let-7a	CCA	↓	RAS	Progression	[21]
hsa-miR-370	CCA	↓	MAP3K8	Inflammation pTNM	[31]
hsa-miR-29b	CCA	↓	C-MYC	Apoptosis	[32]
hsa-miR-101	CCA	↓	VEGF COX-2	Angiogenesis	[33]
hsa-miR-200b/c	CCA	↓	ROCK2	Migration	[28]
hsa-miR-138	CCA	↓	RHOC	Migration	[34]
hsa-miR-376c	CCA	↓	GRB2	Migration	[35]
hsa-miR-124	CCA	↓	SMYD3	Migration	[36]
hsa-miR-204	CCA	↓	SLUG	Migration	[37]
hsa-miR-214	CCA	↓	TWIST	Migration	[38]
hsa-miR-200c	CCA	↓	NCAM1	Migration	[39]
hsa-miR-200b	CCA	↑	PTPN12	Chemoresistance	[14]
hsa-miR-29b	CCA	↓	PIK3R1 MMP2	Chemoresistance	[40]
hsa-miR-205	CCA	↓	—	Chemoresistance	
hsa-miR-221	CCA	↓	PIK3R1	Chemoresistance	
hsa-miR-182	GBC	↑	CADM1	Invasion Migration Metastasis	[27]

TABLE 1: Continued.

miRNA	Tumor	Expression	Target	Roles in BTCs	Reference
hsa-miR-155	GBC	↑	SMAD7	Invasion Lymph node metastasis Proliferation Prognosis	[41]
hsa-miR-130a	GBC	↓	HOTAIR	Invasion Proliferation	[42]
hsa-miR-26a	GBC	↓	HMGA2	pTNM Proliferation	[43]
hsa-miR-135a-5p	GBC	↓	VLDLR	pTNM Proliferation	[44]
hsa-miR-218-5p	GBC	↓	BMI1	Invasion Migration Proliferation	[45]
hsa-miR-146-5p	GBC	↓	EGFR	Apoptosis pTNM Proliferation	[46]
hsa-miR-1	GBC	↓	VEGF-A AXL	Apoptosis Proliferation	[47]
hsa-miR-145	GBC		AXL		
hsa-miR-143	GBC	↓	AXL	Lymph node metastasis pTNM stage	
hsa-miR-122 hsa-miR-187	GBC	↑			

in CCA patients. However, bile samples showed hsa-miR-640, hsa-miR-1537, and hsa-miR-3189 downregulation, as well as hsa-miR-412 upregulation in PSC and PSC/CCA patients. These results demonstrated that PSC and CCA patients have distinct miRNA profiles in their bile and serum, which could be used to discriminate these diseases.

A small number of studies have described circulating miRNAs in patients with GBC. Kishimoto et al. [62] demonstrated an increase in the hsa-miR-21 expression levels in plasma from GBC patients before curative resection when compared with postsurgical patients and healthy volunteers. These findings suggest that hsa-miR-21 plasma levels were significantly affected by cancer occurrence and might have the potential to be a diagnostic biomarker for GBC patients.

Recently, Li and Pu [47] described significantly deregulated miRNAs in the peripheral blood samples of GBC patients compared with healthy volunteers. The expression levels of hsa-miR-187, hsa-miR-192, and hsa-miR-202 were upregulated while hsa-miR-143 was downregulated. These results were associated with lymph node metastasis, inflammation, immune reaction, and poor prognosis and could be translated to clinical practice as biomarkers for the early diagnosis, prognosis, and predictive response in patients with GBC.

Although most studies involving circulating miRNAs utilize real-time PCR for detection, Kojima et al. [68] used a highly sensitive microarray denoted as "3D Gene" that was capable of simultaneously analyzing more than 2,500 miRNAs in serum samples from patients with pancreatobiliary cancers. These authors found several significantly dysregulated miRNAs, including 30 upregulated miRNAs

and 36 downregulated miRNAs in BTCs. However, none of these miRNAs could be used as single biomarker for this type of cancer. The best results were achieved with a panel of eight miRNAs (hsa-miR-6075, hsa-miR-4294, hsa-miR-6880-5p, hsa-miR-6799-5p, hsa-miR-125a-3p, hsa-miR-4530, hsa-miR-6836-3p, and hsa-miR-4476).

4. miRNA Single-Nucleotide Polymorphisms in BTCs

In general, aberrations in miRNA expression result from either epigenetic modifications or genomic changes, which include chromosomal rearrangements, mutations, or SNPs [69].

Several SNPs in miRNAs can lead to distinctions in the miRNA expression levels, which can modulate miRNA-target gene expression and, subsequently, affect cancer susceptibility [4, 70]. However, few studies have been performed to identify SNPs in miRNAs in BTCs patients until now.

The SNPs hsa-miR-27a rs895819, hsa-miR-570 rs4143815, and hsa-miR-181a rs12537 have been found to play important roles in many cancer types [71–78], and their contribution in BTCs has been explored. Gupta et al. [70] observed that the combination of hsa-miR-27a rs895819, hsa-miR-570 rs4143815, and hsa-miR-181a rs12537 was the best gene-gene interaction model for predicting the susceptibility and treatment response in GBC patients. Moreover, the SNPs hsa-miR-27a rs895819 and hsa-miR-181a rs12537 were associated with treatment toxicity but had no influence on the survival outcomes of GBC patients with locally advanced and/or metastatic tumors.

TABLE 2: Circulating miRNAs in patients with BTC as potential diagnostic, prognostic, and predictive biomarkers.

miRNA	Expression	Samples	N samples	Potential biomarker	Method	Clinical implication	Reference
hsa-miR-9	↑	Bile	BTCs (9) HV (9)	Diagnostic Prognostic	RT-PCR	Metastasis	[61]
hsa-miR-145	↑	Bile	BTCs (9) HV (9)	Diagnostic	RT-PCR	—	[61]
hsa-miR-21	↑	Plasma	BTCs (94) HV (50) BBD (2)	Diagnostic	qRT-PCR	Inflammatory reaction	[62]
		Peripheral blood	GBC (40) HV (40)	Diagnostic	qRT-PCR	—	[47]
hsa-miR-150	↑	Plasma	iCCA (15)	Diagnostic	qRT-PCR	Tumor progression	[63]
hsa-miR-106a	↓	Serum	CCA (103) HV (20)	Prognostic	qRT-PCR	Lymph node metastasis	[64]
hsa-miR-126	↑	Serum	PSC (40) CCA (31) HV (12)	Diagnostic	RT-PCR	—	[65]
hsa-miR-26a	↑	Serum	PSC (40) CCA (31) HV (12)	Diagnostic	RT-PCR	—	[65]
hsa-miR-30b	↑	Serum	PSC (40) CC (31) HV (12)	Diagnostic	RT-PCR	—	[65]
hsa- miR-122	↑	Serum	PSC (40) CC (31) HV (12)	Diagnostic	RT-PCR	—	[65]
hsa-miR-1281	↑	Serum	PSC (40) CC (31) HV (12)	Diagnostic	RT-PCR	—	[65]
hsa-miR -187	↑	Peripheral blood	GBC (40) HV (40)	Diagnostic Prognostic Predictive	qRT-PCR	Lymph node metastasis Poor prognosis	[47]
hsa-miR-192	↑	Peripheral blood	GBC (40) HV (40)	Diagnostic Prognostic Predictive	qRT-PCR	Inflammatory reaction Immune reaction Lymph node metastasis	[47]
		Serum	iCCA (11) HV (09)	Diagnostic Prognostic	miRNA RT-PCR array	Lymph node metastasis Poor prognosis	[66]
hsa-miR-194	↑	Serum	CCA (70) HV (70)	Diagnostic	qRT-PCR	Tumor progression	[58]
hsa-miR -202	↑	Peripheral blood	GBC (40) HV (40)	Diagnostic Prognostic Predictive	qRT-PCR	Lymph node metastasis	[47]
hsa-let- 7a	↓	Peripheral blood	GBC (40) HV (40)	Diagnostic	qRT-PCR	—	[47]
hsa-miR -143	↓	Peripheral blood	GBC (40) HV (40)	Diagnostic Prognostic Predictive	qRT-PCR	Inflammatory and immune reaction Lymph node metastasis	[47]
hsa-miR-335	↓	Peripheral blood	GBC (40) HV (40)	Diagnostic	qRT-PCR	—	[47]
hsa-miR-1307-3p	↓	Plasma	iCCA (13) HV (5)	Diagnostic	qRT-PCR	—	[67]
hsa-miR-1275	↑	Plasma	iCCA (13) HV (5)	Diagnostic	qRT-PCR	—	[67]

TABLE 2: Continued.

miRNA	Expression	Samples	N samples	Potential biomarker	Method	Clinical implication	Reference
hsa- miR-320b	↑	Plasma	iCCA (13) HVs (5)	Diagnostic	qRT-PCR	—	[67]
hsa-miR-874	↑	Plasma	iCCA (13) HVs (5)	Diagnostic	qRT-PCR	—	[67]
hsa-miR-483-5p	↑	Plasma	iCCA (13) HV (5)	Diagnostic	qRT-PCR	—	[67]
		Serum	CCA (70) HV (70)	Diagnostic	qRT-PCR	Tumor progression	[58]
hsa-miR-885-5p	↑	Plasma	iCCA (13) HV (5)	Diagnostic	qRT-PCR	—	[67]
hsa-miR-92b-3p	↑	Plasma	iCCA (13) HV (5)	Diagnostic	qRT-PCR	—	[67]
hsa-miR-505-3p	↑	Plasma	iCCA (13) HV (5)	Diagnostic	qRT-PCR	—	[67]
hsa-miR-6836-3p	↑	Serum	BTCs (98) HV (150)	Diagnostic	3D-Gene	—	[68]
hsa-miR-6075	↑	Serum	BTCs (98) HV (150)	Diagnostic	3D-Gene	—	[68]
hsa- miR-4634	↑	Serum	BTCs (98) HV (150)	Diagnostic	3D-Gene	—	[68]
hsa-miR-4294	↓	Serum	BTCs (98) HV (150)	Diagnostic	3D-Gene	—	[68]
hsa-miR-6880-5p	↓	Serum	BTCs (98) HV (150)	Diagnostic	3D-Gene	—	[68]
hsa-miR-6799-5p	↓	Serum	BTCs (98) HV (150)	Diagnostic	3D-Gene	—	[68]
hsa-miR-125a-3p,	↓	Serum	BTCs (98) HV (150)	Diagnostic	3D-Gene	Tumor progression	[68]
hsa-miR-4530	↓	Serum	BTCs (98) HV (150)	Diagnostic	3D-Gene	—	[68]
hsa-miR-7114-5p	↓	Serum	BTCs (98) HV (150)	Diagnostic	3D-Gene	—	[68]
hsa-miR-4476	↓	Serum	BTCs (98) HV (150)	Diagnostic	3D-Gene	—	[68]

BBD: benign biliary disorders; BTCs: biliary tract cancers; CCA: cholangiocarcinoma; iCCA: intrahepatic cholangiocarcinoma; GBC: gallbladder cancer; HV: heath volunteers; PSC: primary sclerosing cholangitis.

SNPs in pri-miRNAs and pre-miRNAs could also affect miRNA processing, miRNA expression, and cancer susceptibility. Srivastava et al. [79] reported genetic polymorphisms in pre-mir-196a2 rs11614913 (C>T), pre-hsa-mir-196a rs11614913, and pre-hsa-mir-499 rs3746444 (T>C) that were associated with an increased overall risk of developing GBC development. In CCA, Mihalache et al. [80] investigated the G/C variant in pre-hsa-miR-146a rs2910164 and found no significant relationship between genetic susceptibility and CCA.

Additional studies addressing the identification of miRNA SNPs could be useful to assess the individual susceptibility of BTCs and improve our understanding of their potential contribution to the disease as well as aid in the development of potential clinical applications.

5. Conclusion

miRNAs are profoundly involved in tumor onset and progression [81–84]. However, the implications of miRNA for the diagnosis, prognosis, and therapeutic options for patients with BTCs remain unsatisfactory. This review highlighted some miRNAs that are dysregulated in BTCs, their targets, and the possible clinical implications. A better understanding of the therapeutic applications of miRNAs could lead to future clinical trials involving the inhibition of oncomiRs or the promotion of expression of tsmiRs as new approaches against diverse cancer types, including aggressive BTCs.

Here, we also reported several circulating miRNAs as possible diagnostic, prognostic, and/or predictive biomarkers in BTCs. Circulating miRNAs could be promising potential biomarkers for cancers because detectable miRNAs in the bodily fluids are stable and can be measured using noninvasive methods [57]. BTCs are usually asymptomatic; therefore, the use of miRNAs as early diagnostic biomarkers could be a useful tool to improve the long-term survival of BTC patients. However, more studies with clinical outcomes are needed to identify which miRNAs could serve as either a potential therapeutic target or diagnostic and prognostic biomarkers of BTCs.

Moreover, several SNPs in miRNAs can affect the expression of target genes, leading to a cellular disorder and, consequently, tumorigenesis [4, 70]. However, few studies have been performed to identify SNPs in the miRNAs expressed by BTC patients until now; this review emphasizes the need to expand the knowledge in this field of study.

Competing Interests

The authors declare no conflict of interests for this article.

Authors' Contributions

Danielle Queiroz Calcagno conceived the review design; Nina Nayara Ferreira Martins, Kelly Cristina da Silva Oliveira, and Danielle Queiroz Calcagno collected the data; Nina Nayara Ferreira Martins, Kelly Cristina da Silva Oliveira, Amanda Braga Bona, and Danielle Queiroz Calcagno wrote the paper; Marília de Arruda Cardoso Smith and Geraldo Ishak performed corrections and made suggestions; Paulo Pimentel Assumpção and Rommel Rodríguez Burbano critically revised the paper.

Acknowledgments

This study was supported by the Fundação de Amparo à Pesquisa do Estado de São Paulo (FAPESP, to Marília de Arruda Cardoso Smith), the Conselho Nacional de Desenvolvimento Científico e Tecnológico (CNPq, to Marília de Arruda Cardoso Smith and Rommel Rodríguez Burbano), and the Coordenação de Aperfeiçoamento de Pessoal de Nível Superior (CAPES, to Nina Nayara Ferreira Martins and Kelly Cristina da Silva Oliveira).

References

[1] K. H. Yoo, N. K. D. Kim, W. I. Kwon et al., "Genomic alterations in biliary tract cancer using targeted sequencing," *Translational Oncology*, vol. 9, no. 3, pp. 173–178, 2016.

[2] K. K. Ciombor and L. W. Goff, "Advances in the management of biliary tract cancers," *Clinical Advances in Hematology and Oncology*, vol. 11, no. 1, pp. 28–34, 2013.

[3] C. O. Gigek, E. S. Chen, D. Q. Calcagno, F. Wisnieski, R. R. Burbano, and M. A. C. Smith, "Epigenetic mechanisms in gastric cancer," *Epigenomics*, vol. 4, no. 3, pp. 279–294, 2012.

[4] D. Q. Calcagno, M. D. A. Cardoso Smith, and R. R. Burbano, "Cancer type-specific epigenetic changes: gastric cancer," *Methods in Molecular Biology*, vol. 1238, pp. 79–101, 2015.

[5] A. Saumet and C.-H. Lecellier, "MicroRNAs and personalized medicine: evaluating their potential as cancer biomarkers," *Advances in Experimental Medicine and Biology*, vol. 888, pp. 5–15, 2015.

[6] D. Huo, W. M. Clayton, T. F. Yoshimatsu, J. Chen, and O. I. Olopade, "Identification of a circulating MicroRNA signature to distinguish recurrence in breast cancer patients," *Oncotarget*, 2016.

[7] G. Yang, L. Zhang, R. Li, and L. Wang, "The role of microRNAs in gallbladder cancer (Review)," *Molecular and Clinical Oncology*, vol. 5, no. 1, pp. 7–13, 2016.

[8] Y. Lee, M. Kim, J. Han et al., "MicroRNA genes are transcribed by RNA polymerase II," *EMBO Journal*, vol. 23, no. 20, pp. 4051–4060, 2004.

[9] S. Lin and R. I. Gregory, "MicroRNA biogenesis pathways in cancer," *Nature Reviews Cancer*, vol. 15, no. 6, pp. 321–333, 2015.

[10] C. Weber, "MicroRNAs: from basic mechanisms to clinical application in cardiovascular medicine," *Arteriosclerosis, Thrombosis, and Vascular Biology*, vol. 33, no. 2, pp. 168–169, 2013.

[11] J. Zhang, J. Jiao, S. Cermelli et al., "miR-21 inhibition reduces liver fibrosis and prevents tumor development by inducing apoptosis of CD24$^+$ progenitor cells," *Cancer Research*, vol. 75, no. 9, pp. 1859–1867, 2015.

[12] Q. He, L. Cai, L. Shuai et al., "Ars2 is overexpressed in human cholangiocarcinomas and its depletion increases PTEN and PDCD4 by decreasing microRNA-21," *Molecular Carcinogenesis*, vol. 52, no. 4, pp. 286–296, 2013.

[13] Z. Liu, Z.-Y. Jin, C.-H. Liu, F. Xie, X.-S. Lin, and Q. Huang, "MicroRNA-21 regulates biological behavior by inducing EMT in human cholangiocarcinoma," *International Journal of Clinical and Experimental Pathology*, vol. 8, no. 5, pp. 4684–4694, 2015.

[14] F. Meng, R. Henson, M. Lang et al., "Involvement of human micro-RNA in growth and response to chemotherapy in human cholangiocarcinoma cell lines," *Gastroenterology*, vol. 130, no. 7, pp. 2113–2129, 2006.

[15] W. Yang, X. Wang, W. Zheng, K. Li, H. Liu, and Y. Sun, "Genetic and epigenetic alterations are involved in the regulation of TPM1 in cholangiocarcinoma," *International Journal of Oncology*, vol. 42, no. 2, pp. 690–698, 2013.

[16] L. Lu, K. Byrnes, C. Han, Y. Wang, and T. Wu, "MiR-21 targets 15-PGDH and promotes cholangiocarcinoma growth," *Molecular Cancer Research*, vol. 12, no. 6, pp. 890–900, 2014.

[17] P. Chusorn, N. Namwat, W. Loilome et al., "Overexpression of microRNA-21 regulating PDCD4 during tumorigenesis of liver fluke-associated cholangiocarcinoma contributes to tumor growth and metastasis," *Tumor Biology*, vol. 34, no. 3, pp. 1579–1588, 2013.

[18] F. M. Selaru, A. V. Olaru, T. Kan et al., "MicroRNA-21 is overexpressed in human cholangiocarcinoma and regulates programmed cell death 4 and tissue inhibitor of metalloproteinase 3," *Hepatology*, vol. 49, no. 5, pp. 1595–1601, 2009.

[19] C.-Z. Liu, W. Liu, Y. Zheng et al., "PTEN and PDCD4 are bona fide targets of microRNA-21 in human cholangiocarcinoma," *Chinese Medical Sciences Journal*, vol. 27, no. 2, pp. 65–72, 2012.

[20] J. He, Y. Yue, C. Dong, and S. Xiong, "MiR-21 confers resistance against CVB3-induced myocarditis by inhibiting PDCD4-mediated apoptosis," *Clinical and Investigative Medicine*, vol. 36, no. 2, pp. E103–E111, 2013.

[21] N. Namwat, P. Chusorn, W. Loilome et al., "Expression profiles of oncomir miR-21 and tumor suppressor let-7a in the progression of opisthorchiasis-associated cholangiocarcinoma," *Asian*

Pacific Journal of Cancer Prevention, vol. 13, supplement, pp. 65–69, 2012.

[22] Q. Huang, L. Liu, C.-H. Liu et al., "MicroRNA-21 Regulates the invasion and metastasis in cholangiocarcinoma and may be a potential biomarker for cancer prognosis," *Asian Pacific Journal of Cancer Prevention*, vol. 14, no. 2, pp. 829–834, 2013.

[23] A. Karakatsanis, I. Papaconstantinou, M. Gazouli, A. Lyberopoulou, G. Polymeneas, and D. Voros, "Expression of microRNAs, miR-21, miR-31, miR-122, miR-145, miR-146a, miR-200c, miR-221, miR-222, and miR-223 in patients with hepatocellular carcinoma or intrahepatic cholangiocarcinoma and its prognostic significance," *Molecular Carcinogenesis*, vol. 52, no. 4, pp. 297–303, 2013.

[24] Y. Chang, J. Yang, G. Liu et al., "MiR-20a triggers metastasis of gallbladder carcinoma," *Journal of Hepatology*, vol. 59, no. 3, pp. 518–527, 2013.

[25] H. Yang, T. W. H. Li, J. Peng et al., "A mouse model of cholestasis-associated cholangiocarcinoma and transcription factors involved in progression," *Gastroenterology*, vol. 141, no. 1, pp. 378.e4–388.e4, 2011.

[26] K. Jin, Y. Xiang, J. Tang et al., "miR-34 is associated with poor prognosis of patients with gallbladder cancer through regulating telomere length in tumor stem cells," *Tumor Biology*, vol. 35, no. 2, pp. 1503–1510, 2014.

[27] Y. Qiu, X. Luo, T. Kan et al., "TGF-β upregulates miR-182 expression to promote gallbladder cancer metastasis by targeting CADM1," *Molecular BioSystems*, vol. 10, no. 3, pp. 679–685, 2014.

[28] F. Peng, J. Jiang, Y. Yu et al., "Direct targeting of SUZ12/ROCK2 by miR-200b/c inhibits cholangiocarcinoma tumourigenesis and metastasis," *British Journal of Cancer*, vol. 109, no. 12, pp. 3092–3104, 2013.

[29] C. Braconi, N. Huang, and T. Patel, "Microrna-dependent regulation of DNA methyltransferase-1 and tumor suppressor gene expression by interleukin-6 in human malignant cholangiocytes," *Hepatology*, vol. 51, no. 3, pp. 881–890, 2010.

[30] C. Hu, F. Huang, G. Deng, W. Nie, W. Huang, and X. Zeng, "miR-31 promotes oncogenesis in intrahepatic cholangiocarcinoma cells via the direct suppression of RASA1," *Experimental and Therapeutic Medicine*, vol. 6, no. 5, pp. 1265–1270, 2013.

[31] F. Meng, H. Wehbe-Janek, R. Henson, H. Smith, and T. Patel, "Epigenetic regulation of microRNA-370 by interleukin-6 in malignant human cholangiocytes," *Oncogene*, vol. 27, no. 3, pp. 378–386, 2008.

[32] J. L. Mott, S. Kurita, S. C. Cazanave, S. F. Bronk, N. W. Werneburg, and M. E. Fernandez-Zapico, "Transcriptional suppression of mir-29b-1/mir-29a promoter by c-Myc, hedgehog, and NF-kappaB," *Journal of Cellular Biochemistry*, vol. 110, no. 5, pp. 1155–1164, 2010.

[33] J. Zhang, C. Han, H. Zhu, K. Song, and T. Wu, "MiR-101 inhibits cholangiocarcinoma angiogenesis through targeting vascular endothelial growth factor (VEGF)," *American Journal of Pathology*, vol. 182, no. 5, pp. 1629–1639, 2013.

[34] Q. Wang, H. Tang, S. Yin, and C. Dong, "Downregulation of microRNA-138 enhances the proliferation, migrationand invasion of cholangiocarcinoma cells through the upregulation of RhoC/p-ERK/MMP-2/MMP-9," *Oncology Reports*, vol. 29, no. 5, pp. 2046–2052, 2013.

[35] J. Iwaki, K. Kikuchi, Y. Mizuguchi et al., "MiR-376c downregulation accelerates EGF-dependent migration by targeting GRB2 in the HuCCT1 human intrahepatic cholangiocarcinoma cell line," *PLoS ONE*, vol. 8, no. 7, Article ID e69496, 2013.

[36] B. Zeng, Z. Li, R. Chen et al., "Epigenetic regulation of miR-124 by Hepatitis C Virus core protein promotes migration and invasion of intrahepatic cholangiocarcinoma cells by targeting SMYD3," *FEBS Letters*, vol. 586, no. 19, pp. 3271–3278, 2012.

[37] Y.-H. Qiu, Y.-P. Wei, N.-J. Shen et al., "MiR-204 Inhibits epithelial to mesenchymal transition by targeting slug in intrahepatic cholangiocarcinoma cells," *Cellular Physiology and Biochemistry*, vol. 32, no. 5, pp. 1331–1341, 2013.

[38] B. Li, Q. Han, Y. Zhu, Y. Yu, J. Wang, and X. Jiang, "Downregulation of miR-214 contributes to intrahepatic cholangiocarcinoma metastasis by targeting Twist," *FEBS Journal*, vol. 279, no. 13, pp. 2393–2398, 2012.

[39] N. Oishi, M. R. Kumar, S. Roessler et al., "Transcriptomic profiling reveals hepatic stem-like gene signatures and interplay of miR-200c and epithelial-mesenchymal transition in intrahepatic cholangiocarcinoma," *Hepatology*, vol. 56, no. 5, pp. 1792–1803, 2012.

[40] K. Okamoto, K. Miyoshi, and Y. Murawaki, "miR-29b, miR-205 and miR-221 enhance chemosensitivity to gemcitabine in HuH28 human cholangiocarcinoma cells," *PLoS ONE*, vol. 8, no. 10, Article ID e77623, 2013.

[41] H. Kono, M. Nakamura, T. Ohtsuka et al., "High expression of microRNA-155 is associated with the aggressive malignant behavior of gallbladder carcinoma," *Oncology reports*, vol. 30, no. 1, pp. 17–24, 2013.

[42] M.-Z. Ma, C.-X. Li, Y. Zhang et al., "Long non-coding RNA HOTAIR, a c-Myc activated driver of malignancy, negatively regulates miRNA-130a in gallbladder cancer," *Molecular Cancer*, vol. 13, no. 1, article no. 156, 2014.

[43] H. Zhou, W. Guo, Y. Zhao et al., "MicroRNA-26a acts as a tumor suppressor inhibiting gallbladder cancer cell proliferation by directly targeting HMGA2," *International Journal of Oncology*, vol. 45, no. 6, pp. 2050–2058, 2014.

[44] H. Zhou, W. Guo, Y. Zhao et al., "MicroRNA-135a acts as a putative tumor suppressor by directly targeting very low density lipoprotein receptor in human gallbladder cancer," *Cancer Science*, vol. 105, no. 8, pp. 956–965, 2014.

[45] M.-Z. Ma, B.-F. Chu, Y. Zhang et al., "Long non-coding RNA CCAT1 promotes gallbladder cancer development via negative modulation of miRNA-218-5p," *Cell Death and Disease*, vol. 6, no. 1, Article ID e1583, 2015.

[46] J. Cai, L. Xu, Z. Cai, J. Wang, B. Zhou, and H. Hu, "MicroRNA-146b-5p inhibits the growth of gallbladder carcinoma by targeting epidermal growth factor receptor," *Molecular Medicine Reports*, vol. 12, no. 1, pp. 1549–1555, 2015.

[47] G. Li and Y. Pu, "MicroRNA signatures in total peripheral blood of gallbladder cancer patients," *Tumor Biology*, vol. 36, no. 9, pp. 6985–6990, 2015.

[48] T. Kitamura, K. Connolly, L. Ruffino et al., "The therapeutic effect of histone deacetylase inhibitor PCI-24781 on gallbladder carcinoma in BK5.erbB2 mice," *Journal of Hepatology*, vol. 57, no. 1, pp. 84–91, 2012.

[49] L.-J. Wang, C.-C. He, X. Sui et al., "MiR-21 promotes intrahepatic cholangiocarcinoma proliferation and growth in vitro and in vivo by targeting PTPN14 and PTEN," *Oncotarget*, vol. 6, no. 8, pp. 5932–5946, 2015.

[50] S. Sekine, Y. Shimada, T. Nagata et al., "Role of aquaporin-5 in gallbladder carcinoma," *European Surgical Research*, vol. 51, no. 3-4, pp. 108–117, 2013.

[51] R. Bao, Y. Shu, Y. Hu et al., "miR-101 targeting ZFX suppresses tumor proliferation and metastasis by regulating the

MAPK/Erk and smad pathways in gallbladder carcinoma," *Oncotarget*, 2016.

[52] P. Y. Wu, X. D. Zhang, J. Zhu, X. Y. Guo, and J. F. Wang, "Low expression of microRNA-146b-5p and microRNA-320d predicts poor outcome of large B-cell lymphoma treated with cyclophosphamide, doxorubicin, vincristine, and prednisone," *Human Pathology*, vol. 45, no. 8, pp. 1664–1673, 2014.

[53] C. Shen, H. Yang, H. Liu, X. Wang, Y. Zhang, and R. Xu, "Inhibitory effect and mechanisms of microRNA-146b-5p on the proliferation and metastatic potential of Caski human cervical cancer cells," *Molecular Medicine Reports*, vol. 11, no. 5, pp. 3955–3961, 2015.

[54] Z. Dang, W.-H. Xu, P. Lu et al., "MicroRNA-135a inhibits cell proliferation by targeting Bmi1 in pancreatic ductal adenocarcinoma," *International Journal of Biological Sciences*, vol. 10, no. 7, pp. 733–745, 2014.

[55] J.-Y. Shin, Y.-I. Kim, S.-J. Cho et al., "MicroRNA 135a suppresses lymph node metastasis through down-regulation of ROCK1 in early gastric cancer," *PLoS ONE*, vol. 9, no. 1, Article ID e85205, 2014.

[56] W. Tang, Y. Jiang, X. Mu, L. Xu, W. Cheng, and X. Wang, "MiR-135a functions as a tumor suppressor in epithelial ovarian cancer and regulates HOXA10 expression," *Cellular Signalling*, vol. 26, no. 7, pp. 1420–1426, 2014.

[57] I. Igaz and P. Igaz, "Diagnostic relevance of microRNAs in other body fluids including urine, feces, and saliva," *EXS*, vol. 106, pp. 245–252, 2015.

[58] F. Bernuzzi, F. Marabita, A. Lleo et al., "Serum microRNAs as novel biomarkers for primary sclerosing cholangitis and cholangiocarcinoma," *Clinical & Experimental Immunology*, vol. 185, no. 1, pp. 61–71, 2016.

[59] K. Piontek and F. M. Selaru, "MicroRNAs in the biology and diagnosis of cholangiocarcinoma," *Seminars in Liver Disease*, vol. 35, no. 1, pp. 55–62, 2015.

[60] P. Letelier, I. Riquelme, A. Hernández, N. Guzmán, J. Farías, and J. Roa, "Circulating MicroRNAs as biomarkers in biliary tract cancers," *International Journal of Molecular Sciences*, vol. 17, no. 5, p. 791, 2016.

[61] K. Shigehara, S. Yokomuro, O. Ishibashi et al., "Real-time PCR-based analysis of the human bile micrornaome identifies miR-9 as a potential diagnostic biomarker for biliary tract cancer," *PLoS ONE*, vol. 6, no. 8, Article ID e23584, 2011.

[62] T. Kishimoto, H. Eguchi, H. Nagano et al., "Plasma miR-21 is a novel diagnostic biomarker for biliary tract cancer," *Cancer Science*, vol. 104, no. 12, pp. 1626–1631, 2013.

[63] S. Wang, J. Yin, T. Li et al., "Upregulated circulating miR-150 is associated with the risk of intrahepatic cholangiocarcinoma," *Oncology Reports*, vol. 33, no. 2, pp. 819–825, 2015.

[64] Q. Cheng, F. Feng, L. Zhu et al., "Circulating miR-106a is a novel prognostic and lymph node metastasis indicator for cholangiocarcinoma," *Scientific Reports*, vol. 5, Article ID 16103, 2015.

[65] T. Voigtländer, S. K. Gupta, S. Thum et al., "MicroRNAs in serum and bile of patients with primary sclerosing cholangitis and/or cholangiocarcinoma," *PLoS ONE*, vol. 10, no. 10, Article ID e0139305, 2015.

[66] R. Silakit, W. Loilome, P. Yongvanit et al., "Circulating miR-192 in liver fluke-associated cholangiocarcinoma patients: a prospective prognostic indicator," *Journal of Hepato-Biliary-Pancreatic Sciences*, vol. 21, no. 12, pp. 864–872, 2014.

[67] J. Plieskatt, G. Rinaldi, Y. Feng et al., "A microRNA profile associated with Opisthorchis viverrini-induced cholangiocarcinoma in tissue and plasma," *BMC Cancer*, vol. 15, no. 1, article no. 309, 2015.

[68] M. Kojima, H. Sudo, J. Kawauchi et al., "MicroRNA markers for the diagnosis of pancreatic and biliary-tract cancers," *PLoS ONE*, vol. 10, no. 2, Article ID e0118220, 2015.

[69] A. Chandra, A. Ray, S. Senapati, and R. Chatterjee, "Genetic and epigenetic basis of psoriasis pathogenesis," *Molecular Immunology*, vol. 64, no. 2, pp. 313–323, 2015.

[70] A. Gupta, A. Sharma, A. Yadav et al., "Evaluation of miR-27a, miR-181a, and miR-570 genetic variants with gallbladder cancer susceptibility and treatment outcome in a north indian population," *Molecular Diagnosis and Therapy*, vol. 19, no. 5, pp. 317–327, 2015.

[71] Q. Sun, H. Gu, Y. Zeng et al., "Hsa-mir-27a genetic variant contributes to gastric cancer susceptibility through affecting miR-27a and target gene expression," *Cancer Science*, vol. 101, no. 10, pp. 2241–2247, 2010.

[72] J. Xu, Z. Yin, H. Shen et al., "A genetic polymorphism in pre-miR-27a confers clinical outcome of non-small cell lung cancer in a Chinese population," *PLoS ONE*, vol. 8, no. 11, Article ID e79135, 2013.

[73] Z. Wang, J. Lai, Y. Wang, W. Nie, and X. Guan, "The Hsa-miR-27a rs895819 (A>G) polymorphism and cancer susceptibility," *Gene*, vol. 521, no. 1, pp. 87–90, 2013.

[74] Y. Lin, Y. Nie, J. Zhao et al., "Genetic polymorphism at miR-181a binding site contributes to gastric cancer susceptibility," *Carcinogenesis*, vol. 33, no. 12, pp. 2377–2383, 2012.

[75] J.-Y. Ma, H.-J. Yan, Z.-H. Yang, and W. Gu, "Rs895819 within miR-27a might be involved in development of non small cell lung cancer in the Chinese Han population," *Asian Pacific Journal of Cancer Prevention*, vol. 16, no. 5, pp. 1939–1944, 2015.

[76] Z. Wang, X. Sun, Y. Wang, X. Liu, Y. Xuan, and S. Hu, "Association between miR-27a genetic variants and susceptibility to colorectal cancer," *Diagnostic Pathology*, vol. 9, no. 1, article no. 146, 2014.

[77] Y. Deng, H. Bai, and H. Hu, "rs11671784 G/A variation in miR-27a decreases chemo-sensitivity of bladder cancer by decreasing miR-27a and increasing the target RUNX-1 expression," *Biochemical and Biophysical Research Communications*, vol. 458, no. 2, pp. 321–327, 2015.

[78] D. Shi, P. Li, L. Ma et al., "A genetic variant in pre-miR-27a is associated with a reduced renal cell cancer risk in a Chinese population," *PLoS ONE*, vol. 7, no. 10, Article ID e46566, 2012.

[79] K. Srivastava, A. Srivastava, and B. Mittal, "Common genetic variants in pre-microRNAs and risk of gallbladder cancer in North Indian population," *Journal of Human Genetics*, vol. 55, no. 8, pp. 495–499, 2010.

[80] F. Mihalache, A. Höblinger, M. Acalovschi, T. Sauerbruch, F. Lammert, and V. Zimmer, "A common variant in the precursor miR-146a sequence does not predispose to cholangiocarcinoma in a large european cohort," *Hepatobiliary and Pancreatic Diseases International*, vol. 11, no. 4, pp. 412–417, 2012.

[81] A. Shinozaki, T. Sakatani, T. Ushiku et al., "Downregulation of MicroRNA-200 in EBV-associated gastric carcinoma," *Cancer Research*, vol. 70, no. 11, pp. 4719–4727, 2010.

[82] M. Zhou, Z. Liu, Y. Zhao et al., "MicroRNA-125b confers the resistance of breast cancer cells to paclitaxel through suppression of pro-apoptotic Bcl-2 antagonist killer 1 (Bak1) expression," *Journal of Biological Chemistry*, vol. 285, no. 28, pp. 21496–21507, 2010.

[83] C.-C. Lin, W. Jiang, R. Mitra, F. Cheng, H. Yu, and Z. Zhao, "Regulation rewiring analysis reveals mutual regulation between STAT1 and miR-155-5p in tumor immunosurveillance in seven major cancers," *Scientific Reports*, vol. 5, Article ID 12063, 2015.

[84] J. H. Hwang, J. Voortman, E. Giovannetti et al., "Identification of microRNA-21 as a biomarker for chemoresistance and clinical outcome following adjuvant therapy in resectable pancreatic cancer," *PLoS ONE*, vol. 5, no. 5, Article ID e10630, 2010.

21

Early Diagnosis of *Helicobacter pylori* Infection in Vietnamese Patients with Acute Peptic Ulcer Bleeding

Duc Trong Quach,[1,2] **Mai Ngoc Luu,**[1,2] **Toru Hiyama,**[3]
Thuy-HuongThi To,[4] **Quy Nhuan Bui,**[4] **Tuan Anh Tran,**[4] **Binh Duy Tran,**[4]
Minh-Cong Hong Vo,[2] **Shinji Tanaka,**[5] **and Naomi Uemura**[6]

[1]*Department of Internal Medicine, University of Medicine and Pharmacy, Ho Chi Minh, Vietnam*
[2]*Department of Gastroenterology, Gia Dinh People's Hospital, Ho Chi Minh City, Vietnam*
[3]*Health Service Center, Hiroshima University, Higashihiroshima, Japan*
[4]*Department of Endoscopy, Gia Dinh People's Hospital, Ho Chi Minh City, Vietnam*
[5]*Department of Endoscopy, Hiroshima University Hospital, Hiroshima, Japan*
[6]*Department of Gastroenterology and Hepatology, National Center for Global Health and Medicine, Ichikawa, Japan*

Correspondence should be addressed to Toru Hiyama; tohiyama@hiroshima-u.ac.jp

Academic Editor: Ford Bursey

Aims. To investigate *H. pylori* infection rate and evaluate a combined set of tests for *H. pylori* diagnosis in Vietnamese patients with acute peptic ulcer bleeding (PUD). *Methods.* Consecutive patients with acute PUB were enrolled prospectively. Rapid urease test (RUT) with 3 biopsies was carried out randomly. Patients without RUT or with negative RUT received urea breath test (UBT) and serological and urinary *H. pylori* antibody tests. *H. pylori* was considered positive if RUT or any noninvasive test was positive. Patients were divided into group A (RUT plus noninvasive tests) and group B (only noninvasive tests). *Results.* The overall *H. pylori* infection rate was 94.2% (161/171). Groups A and B had no differences in demographic characteristics, bleeding severity, endoscopic findings, and proton pump inhibitor use. *H. pylori*-positive rate in group A was significantly higher than that in group B (98.2% versus 86.7%, $p = 0.004$). The positive rate of RUT was similar at each biopsy site but significantly increased if RUT results from 2 or 3 sites were combined ($p < 0.05$). *Conclusions.* *H. pylori* infection rate in Vietnamese patients with acute PUB is high. RUT is an excellent test if at least 2 biopsies are taken.

1. Introduction

Helicobacter pylori (*H. pylori*) is one of the leading causes of peptic ulcer disease, which may lead to severe complications such as peptic ulcer bleeding (PUB) or perforation. Diagnosis and successful *H. pylori* eradication have been shown to prevent recurrent PUB [1, 2]. Recently, the importance of early diagnosis and eradication of *H. pylori* during admission period of patients with PUB has been further emphasized because the rate of recurrent PUB has been reduced with such strategy [3]. A recent study reported that up to 40% of PUB patients with *H. pylori* infection did not receive *H. pylori* eradication therapy and were lost to follow-up if diagnostic tests were performed after discharge [4]. Another study

showed that less than 50% of patients with PUB received *H. pylori* testing and less than 10% had any *H. pylori* testing after discharge [5].

The fact that many diagnostic tests for *H. pylori* are not so highly sensitive and have high false-negative value during acute bleeding period creates a clinical challenge [6–8]. As a consequence, the diagnosis of *H. pylori* infection during acute bleeding situations has been reported to be lower than the true number [9]. A combination of diagnostic tests may help to document more correctly the prevalence of *H. pylori* infection among patients with PUB. The rates of *H. pylori* infection among Vietnamese patients with upper gastrointestinal symptoms were reported of 55.5%–65.5% in previous studies [10, 11]. But there have been no studies on the prevalence of *H. pylori* in Vietnamese patients with acute PUB. The Maastricht IV consensus recommended that *H. pylori* eradication treatment should be started at reintroduction of oral feeding in cases of bleeding ulcer as delaying treatment after discharge leads to reduced compliance or loss to follow-up without receiving treatment [12]. In addition, validated IgG antibody can be used to diagnose *H. pylori* infection in patients with no prior history of *H. pylori* eradication. In clinical practice, therefore, only one positive test is enough to initiate *H. pylori* eradication therapy in patients with bleeding peptic ulcers. In this study, we imitate the real clinical scenario of peptic ulcer bleeding, when sometimes invasive diagnostic tests for *H. pylori* (rapid urease test, histology, and culture) could not be done. This study aimed to assess the prevalence of *H. pylori* infection and evaluate the role of a combined set of tests for *H. pylori* early diagnosis in Vietnamese patients with acute PUB. We did not assess the sensitivity and specificity of each diagnostic test, which has been very nicely reported in a previous meta-analysis [7], but try to identify the testing strategy which has the high possibility of early detecting *H. pylori* infection in this setting.

2. Methods

2.1. Patients. From August 2015 to April 2016, consecutive patients aged ≥ 18 years, hospitalized with acute upper gastrointestinal bleeding, and endoscopically diagnosed with gastric and/or duodenal ulcers at Gia Dinh People's Hospital, Ho Chi Minh, Vietnam, were recruited prospectively. Patients with prior history of gastrectomy were excluded. The study protocol was approved by the Ethics Committee of Gia Dinh People's Hospital.

2.2. Data Collection. Patients admitted with the presentation of upper gastrointestinal bleeding (hematemesis, melena, or hematochezia) were resuscitated and prepared for upper gastrointestinal endoscopy. During endoscopy, the presence of blood in the upper gastrointestinal tract and the recent stigmata of bleeding ulcers were recorded. Endoscopic intervention was performed if high-risk lesions (*i.e.*, spurting or oozing, visible vessels, or blood clot adhered to the ulcer base) were identified. When patients were stabilized after endoscopy, they were asked to fill out a questionnaire that included questions regarding demographic data, history of administration of nonsteroidal anti-inflammatory drugs (NSAIDs), proton pump inhibitors (PPIs), and antibiotics, peptic ulcer, and *H. pylori* eradication therapy. The hemodynamic instability at admission and preendoscopic PPI use were also recorded.

2.3. Helicobacter pylori Tests. *H. pylori* tests which were used in this study included rapid urease test (RUT), urea breath test (UBT), and serological and urinary *H. pylori* antibody tests. Patients without RUT or with negative RUT result then received noninvasive tests, which included UBT, and serological and urinary *H. pylori* antibody tests.

2.3.1. Rapid Urease Test. RUT (PyloriTek, Serim Research Corp., Elkhart, Ind., USA) was carried out randomly (2:1 basis). Three biopsy specimens were taken and tested separately from each patient: the midantrum in the greater curvature (site 1), the lower corpus (site 2), and the midcorpus (site 3) in the greater curvature. The results were read after 1 hour as recommended by the manufacturer and considered to be positive when blue spots appeared over at least one specimen to the same color level as that of the positive control and negative when color changes were absent.

2.3.2. Urea Breath Test. UBT was performed once patients were allowed to drink and eat again. It was done using a commercially available diagnostic method (Helicobacter Test INFAI, INFAI GmbH, Cologne, Germany), with ^{13}C labelled urea to detect urease activity, indicating the presence of *H. pylori* [13, 14].

2.3.3. Serological Helicobacter pylori Antibody Test. Qualitative serological detection of specialized human immunoglobulin G (IgG) antibodies to *H. pylori* was done with *Instant-View® H. pylori Rapid Test* (Alfa Scientific Designs Inc., Poway, CA, USA).

2.3.4. Urinary Helicobacter pylori Antibody Test. Urinary *H. pylori* antibody status was determined with a rapid urinary test (Rapirun® H. Pylori Antibody Stick, Otsuka Pharmaceutical Co., Ltd, Tokyo, Japan). The test measures human IgG antibody against *H. pylori* in urine using the principle of immunochromatography [10].

2.3.5. Definition of Helicobacter pylori-Positive. *H. pylori* infection was diagnosed when RUT was positive at any biopsy site or at least one other *H. pylori* test was positive.

2.4. Statistical Analysis. Baseline characteristics were presented as mean ± standard deviation (SD) for continuous variables and as a frequency (percentage) for all variables. The recruited patients were divided into 2 groups according to the tests that used for *H. pylori* infection diagnosis: group A (RUT plus noninvasive *H. pylori* tests) and group B (only noninvasive *H. pylori* tests).

The chi-square and two-tailed Fisher's exact test were performed to evaluate whether the demographic, clinical characteristics, endoscopic findings, and *H. pylori* infection rate were different between groups A and B. In addition, McNemar's test was used to assess the differences in *H. pylori* infection rates among different RUT biopsy sites.

3. Results

3.1. Patient Characteristics. During the study period, there were 177 consecutive patients with acute PUB admitted to Gia Dinh People's Hospital. Six patients with prior history of gastrectomy were excluded. The mean age of 171 patients recruited in the study was 55.4 ± 17.3. Forty-two (24.6%) patients had prior history of gastroduodenal ulcers, including

Early Diagnosis of Helicobacter pylori Infection in Vietnamese Patients with Acute Peptic Ulcer Bleeding...

171

TABLE 1: Demographics and clinical characteristics ($n = 171$).

Demographics and clinical characteristics	n (%)
Age (mean ± SD)	55.4 ± 17.3
Male	131 (76.6)
Medical use before admission	
NSAIDs	43 (25.1)
PPIs ≤ 2 weeks	28 (16.4)
Antibiotics ≤ 4 weeks	13 (7.6)
Prior history of peptic ulcers	42 (24.6)
Prior history of H. pylori eradication	12 (7.0)
Presenting symptoms	
Hematemesis	88 (51.5)
Melena	77 (45)
Hematochezia	6 (3.5)
Preendoscopic PPIs use	
High-dose, intravenous	133 (77.8)
Low-dose, intravenous	8 (4.6)
Oral	3 (1.8)
None	27 (15.8)
Hemodynamic instability at admission (heart rate > 100 beats per minute and/or systemic blood pressure < 100 mmHg)	47 (27.5)
Transfusion requirement	47 (27.5)

TABLE 2: Endoscopic setting and findings ($n = 171$).

Endoscopic setting and findings	n (%)
Timing	
<12 h	138 (80.7)
12–24 h	16 (9.4)
>24 h	17 (9.9)
Presence of blood in gastrointestinal tract	75 (43.9)
Location of ulcer	
Gastric	73 (42.7)
Duodenal	84 (49.1)
Gastric and duodenal	14 (8.2)
Endoscopic stigmata	
Spurting	1 (0.6)
Oozing	19 (11.1)
Visible vessel	25 (14.6)
Adherent clot	56 (32.7)
Red spot	17 (9.9)
Clean-based	53 (31.0)

six with perforated peptic ulcer managed by simple suture operation. Twelve (7.0%) patients had been diagnosed with *H. pylori* infection and received eradication therapy. Forty-three (25.1%) patients used NSAIDs before admission. The number of patients using PPIs within 2 weeks and antibiotics within 4 weeks before admission was 28 (16.4%) and 13 (7.6%), respectively. Preendoscopy high-dose proton pump inhibitors were prescribed in 133 (77.8%) patients. The detailed characteristics of patients in this study are presented in Table 1.

3.2. Endoscopic Setting and Findings. Upper gastrointestinal endoscopy was performed within 12 hours in 138 (80.7%), within 12–24 hours in 16 (9.4%), and within more than 24 hours after admission in 17 (9.9%) patients. Blood was present in the gastrointestinal tract in 75 (43.9%) patients. The proportions of gastric ulcer, duodenal ulcer, and gastroduodenal ulcer were 42.7%, 49.1%, and 8.2%, respectively. The high-risk stigmata of ulcer in this study included spurting/oozing (11.7%), visible vessel (14.6%), and adherent clot (32.7%) (Table 2).

3.3. Helicobacter pylori Tests. RUT was performed in 111 patients (group A) and not performed in 60 patients (group B). No patients in group A required intervention for bleeding related to gastric mucosal biopsy for RUT. There were 8 patients in group A and 4 patients in group B who had prior history of *H. pylori* eradication therapy.

All patients with *H. pylori* infection in group A were diagnosed by RUT. Additional testing with serological and urinary tests and UBT identified no additional *H. pylori* infected patients (Figure 1). Patients without RUT or with negative RUT result then received noninvasive tests including serological and urinary tests and UBT. In group A, RUT was positive in 98.2% (109/111) patients including 6 of the 8 who had prior history of *H. pylori* eradication therapy. Two patients with negative RUT (both had no prior history of *H. pylori* eradication therapy) were tested with serological and urinary tests and UBT, which were all negative. In group B, 56 (93.3%) patients without prior history of *H. pylori* eradication therapy were tested with serological and urinary tests and UBT, which showed 50 patients with *H. pylori* infection. Four (6.6%) patients had prior history of *H. pylori* eradication therapy, and 2 of them were *H. pylori*-positive. *H. pylori* infection rate in group A was significantly higher than that in group B (98.2% versus 86.7%, $p = 0.004$) while the other characteristics between the 2 groups were not significantly different (Table 3).

The detection rates of *H. pylori* infection by RUT with each single biopsy taken from site 1 (83.8%), site 2 (90.1%), and site 3 (85.6%) were not significantly different ($p = 0.284$) (Table 4). The detection rates by combined results from 2 biopsy sites: site 1 and site 2 (97.3%), site 1 and site 3 (94.6%), and site 2 and site 3 (95.5%) were also not different from each other but significantly increased when compared with each single biopsy site (Figure 2). The detection rate combined result from 3 biopsy sites was the highest, 98.2%.

4. Discussion

Accurately detecting *H. pylori* and subsequently eradicating the organism in infected patients with PUB are important to avoid recurrent bleeding. The recurrence rate has been reported in only 3% of the patients who received eradication

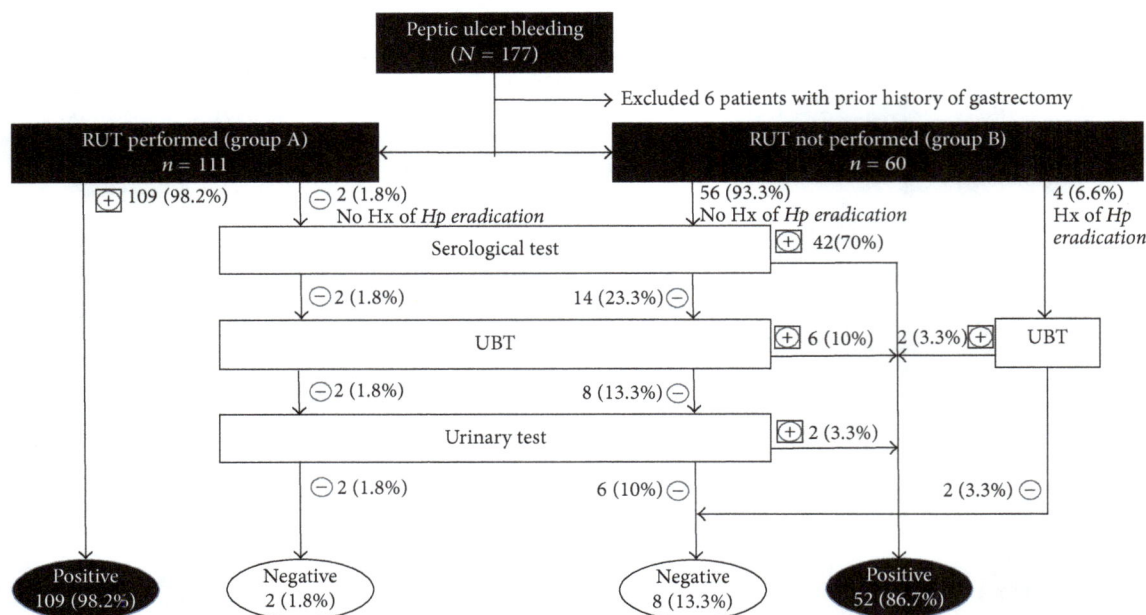

FIGURE 1: *H. pylori* testing in Vietnamese patients with acute peptic ulcer bleeding.

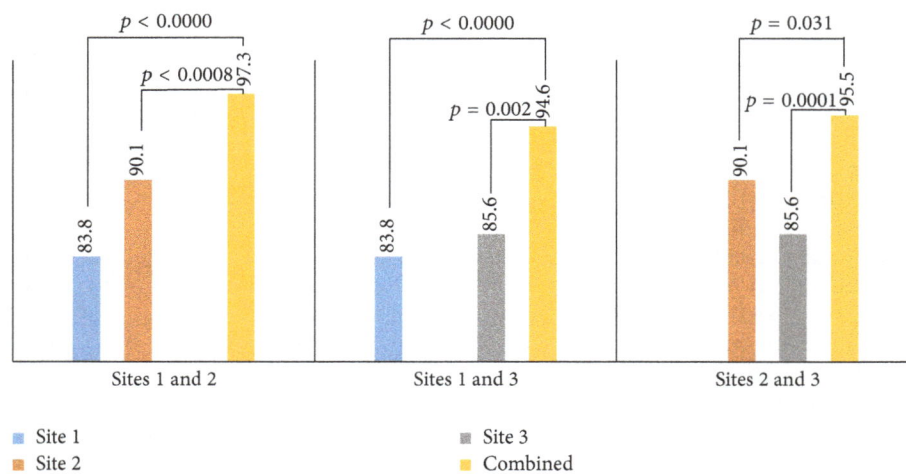

FIGURE 2: RUT results from single specimen versus combined specimens from two biopsy sites.

treatment but 20% in those treated with antisecretory non-eradicating therapy (without subsequent long-term maintenance antisecretory therapy) [15, 16]. The challenge is that many diagnostic tests including RUT, histology, and culture have been reported to have low sensitivity in patients with acute PUB [7]. In a metaregression analysis, the infection rate was significantly higher when diagnostic testing was delayed until at least 4 weeks following the bleeding event, suggesting that retesting *H. pylori* at a later time in PUB patients with initially negative test results was necessary [9]. However, late diagnosis of *H. pylori* infection in PUB patients leads to significant number of those with *H. pylori* infection who did not receive eradication therapy [4]. Therefore, increasing the sensitivity of tests for early diagnosis of *H. pylori* infection during admission period of PUB is crucial.

Regarding first-choice diagnostic tests for *H. pylori*, the American College of Gastroenterology recommended biopsy-based tests [17]. Among these, RUT is the most popular test in clinical practice but has high variable number of false-negative results according to a meta-analysis [7]. Sixteen studies included in this study showed a high degree of heterogeneity with sensitivities ranging between 0.41 and 0.94. When subanalysis of the biopsy sites for RUT was performed with only samples obtained from both the antrum and corpus which were considered, heterogeneity among sensitivities substantially decreased and pooled sensitivity increased. The results of our study help clarify this issue. The number and location of biopsy specimens are among key factors to increase RUT sensitivity. The detection rates of *H. pylori* infection by RUT with specimen taken from each

TABLE 3: The characteristics of patients in groups A and B.

Characteristics	Group A (n = 111) n (%)	Group B (n = 60) n (%)	p
Age (mean ± SD)	54.7 ± 17.6	56.1 ± 16.8	0.696
Male	84 (75.7)	47 (78.3)	0.695
Prior history of gastroduodenal ulcers	28 (25.2)	14 (23.3)	0.784
Prior history of H. pylori eradication	8 (7.2)	4 (6.7)	1.000
Medical use before admission			
NSAIDs	28 (25.2)	15 (25.0)	0.974
PPIs within 2 weeks	21 (18.9)	7 (11.7)	0.221
Antibiotics within 4 weeks	10 (9.0)	3 (5.0)	0.547
Hemodynamic instability at admission (heart rate > 100 beats per minute or systemic blood pressure < 100 mmHg)	29 (26.1)	18 (30.0)	0.219
Preendoscopic PPIs use			
High-dose, intravenous	89 (80.2)	44 (73.3)	
Low-dose, intravenous	6 (5.4)	2 (3.3)	0.136
Oral	3 (2.7)	0 (0)	
None	13 (11.7)	14 (23.3)	
Timing of endoscopy			
<12 h	84 (75.7)	54 (90.0)	
12–24 h	13 (11.7)	3 (5.0)	0.077
>24 h	14 (12.6)	3 (5.0)	
Presence of blood in endoscopy	52 (46.8)	23 (38.3)	0.284
Location of ulcer			
Gastric	49 (44.1)	24 (40.0)	
Duodenal	54 (48.6)	30 (50.0)	0.763
Gastric and duodenal	8 (7.2)	6 (10.0)	
Endoscopic stigmata			
Spurting	1 (0.9)	0 (0)	
Oozing	13 (11.7)	6 (10.0)	
Visible vessel	20 (18.0)	5 (8.3)	0.448
Adherent clot	33 (29.7)	23 (38.3)	
Red spot	12 (10.8)	5 (8.3)	
Clean-based	32 (28.8)	21 (35.0)	
H. pylori-positive rates	109 (98.2)	52 (86.7)	0.004

biopsy site in our study were not different, but significantly increased when specimens from 2 biopsy sites were combined (Table 4 and Figure 2). The combined result from 3 biopsy sites helps to detect even more patients with H. pylori infection, showing that negative RUT result from 2 biopsy sites is still not enough to exclude H. pylori infection and additional diagnostic tests or delaying diagnostic tests should be done.

Because some studies have found that all endoscopic-based diagnostic tests have a lower sensitivity in patients with acute PUB [7], it has been recommended that noninvasive methods should be used in patients who have negative result of endoscopic-based diagnostic tests [17]. Two patients in group A who had negative RUT result were performed serological test, UBT, and urinary test and had negative

results. Therefore, all patients with H. pylori infection in group A were diagnosed by RUT and the total infection rate in this group was 98.2%. As the specificity of RUT during PUB is very high [6, 7], this figure likely represents for the true prevalence of H. pylori in Vietnamese patients with PUB. This is truly first data on Vietnamese population so far. Previous studies in other populations showed a significant lower prevalence of H. pylori in PUB patients. In European studies, the prevalence of H. pylori in PUB patients was lower than that in patients with uncomplicated peptic ulcer disease, varying from 43% to 56%, and was explained by NSAIDs use [18]. In our study, the rate of NSAIDs use was 25.1%. In addition to this, a significant number of patients had prior history of NSAIDs use and were also infected with H. pylori. These 2 factors have been confirmed as independent risk

TABLE 4: RUT results with specimens taken from different biopsy sites.

Biopsy sites	H. pylori-positive cases n (%)
Single biopsy site	
1 (midantrum, greater curvature)	93 (83.8)
2 (low-corpus, greater curvature)	100 (90.1)
3 (midcorpus, greater curvature)	95 (85.6)
Two biopsy sites (combined results)	
1 & 2	108 (97.3)
1 & 3	105 (94.6)
2 & 3	106 (95.5)
Three biopsy sites (combined result)	
1, 2, and 3	109 (98.2)

factors for the development of peptic ulcer disease, associated bleeding, and the risk was significantly augmented when both factors presented [19]. Therefore, patients with PUB who have a single negative H. pylori test and a prior history of NSAIDs use should not be simply referred to as NSAIDs-induced PUB. Further diagnostic tests should be done to detect H. pylori infection.

The difference in infection rate of H. pylori between our study and other studies may be explained by many reasons, such as the different infection rate of H. pylori in each population, the differences in biopsy protocol for RUT, the endoscopy timing, and the types of RUT kit among studies. Many other studies used CLOtest® while we used PyloriTek® [6, 7]. Previous studies showed that results of the PyloriTek at 1 hour and CLOtest at 24 hours are comparable [20, 21], but there have been no direct comparison of the 2 kits in the setting of PUB patients, which is a research question of our future study.

Although biopsy-based tests for H. pylori are recommended as preferred diagnostic tests in PUB patients, they could not be performed in some situations because endoscopic treatment may have already made the procedure too long or patients were not hemodynamically stable during the procedure. In some developing countries, upper gastrointestinal endoscopy is performed under local anesthesia and patients' cooperation with prolonged procedure may be difficult. Therefore, noninvasive tests for H. pylori diagnosis are still required. According to a meta-analysis, H. pylori infection was accurately diagnosed by serological test in patients with PUB [7]. In our study, the test was the first choice among noninvasive diagnostic tests as it is widely available. In addition, UBT was used if serological test was negative. And urinary test was also used as it was locally validated in Vietnam with acceptable accuracy [10]. Although the specificity of this noninvasive approach is not as good as that of RUT in the setting of recent gastrointestinal bleeding [7], we try to combine this set of noninvasive tests in order to early detect all possibly H. pylori infection during admission time. But in spite of combining these three noninvasive tests, the total positive rate of H. pylori infection in group

B was still significantly lower than that in group A. As other characteristics between the 2 groups were not different (Table 3), this result clearly shows that RUT with at least 2 biopsy sites is an important test for H. pylori diagnosis in patients with PUD.

Our study has several weak points. First, number of patients included in this study was relatively limited. Studies with much more patients are needed to verify our results. Second, the definition of H. pylori-positive was based on only one diagnostic test. One false-positive finding may affect the diagnosis. And third, diagnostic tests for H. pylori infection such as histological, cultural, and fecal antigen tests were not included in the design of this study. If these tests were included in this study, the results might differ.

In conclusion, our study shows that the H. pylori infection rate in Vietnamese patients with acute PUB is high. RUT is an excellent test for detecting H. pylori infection in this setting if at least 2 specimens from different biopsy sites are taken. In case that RUT is not performed, late H. pylori retesting may be required even when a combined set of noninvasive tests have shown negative results.

Competing Interests

The authors declare that they have no competing interests.

Authors' Contributions

Dr. Naomi Uemura took responsibility for the integrity of the work as a whole, from inception to published article. Duc Trong Quach, Toru Hiyama, and Shinji Tanaka designed the research study. Duc Trong Quach, Mai Ngoc Luu, Thuy-HuongThi To, Quy Nhuan Bui, Binh Duy Tran, and Minh-Cong Hong Vo performed the research and collected data. Mai Ngoc Luu and Duc Trong Quach analysed the data. Duc Trong Quach, Toru Hiyama, and Naomi Uemura wrote the paper. All authors approved the final version of the manuscript.

Acknowledgments

The authors thank Drs. Phong Ha and Hung Le for their kindly advice to prepare the manuscript.

References

[1] J. P. Gisbert, X. Calvet, F. Feu et al., "Eradication of Helicobacter pylori for the prevention of peptic ulcer rebleeding," Helicobacter, vol. 12, no. 4, pp. 279–286, 2007.

[2] J. P. Gisbert, X. Calvet, A. Cosme et al., "Long-term follow-up of 1,000 patients cured of Helicobacter pylori infection following an episode of peptic ulcer bleeding," The American Journal of Gastroenterology, vol. 107, no. 8, pp. 1197–1204, 2012.

[3] S. S. Chang and H.-Y. Hu, "Helicobacter pylori eradication within 120 days is associated with decreased complicated recurrent peptic ulcers in peptic ulcer bleeding patients," Gut and Liver, vol. 9, no. 3, pp. 346–352, 2015.

[4] H. Yoon, D. H. Lee, E. S. Jang et al., "Optimal initiation of Helicobacter pylori eradication in patients with peptic ulcer

bleeding," *World Journal of Gastroenterology*, vol. 21, no. 8, pp. 2497–2503, 2015.

[5] J. J. Kim, J. S. Lee, S. Olafsson, and L. Laine, "Low adherence to helicobacter pylori testing in hospitalized patients with bleeding peptic ulcer disease," *Helicobacter*, vol. 19, no. 2, pp. 98–104, 2014.

[6] Y. J. Choi, N. Kim, J. Lim et al., "Accuracy of diagnostic tests for *Helicobacter pylori* in patients with peptic ulcer bleeding," *Helicobacter*, vol. 17, no. 2, pp. 77–85, 2012.

[7] J. P. Gisbert and V. Abraira, "Accuracy of Helicobacter pylori diagnostic tests in patients with bleeding peptic ulcer: a systematic review and meta-analysis," *American Journal of Gastroenterology*, vol. 101, no. 4, pp. 848–863, 2006.

[8] J.-H. Tang, N.-J. Liu, H.-T. Cheng et al., "Endoscopic diagnosis of Helicobacter pylori infection by rapid urease test in bleeding peptic ulcers: a prospective case-control study," *Journal of Clinical Gastroenterology*, vol. 43, no. 2, pp. 133–139, 2009.

[9] J. Sánchez-Delgado, E. Gené, D. Suárez et al., "Has H. pylori prevalence in bleeding peptic ulcer been underestimated? a meta-regression," *American Journal of Gastroenterology*, vol. 106, no. 3, pp. 398–405, 2011.

[10] D. T. Quach, T. Hiyama, F. Shimamoto et al., "Value of a new stick-type rapid urine test for the diagnosis of *Helicobacter pylori* infection in the Vietnamese population," *World Journal of Gastroenterology*, vol. 20, no. 17, pp. 5087–5091, 2014.

[11] T. L. Nguyen, T. Uchida, Y. Tsukamoto et al., "Helicobacter pylori infection and gastroduodenal diseases in Vietnam: a cross-sectional, hospital-based study," *BMC Gastroenterology*, vol. 10, article no. 114, 2010.

[12] P. Malfertheiner, F. Megraud, C. A. O'Morain et al., "Management of *Helicobacter pylori* infection—the Maastricht IV/Florence Consensus Report," *Gut*, vol. 61, no. 5, pp. 646–664, 2012.

[13] K. E. L. McColl, L. S. Murray, D. Gillen et al., "Randomised trial of endoscopy with testing for Helicobacter pylori compared with non-invasive H pylori testing alone in the management of dyspepsia," *British Medical Journal*, vol. 324, no. 7344, pp. 999–1002, 2002.

[14] H. Alberti, "Gastro-oesophageal reflux disease in general practice. Utility and acceptability of Infai C13-urea breath test has been shown," *British Medical Journal*, vol. 324, no. 7335, pp. 485–486, 2002.

[15] J. P. Gisbert, S. Khorrami, F. Carballo, X. Calvet, E. Gené, and J. E. Dominguez-Muñoz, "H. pylori eradication therapy vs. antisecretory non-eradication therapy (with or without long-term maintenance antisecretory therapy) for the prevention of recurrent bleeding from peptic ulcer," *The Cochrane Database of Systematic Reviews*, no. 2, Article ID CD004062, 2004.

[16] J. P. Gisbert, S. Khorrami, F. Carballo, X. Calvet, E. Gene, and E. Dominguez-Muñoz, "Meta-analysis: Helicobacter pylori eradication therapy vs. antisecretory non-eradication therapy for the prevention of recurrent bleeding from peptic ulcer," *Alimentary Pharmacology and Therapeutics*, vol. 19, no. 6, pp. 617–629, 2004.

[17] L. Laine and D. M. Jensen, "Management of patients with ulcer bleeding," *American Journal of Gastroenterology*, vol. 107, no. 3, pp. 345–360, 2012.

[18] M. E. van Leerdam, "Epidemiology of acute upper gastrointestinal bleeding," *Best Practice and Research: Clinical Gastroenterology*, vol. 22, no. 2, pp. 209–224, 2008.

[19] J.-Q. Huang, S. Sridhar, and R. H. Hunt, "Role of Helicobacter pylori infection and non-steroidal anti-inflammatory drugs in

peptic-ulcer disease: a meta-analysis," *The Lancet*, vol. 359, no. 9300, pp. 14–22, 2002.

[20] T. Puetz, N. Vakil, S. Phadnis, B. Dunn, and J. Robinson, "The Pyloritek test and the CLO test: accuracy and incremental cost analysis," *American Journal of Gastroenterology*, vol. 92, no. 2, pp. 254–257, 1997.

[21] Y. Elitsur, I. Hill, S. N. Lichtman, and A. J. Rosenberg, "Prospective comparison of rapid urease tests (PyloriTek, CLO test) for the diagnosis of Helicobacter pylori infection in symptomatic children: A Pediatric Multicenter Study," *American Journal of Gastroenterology*, vol. 93, no. 2, pp. 217–219, 1998.

22

Fatty Liver Index and Lipid Accumulation Product Can Predict Metabolic Syndrome in Subjects without Fatty Liver Disease

Yuan-Lung Cheng,[1,2] Yuan-Jen Wang,[2,3] Keng-Hsin Lan,[2,4,5] Teh-Ia Huo,[4,5] Yi-Hsiang Huang,[4,6] Chien-Wei Su,[2,4] Wei-Yao Hsieh,[4] Ming-Chih Hou,[2,4] Han-Chieh Lin,[2,4] Fa-Yauh Lee,[2,4] Jaw-Ching Wu,[6,7] and Shou-Dong Lee[2,8]

[1]Taipei Municipal Gan-Dau Hospital, Taipei, Taiwan
[2]Faculty of Medicine, School of Medicine, National Yang-Ming University, Taipei, Taiwan
[3]Healthcare Center, Taipei Veterans General Hospital, Taipei, Taiwan
[4]Division of Gastroenterology and Hepatology, Department of Medicine, Taipei Veterans General Hospital, Taipei, Taiwan
[5]Department and Institute of Pharmacology, National Yang-Ming University, Taipei, Taiwan
[6]Institute of Clinical Medicine, School of Medicine, National Yang-Ming University, Taipei, Taiwan
[7]Division of Translational Research, Department of Medical Research, Taipei Veterans General Hospital, Taipei, Taiwan
[8]Division of Gastroenterology, Department of Medicine, Cheng Hsin General Hospital, Taipei, Taiwan

Correspondence should be addressed to Chien-Wei Su; cwsu2@vghtpe.gov.tw

Academic Editor: Kazuhiko Uchiyama

Background. Fatty liver index (FLI) and lipid accumulation product (LAP) are indexes originally designed to assess the risk of fatty liver and cardiovascular disease, respectively. Both indexes have been proven to be reliable markers of subsequent metabolic syndrome; however, their ability to predict metabolic syndrome in subjects without fatty liver disease has not been clarified. *Methods*. We enrolled consecutive subjects who received health check-up services at Taipei Veterans General Hospital from 2002 to 2009. Fatty liver disease was diagnosed by abdominal ultrasonography. The ability of the FLI and LAP to predict metabolic syndrome was assessed by analyzing the area under the receiver operating characteristic (AUROC) curve. *Results*. Male sex was strongly associated with metabolic syndrome, and the LAP and FLI were better than other variables to predict metabolic syndrome among the 29,797 subjects. Both indexes were also better than other variables to detect metabolic syndrome in subjects without fatty liver disease (AUROC: 0.871 and 0.879, resp.), and the predictive power was greater among women. *Conclusion*. Metabolic syndrome increases the cardiovascular disease risk. The FLI and LAP could be used to recognize the syndrome in both subjects with and without fatty liver disease who require lifestyle modifications and counseling.

1. Introduction

Metabolic syndrome comprises risk factors of cardiovascular disease and type 2 diabetes mellitus (DM), including central obesity, dyslipidemia, and high blood pressure and fasting glucose [1]. Nonalcoholic fatty liver disease (NAFLD) used to be considered an incidental pathologic finding in type 2 DM and obesity but was found to be strongly associated with features of subsequent metabolic syndrome and was even included in the definition of metabolic syndrome [2, 3].

Using data from the general population of northern Italy, the fatty liver index (FLI), an algorithm based on triglyceride (TG) concentration, gamma-glutamyl transferase (GGT) level, body mass index (BMI), and waist circumference (WC), was developed to predict the risk of fatty liver disease in the general population [4]. The FLI has been validated by several studies and has been proven to have a strong association with hypertension and type 2 DM [5–9]. As cardiovascular disease, NAFLD, and metabolic syndrome are closely related, the FLI

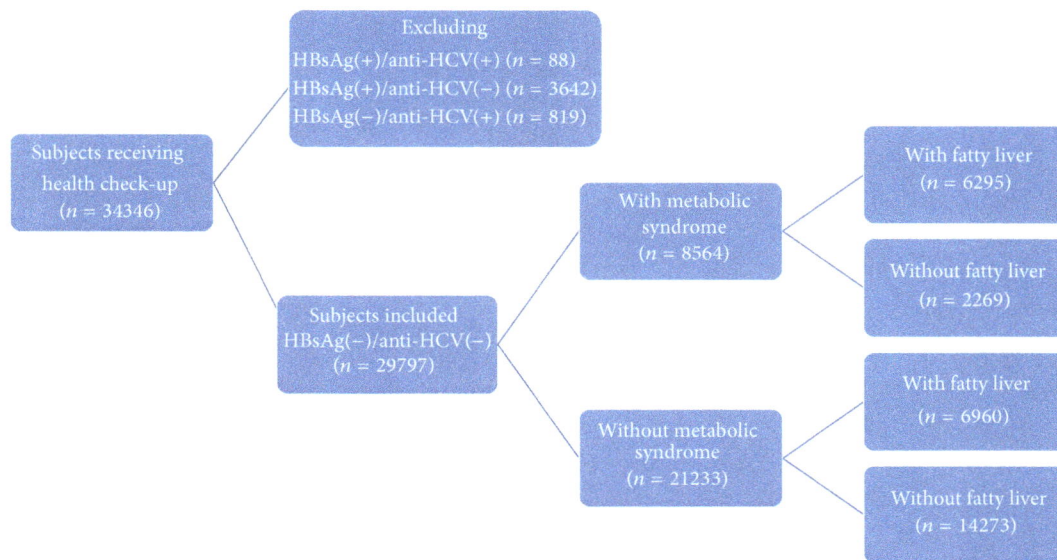

FIGURE 1: The algorithm for patient selection.

was also found to have a strong association with metabolic syndrome [10, 11].

The lipid accumulation product (LAP) is an index based on two components, WC and TG concentration, and was designed to indicate the risk of cardiovascular disease. As the LAP shares two of the five components of metabolic syndrome, it has been found to be a reliable tool to detect metabolic syndrome as well [12–14].

However, the ability of the FLI and LAP to predict metabolic syndrome in subjects without fatty liver disease, a group of people with cardiovascular risk as well, has not been clarified. Therefore, the present study aimed to determine the association between the two indexes and metabolic syndrome and to further explore their ability to predict metabolic syndrome in subjects without fatty liver disease in a large-scale cohort in Taiwan.

2. Materials and Methods

2.1. Study Population. In total, 34,346 subjects received health check-up services provided by internists in the Healthcare Center without hospitalization at the Taipei Veterans General Hospital from 2002 to 2009 [15–18]. Those with hepatitis B virus (HBV) infection, hepatitis C virus (HCV) infection, or HBV/HCV dual infections were excluded, and the remaining subjects were analyzed (Figure 1). All the subjects underwent complete clinical evaluations, laboratory examinations, and abdominal ultrasonography. The BMI was calculated as body weight (in kilograms) divided by the square of body height (in meters). Blood pressure (BP) was measured after the subjects had been seated for more than 5 minutes. The means of three consecutive readings were recorded as the systolic and diastolic BP with a difference in systolic BP < 10 mmHg. A diagnosis of metabolic syndrome was made when three of the following five abnormal findings were met according to the joint interim statement of the International Diabetes Federation Task Force on Epidemiology and Prevention [1]: elevated waist circumference (WC, men ≥ 90 cm or women ≥ 80 cm); TG ≥ 150 mg/dL; low high-density lipoprotein cholesterol (men < 40 mg/dL or women < 50 mg/dL); systolic BP ≥ 130 mmHg and/or diastolic BP ≥ 85 mmHg; and fasting glucose ≥ 100 mg/dL. Impaired fasting glucose (IFG) was defined as an elevated fasting plasma glucose concentration between 100 and 126 mg/dL [19]. Normal or lean subjects were defined as those with a BMI < 23 kg/m^2 and overweight and obese subjects were defined as those with a BMI ≥ 23 kg/m^2 [20]. Ultrasonography with Aloka SSD 4000 and 5000 and Philips HD15 was used to diagnose fatty liver disease according to the practice guideline of the American Gastroenterological Association [21]. The FLI was calculated using the following formula: FLI = (e 0.953 ∗ loge (TG) + 0.139 ∗ BMI + 0.718 ∗ loge (GGT) + 0.053 ∗ WC − 15.745)/(1 + e 0.953 ∗ loge (TG) + 0.139 ∗ BMI + 0.718 ∗ loge (GGT) + 0.053 ∗ WC − 15.745) ∗ 100 [4]. The LAP was calculated using the following formula: LAP = (waist circumference (cm) − 65) × triglycerides (mmol/L) for men and LAP = (waist circumference (cm) − 58) × triglycerides (mmol/L) for women [12].

This study followed the standards of the Declaration of Helsinki and was approved by the Institutional Review Board of Taipei Veterans General Hospital.

2.2. Biochemical and Serological Markers. Venous blood samples were collected after an overnight fast. Serum HBV surface antigen was tested by radioimmunoassay (Abbott Laboratories, North Chicago, IL, USA), and HCV antibodies were tested by a second-generation enzyme immunoassay. The serum biochemical markers were measured with a Roche/Hitachi Modular Analytics System (Roche Diagnostics GmbH, Mannheim, Germany).

TABLE 1: Characteristics of subjects with and without metabolic syndrome.

	All ($n = 29{,}797$)	With metabolic syndrome ($n = 8564$)	Without metabolic syndrome ($n = 21{,}233$)	P value
BMI, kg/m^2*	23.81 ± 3.58	26.23 ± 3.31	22.84 ± 3.21	<0.001
Age, years*	52.2 ± 13.3	56.3 ± 12.5	50.6 ± 13.2	<0.001
Sex (M/F) (%)	16,098/13,699 (54.0/46.0)	6525/2039 (76.2/23.8)	9573/11,660 (45.1/54.9)	<0.001
WC, cm*	83.8 ± 10.3	91.5 ± 8.4	80.7 ± 9.3	<0.001
SBP, mmHg*	124.3 ± 18.6	134.9 ± 17.2	120.0 ± 17.4	<0.001
DBP, mmHg*	77.5 ± 14.3	83.7 ± 17.5	75.0 ± 11.8	<0.001
Fasting glucose, mg/dL*	95.5 ± 24.8	110.4 ± 35.3	89.5 ± 15.3	<0.001
Cholesterol, mg/dL*	199.2 ± 37.0	203.1 ± 38.1	197.6 ± 36.5	<0.001
HDL, mg/dL*	53.7 ± 15.0	42.9 ± 10.12	58.0 ± 14.5	<0.001
LDL, mg/dL*	125.3 ± 32.9	129.0 ± 33.3	123.8 ± 32.6	<0.001
TG, mg/dL*	130.4 ± 88.1	201.3 ± 111.5	101.8 ± 55.1	<0.001
AST, IU/L*	23.1 ± 13.2	26.0 ± 18.2	21.9 ± 10.3	<0.001
ALT, IU/L*	27.0 ± 22.2	35.1 ± 29.1	23.8 ± 17.6	<0.001
GGT, IU/L*	24.8 ± 36.8	34.2 ± 50.9	21.0 ± 28.4	<0.001
Platelet, 1000/mm^3*	249.8 ± 60.3	247.5 ± 62.0	250.8 ± 59.6	<0.001
Fatty liver (yes/no) (%)	13,255/16,542 (44.5/55.5)	6295/2269 (73.5/26.5)	6960/14,273 (32.8/67.2)	<0.001
FLI	27.24 ± 24.18	50.22 ± 22.81	17.97 ± 17.65	<0.001
LAP	35.28 ± 33.59	64.22 ± 43.52	23.61 ± 18.57	<0.001

*Expressed as mean ± standard deviation.
BMI, body mass index; M, male; F, female; WC, waist circumference; SBP, systolic blood pressure; DBP, diastolic blood pressure; HDL, high-density lipoprotein; LDL, low-density lipoprotein; TG, triglyceride; AST, aspartate aminotransferase; ALT, alanine aminotransferase; GGT, gamma-glutamyl transferase; FLI, fatty liver index; LAP, lipid accumulation product.

2.3. Statistical Analysis. The study cohort was first divided by metabolic syndrome, and subjects without ultrasonographic fatty liver disease were selected for further analysis. Pearson's chi-squared test and Student's t-test were performed to compare categorical and continuous variables with two samples, respectively. Variables with statistical significance ($P < 0.05$) or proximate to it ($P < 0.1$) in univariate analysis were further included in the multivariate analysis using a logistic regression model with the forward stepwise selection procedure. The ability of serum markers to detect ultrasonographic fatty liver disease was examined using the area under the receiver operator characteristic (AUROC) curves. A P value less than 0.05 was considered to be statistically significant. All statistical analyses were performed using SPSS 17.0 for Windows (SPSS Inc., Chicago, IL, USA).

3. Results

3.1. Subject Characteristics Stratified by Metabolic Syndrome. The demographic data of all subjects are summarized in Table 1. The mean age of the population was 52.2 years and 54% was male. Metabolic syndrome was diagnosed in 28.7% of the population. Subjects with metabolic syndrome tended to be older in age, be male, have a higher BMI, serum total cholesterol, low-density lipoprotein cholesterol (LDL-c), alanine aminotransferase (ALT), aspartate aminotransferase (AST), GGT, and fatty liver prevalence, and have lower

platelet counts. The FLI averages of subjects with and without metabolic syndrome were 50.2 and 18.0, respectively, while the LAP averages in subjects with and without metabolic syndrome were 64.2 and 23.6, respectively.

We performed a correlation test between total cholesterol and LDL and between ALT and AST. The result showed that the correlation between the sets of data was very high ($r^2 = 0.841$ and 0.659, resp.). As the collinearity could affect the calculation of individual predictors even though the whole bundle of predictors could still predict the outcome well, we included only total cholesterol and ALT but not LDL and AST in the multivariate analysis to avoid the condition.

By multivariate analysis, ultrasonographic fatty liver disease and male sex were strongly associated with metabolic syndrome (odds ratio: 2.499 and 3.005, resp.), while higher BMI, older age, and higher ALT and GGT were also associated with metabolic syndrome (Table 2). After subjects were divided by ultrasonographic fatty liver disease, the presence of ultrasonographic fatty liver disease was strongly associated with metabolic syndrome as shown in Figure 2(a). We further stratified subjects by age and sex, and the result revealed that male subjects had higher prevalence of metabolic syndrome, and the prevalence of metabolic syndrome increased with age (Figure 2(b)).

3.2. Validation of the FLI and LAP for Identifying Metabolic Syndrome. The discriminative ability of the FLI and LAP to

TABLE 2: Factors associated with metabolic syndrome by multivariate analysis.

	Odds ratio	95% confidence interval	P value
All subjects			
BMI	1.272	1.258–1.285	<0.001
Age	1.041	1.038–1.043	<0.001
ALT	1.006	1.005–1.008	<0.001
GGT	1.005	1.004–1.006	<0.001
Platelet	1.002	1.001–1.002	<0.001
Fatty liver	2.499	2.339–2.670	<0.001
Male gender	3.005	2.811–3.214	<0.001
Females			
BMI	1.311	1.288–1.335	<0.001
Age	1.065	1.059–1.071	<0.001
ALT	1.007	1.004–1.009	<0.001
GGT	1.004	1.002–1.005	<0.001
Platelet	1.001	1.001–1.002	0.002
Fatty liver	3.275	2.888–3.714	<0.001
Males			
BMI	1.242	1.225–1.259	<0.001
Age	1.032	1.029–1.035	<0.001
ALT	1.006	1.004–1.008	<0.001
GGT	1.005	1.004–1.007	<0.001
Platelet	1.002	1.001–1.002	<0.001
Fatty liver	2.205	2.040–2.384	<0.001

BMI, body mass index; ALT, alanine aminotransferase; GGT, gamma-glutamyl transferase.

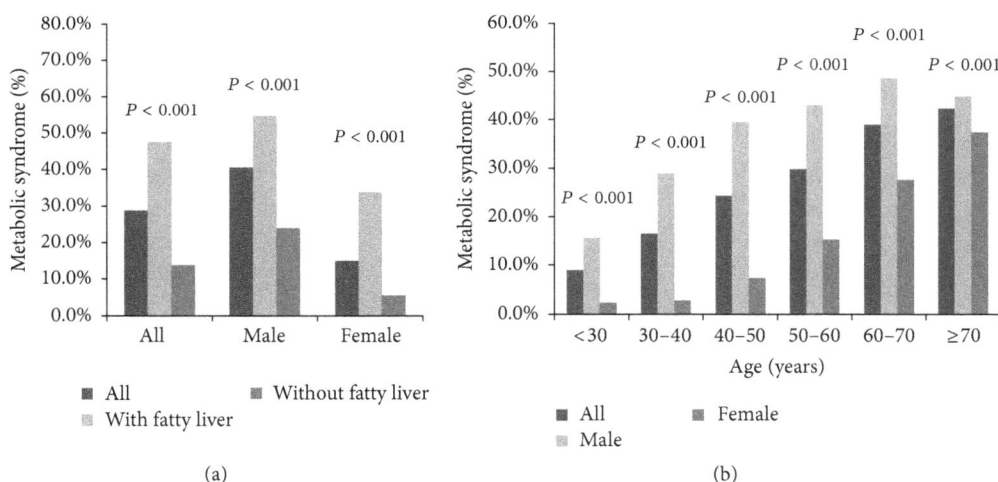

FIGURE 2: (a) The prevalence of metabolic syndrome divided by the status of fatty liver. (b) The prevalence of metabolic syndrome stratified by age and gender.

identify metabolic syndrome was determined by comparing their AUROC values. The AUROC curve values of the LAP and FLI for the prediction of metabolic syndrome were 0.884 and 0.875, respectively (Table 3). After the subjects were stratified by sex, the AUROC curve values of the LAP and FLI were 0.927 and 0.916, respectively, in women and 0.856 and 0.818, respectively, in men. These values were higher than those of other variables such as BMI, fasting glucose,

ALT, GGT, and TG to predict the presence of the metabolic syndrome.

3.3. Subject Characteristics Stratified by the IFG and Validation of the FLI and LAP for Identifying IFG. IFG was diagnosed in 21.8% of the population. Subjects with IFG had similar characteristics to those with metabolic syndrome. They tended to be older in age, be male, have a higher BMI, ALT, GGT, and

TABLE 3: Comparison of AUROC curve values among noninvasive markers for predicting metabolic syndrome.

	AUROC	95% confidence interval	Standard error	P value
All subjects				
LAP	0.884	0.893–0.901	0.002	<0.001
FLI	0.875	0.871–0.879	0.002	<0.001
TG	0.853	0.849–0.858	0.002	<0.001
HDL	0.820	0.815–0.825	0.003	<0.001
WC	0.817	0.812–0.821	0.002	<0.001
BMI	0.785	0.779–0.790	0.003	<0.001
Fasting glucose	0.775	0.769–0.781	0.003	<0.001
GGT	0.724	0.717–0.730	0.003	<0.001
Fatty liver	0.704	0.697–0.710	0.003	<0.001
ALT	0.691	0.684–0.698	0.003	<0.001
LDL	0.548	0.541–0.556	0.004	<0.001
Cholesterol	0.543	0.536–0.550	0.004	<0.001
Female subjects				
LAP	0.927	0.922–0.933	0.003	<0.001
FLI	0.916	0.910–0.922	0.003	<0.001
TG	0.874	0.866–0.882	0.004	<0.001
WC	0.853	0.845–0.862	0.004	<0.001
Fasting glucose	0.850	0.840–0.860	0.005	<0.001
BMI	0.833	0.824–0.842	0.005	<0.001
HDL	0.825	0.816–0.835	0.005	<0.001
Fatty liver	0.747	0.736–0.759	0.006	<0.001
GGT	0.733	0.721–0.744	0.006	<0.001
ALT	0.693	0.681–0.706	0.006	<0.001
LDL	0.591	0.577–0.604	0.007	<0.001
Cholesterol	0.575	0.562–0.589	0.007	<0.001
Male subjects				
LAP	0.856	0.850–0.862	0.003	<0.001
TG	0.825	0.818–0.831	0.003	<0.001
FLI	0.818	0.812–0.825	0.003	<0.001
HDL	0.780	0.773–0.788	0.004	<0.001
Fasting glucose	0.744	0.736–0.752	0.004	<0.001
WC	0.741	0.733–0.748	0.004	<0.001
BMI	0.723	0.716–0.731	0.004	<0.001
GGT	0.659	0.650–0.667	0.004	<0.001
ALT	0.634	0.625–0.643	0.004	<0.001
Fatty liver	0.658	0.650–0.667	0.004	<0.001
Cholesterol	0.542	0.533–0.551	0.005	<0.001
LDL	0.518	0.508–0.527	0.005	<0.001

AUROC, area under the receiver operating characteristic; LAP, lipid accumulation product; FLI, fatty liver index; TG, triglyceride; HDL, high-density lipoprotein; WC, waist circumference; BMI, body mass index; GGT, gamma-glutamyl transferase; ALT: alanine aminotransferase; LDL, low-density lipoprotein.

fatty liver prevalence, and have lower platelet counts. The FLI averages of subjects with and without IFG were 38.15 and 23.3, respectively, while the LAP averages were 46.51 and 30.69, respectively (Table 4). The discriminative ability of FLI and LAP to identify IFG was better in subjects without fatty liver disease (0.669 and 0.643, respectively) than in subjects with fatty liver disease. The FLI and LAP also predicted IFG in subjects with lower BMI (0.673 and 0.642, resp.) (Table 5).

3.4. Characteristics of Subjects without Ultrasonographic Fatty Liver Disease Stratified by Metabolic Syndrome. The demographics of subjects without ultrasonographic fatty liver disease are summarized in Table 6. The average age of the subjects was 50.9 years and 45% were male. Subjects with metabolic syndrome tended to be older in age, be male, have higher BMI, ALT, and GGT, and have lower platelet counts. The FLI and LAP were 37 and 47, respectively, in subjects with

TABLE 4: Characteristics of subjects with IFG.

	IFG (n = 5001)	Non-IFG (n = 22,970)	P value
BMI, kg/m²*	25.28 ± 3.48	23.34 ± 3.44	<0.001
Age, years*	57.7 ± 11.8	50.3 ± 13.1	<0.001
Sex (M/F) (%)	3036/1965 (60.7/39.3)	11,859/11,111 (51.6/48.4)	<0.001
WC, cm*	88.2 ± 9.4	82.3 ± 9.9	<0.001
SBP, mmHg*	131.8 ± 18.5	121.7 ± 17.8	<0.001
DBP, mmHg*	81.2 ± 15.5	76.4 ± 13.3	<0.001
Fasting glucose, mg/dL*	107.6 ± 6.8	87 ± 7.6	<0.001
Cholesterol, mg/dL*	203.8 ± 37.6	197.9 ± 36.5	<0.001
HDL, mg/dL*	50.4 ± 13.4	55 ± 15.3	<0.001
LDL, mg/dL*	129 ± 32.7	124.4 ± 32.7	<0.001
TG, mg/dL*	152.3 ± 90	120.9 ± 80.8	<0.001
AST, IU/L*	25.2 ± 19	22.3 ± 10.5	<0.001
ALT, IU/L*	31.6 ± 28.9	25.4 ± 19.2	<0.001
GGT, IU/L*	30.7 ± 51.4	22.4 ± 27.3	<0.001
Platelet, 1000/mm³*	245.3 ± 60.1	251.4 ± 59.9	<0.001
Fatty liver (yes/no) (%)	3150/1851 (63.0/37.0)	8737/14,233 (38.0/62.0)	<0.001
FLI	38.15 ± 25.02	23.3 ± 22.28	<0.001
LAP	46.51 ± 35.15	30.69 ± 29.6	<0.001

*Expressed as mean ± standard deviation.
IFG, impaired fasting glucose; BMI, body mass index; M, male; F, female; WC, waist circumference; SBP, systolic blood pressure; DBP, diastolic blood pressure; HDL, high-density lipoprotein; LDL, low-density lipoprotein; TG, triglyceride; AST, aspartate aminotransferase; ALT, alanine aminotransferase; GGT, gamma-glutamyl transferase; LAP, lipid accumulation product.

TABLE 5: Comparison of AUROC curve values among noninvasive markers for predicting IFG.

	AUROC	95% confidence interval	Standard error	P value
All				
FLI	0.689	0.004	0.682–0.697	<0.001
LAP	0.675	0.004	0.667–0.683	<0.001
With fatty liver				
FLI	0.609	0.006	0.598–0.62	<0.001
LAP	0.602	0.006	0.591–0.613	<0.001
Without fatty liver				
FLI	0.669	0.006	0.656–0.681	<0.001
LAP	0.643	0.007	0.629–0.656	<0.001
BMI (lean and normal)				
FLI	0.673	0.008	0.658–0.688	<0.001
LAP	0.642	0.008	0.626–0.659	<0.001
BMI (overweight and obesity)				
FLI	0.616	0.005	0.606–0.627	<0.001
LAP	0.605	0.005	0.595–0.615	<0.001

IFG, impaired fasting glucose; AUROC, area under the receiver operating characteristic; FLI, fatty liver index; LAP, lipid accumulation product; BMI, body mass index.

metabolic syndrome and 12 and 18, respectively, in subjects without metabolic syndrome. By multivariate analysis, older age, male sex, and higher BMI, ALT, and GGT were still associated with metabolic syndrome in subjects without fatty liver disease (Table 7). We further stratified subjects by age and sex, and the result revealed that male subjects had higher prevalence of metabolic syndrome, and the prevalence of metabolic syndrome increased with age (Figure 3).

TABLE 6: Characteristics of non-fatty liver subjects with and without metabolic syndrome.

	All (n = 16,542)	With metabolic syndrome (n = 2269)	Without metabolic syndrome (n = 14,273)	P value
BMI, kg/m^2*	22.32 ± 2.90	24.79 ± 2.72	21.93 ± 2.73	<0.001
Age, years*	50.9 ± 14.1	58.6 ± 13.8	49.6 ± 13.8	<0.001
Sex (M/F) (%)	7388/9154 (44.7/55.3)	1765/504 (77.8/22.2)	5623/8650 (39.4/60.6)	<0.001
WC, cm*	79.5 ± 8.9	88.4 ± 7.3	78.1 ± 8.4	<0.001
SBP, mmHg*	121.1 ± 18.5	136.0 ± 17.6	118.8 ± 17.6	<0.001
DBP, mmHg*	75.3 ± 11.6	82.6 ± 11.1	74.1 ± 11.3	<0.001
Fasting glucose, mg/dL*	90.7 ± 19.1	107.1 ± 32.7	88.1 ± 14.2	<0.001
Cholesterol, mg/dL*	194.5 ± 36.0	195.8 ± 37.7	194.3 ± 35.7	0.058
HDL, mg/dL*	58.2 ± 15.5	44.2 ± 11.4	60.4 ± 14.9	<0.001
LDL, mg/dL*	120.5 ± 31.7	124.2 ± 32.3	119.9 ± 31.6	<0.001
TG, mg/dL*	101.0 ± 57.2	168.0 ± 81.5	90.3 ± 43.7	<0.001
AST, IU/L*	21.1 ± 11.4	23.1 ± 23.9	20.8 ± 7.7	<0.001
ALT, IU/L*	21.2 ± 17.2	26.2 ± 33.2	20.4 ± 12.7	<0.001
GGT, IU/L*	20.0 ± 33.9	30.4 ± 66.9	18.3 ± 24.5	<0.001
Platelet, 1000/mm^3*	247.6 ± 60.9	238.7 ± 65.5	249.0 ± 60.0	<0.001
FLI	15.61 ± 16.27	36.99 ± 20.27	12.21 ± 12.54	<0.001
LAP	22.35 ± 18.81	47.10 ± 27.58	18.41 ± 13.27	<0.001

*Expressed as mean ± standard deviation.
BMI, body mass index; M, male; F, female; WC, waist circumference; SBP, systolic blood pressure; DBP, diastolic blood pressure; HDL, high-density lipoprotein; LDL, low-density lipoprotein; TG, triglyceride; AST, aspartate aminotransferase; ALT, alanine aminotransferase; GGT, gamma-glutamyl transferase; FLI, fatty liver index; LAP, lipid accumulation product.

TABLE 7: Risk factors of metabolic syndrome in subjects with non-fatty liver disease by multivariate analysis.

	Odds ratio	95% confidence interval	P value
All subjects			
BMI	1.371	1.346–1.397	<0.001
Age	1.042	1.038–1.046	<0.001
ALT	1.007	1.004–1.010	<0.001
GGT	1.004	1.002–1.006	<0.001
Platelet	1.001	1.001–1.002	0.001
Male gender	4.071	3.628–4.568	<0.001
Female subjects			
BMI	1.382	1.339–1.426	<0.001
Age	1.080	1.070–1.089	<0.001
ALT	1.010	1.005–1.015	<0.001
Platelet	1.002	1.000–1.003	0.028
Male subjects			
BMI	1.351	1.320–1.383	<0.001
Age	1.032	1.028–1.037	<0.001
ALT	1.005	1.001–1.009	0.021
GGT	1.005	1.003–1.007	<0.001
Platelet	1.002	1.001–1.003	0.002

BMI, body mass index; ALT, alanine aminotransferase; GGT, gamma-glutamyl transferase.

3.5. Validation of the FLI and LAP for Identifying Metabolic Syndrome in Subjects without Ultrasonographic Fatty Liver Disease. The predictive ability of FLI and LAP to identify metabolic syndrome was determined by comparing their AUROC curve values (Table 8). The AUROC curve values of the LAP and FLI to predict the presence of metabolic syndrome were 0.871 and 0.879, respectively. After the subjects were stratified by sex, the AUROC curve values of the LAP

TABLE 8: Comparison of AUROC curve values among non-fatty liver subjects with metabolic syndrome.

	AUROC	95% confidence interval	Standard error	P value
All subjects				
FLI	0.879	0.872–0.885	0.003	<0.001
LAP	0.871	0.863–0.879	0.004	<0.001
Triglyceride	0.828	0.818–0.838	0.005	<0.001
WC	0.827	0.819–0.835	0.004	<0.001
HDL	0.822	0.832–0.813	0.005	<0.001
BMI	0.783	0.774–0.792	0.005	<0.001
Fasting glucose	0.774	0.762–0.785	0.006	<0.001
GGT	0.693	0.682–0.704	0.006	<0.001
Age	0.679	0.667–0.691	0.006	<0.001
ALT	0.619	0.607–0.631	0.006	<0.001
LDL	0.543	0.531–0.556	0.006	<0.001
Cholesterol	0.513	0.501–0.526	0.007	0.04
Female subjects				
LAP	0.921	0.909–0.932	0.006	<0.001
FLI	0.909	0.898–0.921	0.006	<0.001
Triglyceride	0.860	0.842–0.878	0.009	<0.001
Fasting glucose	0.841	0.820–0.862	0.011	<0.001
WC	0.830	0.811–0.849	0.010	<0.001
HDL	0.822	0.841–0.803	0.010	<0.001
BMI	0.812	0.792–0.831	0.010	<0.001
Age	0.784	0.765–0.804	0.010	<0.001
GGT	0.673	0.650–0.697	0.012	<0.001
ALT	0.589	0.563–0.615	0.013	<0.001
LDL	0.574	0.548–0.600	0.013	<0.001
Cholesterol	0.547	0.520–0.574	0.014	<0.001
Male subjects				
LAP	0.844	0.834–0.855	0.005	<0.001
FLI	0.814	0.803–0.825	0.005	<0.001
Triglyceride	0.787	0.774–0.801	0.007	<0.001
HDL	0.772	0.786–0.759	0.007	<0.001
WC	0.757	0.745–0.768	0.006	<0.001
Fasting glucose	0.738	0.724–0.753	0.007	<0.001
BMI	0.723	0.711–0.736	0.006	<0.001
Age	0.615	0.601–0.630	0.007	<0.001
GGT	0.615	0.600–0.630	0.008	<0.001
ALT	0.559	0.544–0.575	0.008	<0.001
Cholesterol	0.517	0.502–0.533	0.008	0.029
LDL	0.514	0.499–0.529	0.008	0.074

AUROC, area under the receiver operating characteristic; FLI, fatty liver index; LAP, lipid accumulation product; TG, triglyceride; WC, waist circumference; HDL, high-density lipoprotein; BMI, body mass index; GGT, gamma-glutamyl transferase; ALT, alanine aminotransferase; LDL, low-density lipoprotein.

and FLI were 0.921 and 0.909, respectively, in women and 0.844 and 0.814, respectively, in men.

4. Discussion

The FLI and LAP are indexes originally designed to assess the risk of fatty liver and cardiovascular disease, respectively, and both have been shown to be good markers of metabolic

syndrome [4, 10, 12, 13]. In the present study, fatty liver disease was closely associated with metabolic syndrome, and both the FLI and LAP were predictive of metabolic syndrome. For people without fatty liver, both indexes were still strong predictors of metabolic syndrome.

Twenty-seven percent of the population aged more than 25 years in the US [22] and approximately 12% between 1999 and 2002 in Taiwan have been reported to have metabolic

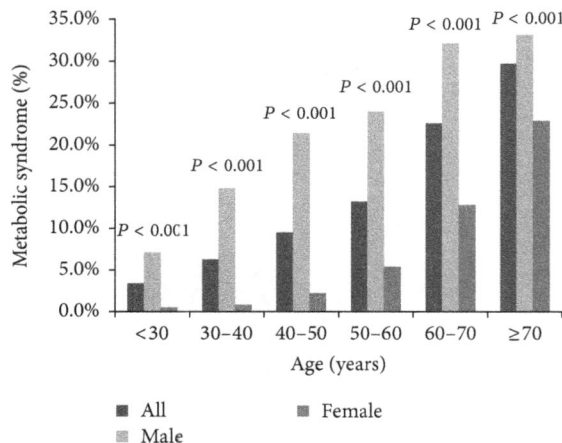

FIGURE 3: The prevalence of metabolic syndrome in subjects without sonographic fatty liver stratified by age and gender.

syndrome [23]. However, the prevalence of metabolic syndrome was much higher in the present study (28%), which may be because of the westernization of diet, greater awareness of the syndrome, or higher socioeconomic status of the subjects. It was noteworthy that the proportion of subjects with metabolic syndrome increased with age and the trend existed in both sexes (Figure 2(b)).

The prevalence of NAFLD, which varies by the diagnostic modality and ethnicity, ranges from 23% to 51% in Asian populations, and the prevalence of fatty liver disease in this study population falls within this range at 44.5% [24, 25]. Fatty liver disease was the strongest factor associated with metabolic syndrome in both sexes (Table 2 and Figure 2(a)). However, metabolic syndrome also exists in subjects without fatty liver disease, a group of subjects who have cardiovascular risk but is rarely focused on. Han et al. observed that 12% of subjects without ultrasonographic fatty liver disease at the end of the study developed metabolic syndrome in South Korea [26]. Up to 26.5% of subjects with mild or absent liver steatosis were also noted to have metabolic syndrome in Italy [27]. Metabolic syndrome can even occur in children without fatty liver disease. Schwimmer et al. defined the absence of NAFLD as the combination of a normal ALT level (<30 U/L) and the absence of hepatomegaly and found that metabolic syndrome exists in 15% of children with a mean age of 12.7 years without NAFLD [28]. After subjects with ultrasonographic fatty liver disease were excluded, the prevalence of metabolic syndrome in our study fell to 13.7%, similar to that in previous studies. Besides, an age-related increasing trend in the prevalence of metabolic syndrome was observed in both subjects with and without fatty liver disease (Figure 3).

Prediabetes has been recognized as a cardiometabolic risk factor and its phenotypes have been thoroughly assessed [29]. In this study, we investigated the role of the FLI and LAP to predict IFG after the subjects were stratified by the diagnosis of fatty liver disease and BMI. Interestingly, the results showed that the FLI and LAP had better predictive abilities for lean subjects and those without fatty liver than their counterparts. These findings suggest that the FLI and LAP

could help clinical physicians identify a high-risk group of cardiometabolic diseases in these two commonly overlooked populations.

Bedogni et al. developed the FLI as an accurate index which correlates well with ultrasonographic fatty liver disease. The FLI has limited utility for the quantification of hepatic steatosis [30–32], but it has been validated by abdominal ultrasonography in several populations with an AUROC curve between 0.930 and 0.840 in Western countries to identify fatty liver disease, though the accuracy is less prominent in Asian countries probably because of variation of ethnicity, dietary, and environmental factors [4, 33].

Furthermore, the FLI is associated with cardiovascular risk factors including hypertension and carotid plaques [9, 34] and can predict cardiovascular and liver-related mortality [35–37]. As cardiovascular disease, obesity, NAFLD, and metabolic syndrome are intertwined, Rogulj et al. suggested that the FLI may be an optimal diagnostic method for metabolic syndrome in terms of sensitivity and specificity [10]. Their findings were comparable with those of the present study in that the FLI was better than other variables to predict metabolic syndrome with an AUROC curve of 0.875. We further analyzed the performance of the FLI to identify metabolic syndrome in subjects without fatty liver disease. Our results showed that the FLI was a reliable tool to predict metabolic syndrome with an AUROC curve of 0.879. Accordingly, subjects without fatty liver disease and a high FLI may also need an intensified counselling plan.

The LAP, which includes TG concentration and WC, was first proposed by Kahn to recognize cardiovascular risk [14, 38]. The LAP was further noticed to have a strong association with insulin resistance [39, 40], glucose dysregulation [40, 41], and type 2 DM [42, 43] and was also associated with the stroke incidence in a 9.2-year prospective Chinese study [44]. Bedogni et al. concluded that the LAP can be a good marker of liver steatosis and the conclusion was validated in Korea although the accuracy is lower in the Asian population [12, 45]. Several studies found that the LAP could be a good indicator of metabolic syndrome with an AUROC curve greater than 0.9 [13, 46–48]. The present study revealed that the LAP was a useful tool to identify subjects with metabolic syndrome, which was comparable to the findings of previous studies. However, in our analysis, the LAP was found to be a better predictor of metabolic syndrome among women, which was different from the results of another Taiwanese study which found that the LAP was better to recognize metabolic syndrome among men [47]. The inclusion of people aged over 50 years and the small sample size may explain the difference in the results. Furthermore, we also found that the LAP could reliably identify metabolic syndrome (AUROC: 0.879) even in subjects without fatty liver, and the predictive power was better among women as well.

TG values already have a high power to predict metabolic syndrome. With the addition of the FLI and LAP, more people with risk of cardiovascular disease can be recognized. The awareness of the risk with further implementation of an intensive counselling plan will be of great importance to prevent cardiovascular disease.

The large sample size and detailed biochemistry data are the strengths of this study. However, there are several noteworthy limitations. First, the study population had a higher socioeconomic status and subjects could afford the expense of a physical check-up, so the results might not represent the general population. Second, alcohol consumption was not evaluated in the present study. However, the prevalence of alcoholism was surveyed to be 1.5% in Taiwanese communities [49], and the impact on our results should be small. Third, liver biopsy is the gold standard for the diagnosis of fatty liver disease. However, the invasiveness of that procedure is not justified for surveillance in the general population. The diagnosis of fatty liver disease was made by at least two of three abnormal findings on abdominal ultrasonography: diffusely increased echogenic liver as compared with the kidney or spleen, vascular blurring, and deep attenuation of the ultrasound signal with sensitivity of 89% and specificity of 93% [50, 51]. Fourth, we could not analyze impaired glucose tolerance, another important phenotype of cardiometabolic risk, because the oral glucose tolerance test was not performed in our cohort. Further studies are warranted to elucidate the correlation between the FLI/LAP and cardiometabolic risk.

In conclusion, metabolic syndrome increases risk of cardiovascular disease, and the FLI and LAP could be used to recognize the syndrome in people without fatty liver disease who also require lifestyle modifications and counseling in addition to their counterparts with fatty liver disease.

Competing Interests

The authors declare that there are no competing interests regarding the publication of this paper.

Acknowledgments

This study was supported by grants from the National Science Council (NSC 101-2314-B-075-014) and Taipei Veterans General Hospital (V102C-151).

References

[1] K. G. M. M. Alberti, R. H. Eckel, S. M. Grundy et al., "Harmonizing the metabolic syndrome: a joint interim statement of the international diabetes federation task force on epidemiology and prevention; national heart, lung, and blood institute; American heart association; world heart federation; international atherosclerosis society; and international association for the study of obesity," *Circulation*, vol. 120, no. 16, pp. 1640–1645, 2009.

[2] G. Musso, R. Gambino, S. Bo et al., "Should nonalcoholic fatty liver disease be included in the definition of metabolic syndrome? A cross-sectional comparison with Adult Treatment Panel III criteria in nonobese nondiabetic subjects," *Diabetes Care*, vol. 31, no. 3, pp. 562–568, 2008.

[3] P. Almeda-Valdes, D. Cuevas-Ramos, and C. A. Aguilar-Salinas, "Metabolic syndrome and non-alcoholic fatty liver disease," *Annals of Hepatology*, vol. 8, no. 1, pp. S18–S24, 2009.

[4] G. Bedogni, S. Bellentani, L. Miglioli et al., "The fatty liver index: a simple and accurate predictor of hepatic steatosis in the general population," *BMC Gastroenterology*, vol. 6, article no. 33, 2006.

[5] C. H. Jung, Y. M. Kang, J. E. Jang et al., "Fatty liver index is a risk determinant of incident type 2 diabetes in a metabolically healthy population with obesity," *Obesity*, vol. 24, no. 6, pp. 1373–1379, 2016.

[6] S. Jäger, S. Jacobs, J. Kröger et al., "Association between the fatty liver index and risk of type 2 diabetes in the EPIC-Potsdam study," *PLoS ONE*, vol. 10, no. 4, Article ID e0124749, 2015.

[7] C. H. Jung, W. J. Lee, J. Y. Hwang et al., "Assessment of the fatty liver index as an indicator of hepatic steatosis for predicting incident diabetes independently of insulin resistance in a Korean population," *Diabetic Medicine*, vol. 30, no. 4, pp. 428–435, 2013.

[8] L. Bozkurt, C. S. Göbl, A. Tura et al., "Fatty liver index predicts further metabolic deteriorations in women with previous gestational diabetes," *PLoS ONE*, vol. 7, no. 2, Article ID e32710, 2012.

[9] J. H. Huh, S. V. Ahn, S. B. Koh et al., "A prospective study of fatty liver index and incident hypertension: the KoGES-ARIRANG study," *PLoS ONE*, vol. 10, no. 11, Article ID e0143560, 2015.

[10] D. Rogulj, P. Konjevoda, M. Milić, M. Mladinić, and A.-M. Domijan, "Fatty liver index as an indicator of metabolic syndrome," *Clinical Biochemistry*, vol. 45, no. 1-2, pp. 68–71, 2012.

[11] E. Lerchbaum, H.-J. Gruber, V. Schwetz et al., "Fatty liver index in polycystic ovary syndrome," *European Journal of Endocrinology*, vol. 165, no. 6, pp. 935–943, 2011.

[12] G. Bedogni, H. S. Kahn, S. Bellentani, and C. Tiribelli, "A simple index of lipid overaccumulation is a good marker of liver steatosis," *BMC Gastroenterology*, vol. 10, article no. 98, 2010.

[13] M. J. Taverna, M. T. Martínez-Larrad, G. D. Frechtel, and M. Serrano-Ríos, "Lipid accumulation product: a powerful marker of metabolic syndrome in healthy population," *European Journal of Endocrinology*, vol. 164, no. 5, pp. 559–567, 2011.

[14] H. S. Kahn, "The 'lipid accumulation product' performs better than the body mass index for recognizing cardiovascular risk: a population-based comparison," *BMC Cardiovascular Disorders*, vol. 5, article 26, 2005.

[15] W.-C. Wu, C.-Y. Wu, Y.-J. Wang et al., "Updated thresholds for serum alanine aminotransferase level in a large-scale population study composed of 34 346 subjects," *Alimentary Pharmacology and Therapeutics*, vol. 36, no. 6, pp. 560–568, 2012.

[16] Y.-L. Cheng, Y.-J. Wang, W.-Y. Kao et al., "Inverse association between hepatitis B virus infection and fatty liver disease: a large-scale study in populations seeking for check-up," *PLoS ONE*, vol. 8, Article ID e72049, 2013.

[17] Y.-L. Cheng, Y.-C. Wang, K.-H. Lan et al., "Anti-hepatitis C virus seropositivity is not associated with metabolic syndrome irrespective of age, gender and fibrosis," *Annals of Hepatology*, vol. 14, no. 2, pp. 181–189, 2015.

[18] B.-L. Yang, W.-C. Wu, K.-C. Fang et al., "External validation of fatty liver index for identifying ultrasonographic fatty liver in a large-scale cross-sectional study in Taiwan," *PLoS ONE*, vol. 10, no. 3, Article ID e0120443, 2015.

[19] D. M. Nathan, M. B. Davidson, R. A. DeFronzo et al., "Impaired fasting glucose and impaired glucose tolerance: implications for care," *Diabetes Care*, vol. 30, no. 3, pp. 753–759, 2007.

[20] W. C. Hsu, M. R. G. Araneta, A. M. Kanaya, J. L. Chiang, and W. Fujimoto, "BMI cut points to identify at-Risk asian americans for type 2 diabetes screening," *Diabetes Care*, vol. 38, no. 1, pp. 150–158, 2015.

[21] N. Chalasani, Z. Younossi, J. E. Lavine et al., "The diagnosis and management of non-alcoholic fatty liver disease: practice guideline by the American Gastroenterological Association, American Association for the Study of Liver Diseases, and American College of Gastroenterology," *Gastroenterology*, vol. 142, no. 7, pp. 1592–1609, 2012.

[22] E. S. Ford, W. H. Giles, and A. H. Mokdad, "Increasing prevalence of the metabolic syndrome among U.S. adults," *Diabetes Care*, vol. 27, no. 10, pp. 2444–2449, 2004.

[23] C.-F. Jan, C.-J. Chen, Y.-H. Chiu et al., "A population-based study investigating the association between metabolic syndrome and hepatitis B/C infection (Keelung Community-based Integrated Screening study No. 10)," *International Journal of Obesity*, vol. 30, no. 5, pp. 794–799, 2006.

[24] J. Y. Lee, K. M. Kim, S. G. Lee et al., "Prevalence and risk factors of non-alcoholic fatty liver disease in potential living liver donors in Korea: a review of 589 consecutive liver biopsies in a single center," *Journal of Hepatology*, vol. 47, no. 2, pp. 239–244, 2007.

[25] X.-H. Hou, Y.-X. Zhu, H.-J. Lu et al., "Non-alcoholic fatty liver disease's prevalence and impact on alanine aminotransferase associated with metabolic syndrome in the Chinese," *Journal of Gastroenterology and Hepatology (Australia)*, vol. 26, no. 4, pp. 722–730, 2011.

[26] E. N. Han, E. S. Cheong, J. I. Lee, M. C. Kim, C. D. Byrne, and K. Sung, "Change in fatty liver status and 5-year risk of incident metabolic syndrome: A Retrospective Cohort Study," *Clinical Hypertension*, vol. 21, no. 1, 2015.

[27] F. Angelico, M. Del Ben, R. Conti et al., "Insulin resistance, the metabolic syndrome, and nonalcoholic fatty liver disease," *Journal of Clinical Endocrinology and Metabolism*, vol. 90, no. 3, pp. 1578–1582, 2005.

[28] J. B. Schwimmer, P. E. Pardee, J. E. Lavine, A. K. Blumkin, and S. Cook, "Cardiovascular risk factors and the metabolic syndrome in pediatric nonalcoholic fatty liver disease," *Circulation*, vol. 118, no. 3, pp. 277–283, 2008.

[29] C. Giraldez-Garcia, F. J. Sangros, A. Diaz-Redondo et al., "Cardiometabolic risk profiles in patients with impaired fasting glucose and/or hemoglobin A1c 5.7% to 6.4%: evidence for a gradient according to diagnostic criteria: the PREDAPS Study," *Medicine (Baltimore)*, vol. 94, no. 44, Article ID e1935, 2015.

[30] D. J. Cuthbertson, M. O. Weickert, D. Lythgoe et al., "External validation of the fatty liver index and lipid accumulation product indices, using ^{1}H-magnetic resonance spectroscopy, to identify hepatic steatosis in healthy controls and obese, insulin-resistant individuals," *European Journal of Endocrinology*, vol. 171, no. 5, pp. 561–569, 2014.

[31] L. Fedchuk, F. Nascimbeni, R. Pais, F. Charlotte, C. Housset, and V. Ratziu, "Performance and limitations of steatosis biomarkers in patients with nonalcoholic fatty liver disease," *Alimentary Pharmacology and Therapeutics*, vol. 40, no. 10, pp. 1209–1222, 2014.

[32] M. A. Borman, F. Ladak, P. Crotty et al., "The Fatty Liver Index has limited utility for the detection and quantification of hepatic steatosis in obese patients," *Hepatology International*, vol. 7, no. 2, pp. 592–599, 2013.

[33] E. Vanni and E. Bugianesi, "Editorial: utility and pitfalls of Fatty Liver Index in epidemiologic studies for the diagnosis of NAFLD," *Alimentary Pharmacology and Therapeutics*, vol. 41, no. 4, pp. 406–407, 2015.

[34] M. Kozakova, C. Palombo, M. P. Eng et al., "Fatty liver index, gamma-glutamyltransferase, and early carotid plaques," *Hepatology*, vol. 55, no. 5, pp. 1406–1415, 2012.

[35] C.-L. Cheung, K. S. L. Lam, I. C. K. Wong, and B. M. Y. Cheung, "Non-invasive score identifies ultrasonography-diagnosed non-alcoholic fatty liver disease and predicts mortality in the USA," *BMC medicine*, vol. 12, p. 154, 2014.

[36] E. Lerchbaum, S. Pilz, T. B. Grammer et al., "The fatty liver index is associated with increased mortality in subjects referred to coronary angiography," *Nutrition, Metabolism and Cardiovascular Diseases*, vol. 23, no. 12, pp. 1231–1238, 2013.

[37] G. Calori, G. Lattuada, F. Ragogna et al., "Fatty liver index and mortality: the cremona study in the 15th year of follow-up," *Hepatology*, vol. 54, no. 1, pp. 145–152, 2011.

[38] I. Wakabayashi and T. Daimon, "A strong association between lipid accumulation product and diabetes mellitus in Japanese women and men," *Journal of Atherosclerosis and Thrombosis*, vol. 21, no. 3, pp. 282–288, 2014.

[39] C. Xia, R. Li, S. Zhang et al., "Lipid accumulation product is a powerful index for recognizing insulin resistance in non-diabetic individuals," *European Journal of Clinical Nutrition*, vol. 66, no. 9, pp. 1035–1038, 2012.

[40] D. Brisson, P. Perron, H. S. Kahn, D. Gaudet, and L. Bouchard, "The lipid accumulation product for the early prediction of gestational insulin resistance and glucose dysregulation," *Journal of Women's Health*, vol. 22, no. 4, pp. 362–367, 2013.

[41] J.-Y. Oh, Y.-A. Sung, and H. J. Lee, "The lipid accumulation product as a useful index for identifying abnormal glucose regulation in young Korean women," *Diabetic Medicine*, vol. 30, no. 4, pp. 436–442, 2013.

[42] H. S. Kahn, "The lipid accumulation product is better than BMI for identifying diabetes: a population-based comparison," *Diabetes Care*, vol. 29, no. 1, pp. 151–153, 2006.

[43] M. Bozorgmanesh, F. Hadaegh, and F. Azizi, "Diabetes prediction, Lipid accumulation product, and adiposity measures; 6-year follow-up: Tehran Lipid and Glucose Study," *Lipids in Health and Disease*, vol. 9, article no. 45, 2010.

[44] C. Zhong, W. Xia, X. Zhong et al., "Lipid accumulation product and hypertension related to stroke: a 9.2-year prospective study among Mongolians in China," *Journal of Atherosclerosis and Thrombosis*, vol. 23, no. 7, pp. 830–838, 2016.

[45] J. H. Kim, S. Y. Kwon, S. W. Lee, and C. H. Lee, "Validation of fatty liver index and lipid accumulation product for predicting fatty liver in Korean population," *Liver International*, vol. 31, no. 10, pp. 1600–1601, 2011.

[46] M. L. Tellechea, F. Aranguren, M. T. Martínez-Larrad, M. Serrano-Ríos, M. J. Taverna, and G. D. Frechtel, "Ability of lipid accumulation product to identify metabolic syndrome in healthy men from Buenos Aires," *Diabetes Care*, vol. 32, article no. e85, 2009.

[47] J.-K. Chiang and M. Koo, "Lipid accumulation product: a simple and accurate index for predicting metabolic syndrome in Taiwanese people aged 50 and over," *BMC Cardiovascular Disorders*, vol. 12, article 78, 2012.

[48] N. Motamed, S. Razmjou, G. Hemmasi, M. Maadi, and F. Zamani, "Lipid accumulation product and metabolic syndrome: a population-based study in northern Iran, Amol," *Journal of Endocrinological Investigation*, vol. 39, no. 4, pp. 375–382, 2016.

[49] M.-C. Huang and C.-C. Chen, "Alcohol dependence in Taiwan: from epidemiology to biomedicine," *Journal of Experimental & Clinical Medicine*, vol. 4, no. 2, pp. 108–112, 2012.

[50] A. E. A. Joseph, S. H. Saverymuttu, S. Al-Sam, M. G. Cook, and J. D. Maxwell, "Comparison of liver histology with ultrasonography in assessing diffuse parenchymal liver disease," *Clinical Radiology*, vol. 43, no. 1, pp. 26–31, 1991.

[51] R. Haring, H. Wallaschofski, M. Nauck, M. Dörr, S. E. Baumeister, and H. Völzke, "Ultrasonographic hepatic steatosis increases prediction of mortality risk from elevated serum gamma-glutamyl transpeptidase levels," *Hepatology*, vol. 50, no. 5, pp. 1403–1411, 2009.

23

Impact of Pressurized Intraperitoneal Aerosol Chemotherapy on Quality of Life and Symptoms in Patients with Peritoneal Carcinomatosis: A Retrospective Cohort Study

Hugo Teixeira Farinha,[1] Fabian Grass,[1] Amaniel Kefleyesus,[1] Chahin Achtari,[2] Benoit Romain,[1,3] Michael Montemurro,[4] Nicolas Demartines,[1] and Martin Hübner[1]

[1]Department of Visceral Surgery, University Hospital of Lausanne (CHUV), Lausanne, Switzerland
[2]Department of Gynecology, University Hospital of Lausanne (CHUV), Lausanne, Switzerland
[3]Department of Digestive Surgery, Strasbourg University, Strasbourg, France
[4]Department of Oncology, University Hospital of Lausanne (CHUV), Lausanne, Switzerland

Correspondence should be addressed to Nicolas Demartines; demartines@chuv.ch

Academic Editor: Guoxiang Cai

Background. Peritoneal cancer treatment aims to prolong survival, but preserving Quality of Life (QoL) under treatment is also a priority. Pressurized Intraperitoneal Aerosol Chemotherapy (PIPAC) is a novel minimally invasive repeatable treatment modality. The aim of the present study was to assess QoL in our cohort of PIPAC patients. *Methods.* Analysis of all consecutive patients included from the start of PIPAC program (January 2015). QoL (0–100: optimal) and symptoms (no symptom: 0–100) were measured prospectively before and after every PIPAC procedure using EORTC QLQ-C30. *Results.* Forty-two patients (M : F = 8 : 34, median age 66 (59–73) years) had 91 PIPAC procedures in total (1 : 4x, 17 : 3x, 12 : 2x, and 12 : 1x). Before first PIPAC, baseline QoL was measured as median of 66 ± 2.64. Prominent complaints were fatigue (32 ± 4.3) and digestive symptoms as diarrhea (17 ± 3.75), constipation (17 ± 4.13), and nausea (7 ± 2.54). Overall Quality of Life was 64 ± 3.75 after PIPAC#1 ($p = 0.57$), 61 ± 4.76 after PIPAC#2 ($p = 0.89$), and 70 ± 6.67 after PIPAC#3 ($p = 0.58$). Fatigue symptom score was 44 ± 4.86 after PIPAC#1 and 47 ± 6.69 and 34 ± 7.85 after second and third applications, respectively ($p = 0.40$). Diarrhea ($p = 0.31$), constipation ($p = 0.76$), and nausea ($p = 0.66$) did not change significantly under PIPAC treatment. *Conclusion.* PIPAC treatment of peritoneal carcinomatosis had no negative impact on patients' overall QoL and its components or on main symptoms. This study was registered online on Research Registry (UIN: 1608).

1. Introduction

Requirements for optimal oncological treatment include oncological efficacy (tumor response, survival) but also low toxicity, few side effects, and no negative impact on Quality of Life (QoL). Peritoneal carcinomatosis (PC) remains a particular challenge with sparse treatment options but high potential for side effects and complications [1, 2].

The effect of systemic chemotherapy remains limited on the peritoneum due to low penetration and relative resistance of peritoneal nodules. Combining several active agents has increased efficacy but was also associated with considerable risk for side effects with negative impact on QoL [3]. Hyperthermic Intraperitoneal Chemotherapy (HIPEC) overcomes some of the pharmacokinetic limitations and improves survival in selected patients [4, 5] at the price of high morbimortality and a negative impact on QoL for months after the procedure [6].

Intraperitoneal Aerosol Chemotherapy (PIPAC) was developed to disperse the active agents inside the peritoneal cavity by laparoscopy without tumor debulking, thus allowing for repeated treatments [7–9]. The few available studies

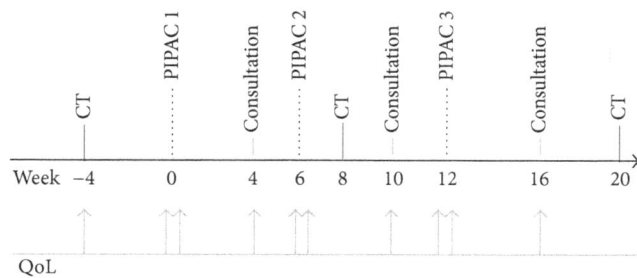

FIGURE 1: Treatment algorithm for Pressurized Intraperitoneal Aerosol Chemotherapy (PIPAC). PIPAC treatment was scheduled as repeated application (3x) at 6-week intervals. Thoracoabdominal computed tomography (CT) was performed 4 weeks prior to PIPAC#1, between PIPAC#2 and PIPAC#3, and after the completion of intraperitoneal treatment to search for extraperitoneal disease. Quality of Life (QoL) was systematically assessed (EORTC QLQ-C30) during every patient encounter: in outpatient consultation, before surgery, and at discharge.

reported encouraging objective tumor response of 50–86% and only little toxicity in patients with therapy-refractory PC of various origins [10–12]. Only one study reported on QoL under PIPAC treatment so far [13].

The present analysis was performed to evaluate QoL and symptoms under PIPAC treatment in a consecutive cohort of patients with PC.

2. Methods

This study included all consecutive patients treated by PIPAC from January 2015 until April 2016. All patients were discussed in the setting of a multidisciplinary tumor board to determine the best treatment option for each patient. PIPAC was considered only in patients with chemoresistant isolated peritoneal carcinomatosis who were not eligible for cytoreductive surgery (CRS) and Hyperthermic Intraperitoneal Chemotherapy (HIPEC) due to medical or surgical contraindications. The study was approved by the Institutional Review Board (Number 2016-00274) and all patients provided written consent prior to surgery. STROBE criteria (http://strobe-statement.org/) were followed for reporting of the study (http://www.researchregistry.com/; UIN: 1608).

2.1. PIPAC Procedure and Treatment Algorithm.
Surgical setup, treatment regimens, and safety checklist were adopted from recommendations by Solaß et al. [9, 17]. Three PIPAC treatments were scheduled at 6-week intervals upon decision of the multidisciplinary tumor board (Figure 1). Systematically, thoracoabdominal computed tomography (CT) was performed not exceeding four weeks prior to first PIPAC and between PIPAC#2 and PIPAC#3 to actively rule out extraperitoneal disease. A third CT was scheduled 2 months after the completed 3 PIPAC cycles. Every patient was seen in outpatient consultation 4 weeks after PIPAC treatment for monitoring of complications and evaluation of contraindications to proceed with further PIPAC. QoL assessment was

performed before surgery, at discharge, and every time when the patient was seen in outpatient consultation (Figure 1).

2.2. Assessment of Quality of Life and Symptoms.
European Organization for Research and Treatment of Cancer (EORTC) generic questionnaire QLQ-C30 (version 3.0) was used to measure QoL and symptoms [14, 18]. QLQ-C30 is a 30-question self-administered questionnaire inquiring about global health status, 9 individual symptoms, and 5 functional scales. Validated versions were provided in French, English, Italian, and German. The EORTC QLQ-C30 scoring manual was followed in terms of scoring QoL data and with regard to missing answers [19]. For statistical analysis, the 30 scores were linearly converted to a 0–100 scale according to EORTC recommendations [19]. Of note, high functional scores indicate a high level of function (optimum: 100), while high symptom scores represented high degree of symptoms (optimum: 0). A mean difference of ±5 was considered to be of no clinical relevance for the patient, while ±5–10 and ±10–20 points represented small and modest clinical differences, respectively [15].

2.3. Data Management.
Pertinent demographic and surgical data was prospectively recorded in coded form in a computerized data base (secuTrial®, IAS GmbH, Berlin). Performance status was assessed according to the Eastern Cooperative Oncology Group (ECOG) [20]. Intraoperative data included peritoneal cancer index (PCI) [16], ascites (mL), adhesiolysis, and operative time (min). Postoperative hospital stay and 30-day complications (Clavien classification [21]) were reported.

2.4. Predefined Subgroup Analyses.
Overall QoL under PIPAC treatment was compared between patients with PC of gynecological versus digestive origin to detect potential differences between those different patient groups and entities.

Reaction to treatment and side effects might be different after first application as compared with consecutive administration. Further, cumulative toxicity might decrease tolerance to repeated application. Therefore, QoL and symptoms were analyzed separately for PIPAC#1 as compared to repeated PIPAC procedures.

A possible direct relationship was assessed between higher intraperitoneal tumor load (measured by PCI) and preoperative QoL. And finally, the hypothesis has tested whether low baseline QoL was correlated with longer hospital stay after PIPAC treatment.

2.5. Statistical Analysis and Interpretation.
Continuous variables were presented as mean with standard error of the mean (SEM) or median with range or interquartile range (IQR) as appropriate. Student's t-test and Mann–Whitney U test were used for statistical comparisons depending on the distribution. Categorical variables were reported as frequencies (%) and compared with chi-square test. Statistical correlations were tested by use of Spearman's rank correlation. A p value < 0.05 was considered to be statistically significant in all tests. Statistical analyses were performed and figures were produced with SPSS v20 statistical software (Chicago, IL,

TABLE 1: Baseline demographics and surgical details of patients treated with Pressurized Intraperitoneal Aerosol Chemotherapy (PIPAC).

		All patients (n = 42)	GYN (n = 21)	Digestive (n = 21)	p value
Demographics	Median age (years)	66 (59–73)	67 (63–74)	62 (55–72)	0.193
	Gender (male)	8 (19%)	—	8	—
	Median BMI (kg/m^2)	22.5 (20–25)	23 (21–28)	22 (19–25)	**0.116**
	BMI < 18.5 kg/m^2	2 (5%)	0	2	—
	ECOG (0-1)	36 (86%)	20 (95%)	76 (90%)	0.077
		All PIPAC (n = 91)	GYN (n = 51)	Digestive (n = 40)	p value
Intra-OP findings	PCI	10 (5–17)	9 (4–14)	15 (7–19)	**0.002**
	Ascites (mL)	50 (0–4000)	0 (0–300)	50 (0–4000)	**0.034**
	Adhesions	15 (16%)	9 (18%)	6 (15%)	0.735
	Operation time (min)	94 (89–108)	91 (87–97)	100 (92–117)	**0.002**

Median (IQR) or number of (%) as appropriate. Statistical significance ($p < 0.05$) is highlighted in bold.
BMI: Body Mass Index; ECOG: Eastern Cooperative Oncology Group performance status [20]; PCI: Peritoneal Cancer Index [16].

USA) and GraphPad Prism 7 (GraphPad Software, Inc., La Jolla, CA, USA).

3. Results

Forty-two consecutive patients were included in the present analysis as detailed in Table 1. Indication was carcinomatosis of gynecological origin in 21 patients. The digestive group included 14 patients with PC of colorectal and 3 of gastric origin (1 each for small bowel, appendicular, pseudomyxoma, and mesothelioma). One out of forty-two patients (2%) had combined systemic chemotherapy. Overall, 91 PIPAC procedures were performed in 42 patients (18 : ≥3, 12 : 2, and 12 : 1). Overall complication rate was 8.8% and median hospital stay was 3 (range 1–20).

3.1. Quality of Life and Symptoms during PIPAC Treatment. Overall QoL score was 66 ± 2.6 at baseline before the start of PIPAC treatment. QoL scores during the treatments cycles are displayed in Figure 2(a). QoL was not significantly different before and after PIPAC#1, PIPAC#2, and PIPAC#3, respectively, and the threshold for small or moderate clinically relevant difference was not reached at any time point (Figure 2(b)). Similarly, no significant changes were noted under PIPAC treatment for the QoL components *cognitive, physical, emotional, role,* and *social functioning*; individual curves are provided as in Figure 3.

Overall QoL was separately analyzed in gynecological and digestive patients (Figure 4). The latter group tended to have lower scores throughout the treatment course with significant differences after PIPAC#1 (discharge: $p = 0.03$; 4 weeks: $p = 0.02$) and after PIPAC#2 (discharge: $p = 0.01$).

Prominent complaints at baseline were fatigue (32 ± 4.3) and the digestive symptoms diarrhea (17 ± 3.4), constipation (17 ± 4.1), and nausea (7 ± 2.5). Digestive symptoms before and after PIPAC are detailed for 1st, 2nd, and 3rd applications. *Nausea/vomiting* increased transitorily after PIPAC#1 ($p = 0.03$), just reaching the defined threshold for a small clinically relevant difference; no significant increase was present after PIPAC#2 and PIPAC#3, respectively (Figure 5(a)). For the

symptoms *appetite loss, constipation,* and *diarrhea,* nonsignificant variation was noted in both directions (Figures 5(b), 5(c), and 5(d)). Nondigestive symptoms *insomnia, fatigue, pain,* and *dyspnea* did not show significant changes throughout PIPAC treatment (Figure 6).

3.2. QoL and Symptoms after First and Repeated PIPAC. Change of overall QoL (Δ before − after) was small and nonsignificant for both 1st and repeated PIPAC procedures ($p = 0.388$) as shown in Figure 7. Performing similar analyses for digestive symptoms, there was a significantly higher symptom score for constipation after PIPAC#1 as compared to repeated PIPAC ($p = 0.030$), while no difference was measured with regard to nausea/vomiting, appetite loss, and diarrhea (Figures 8(a), 8(b), 8(c), and 8(d)).

3.3. Correlation between QoL, Tumor Load, and Hospital Stay (Figure 9). There was no statistical correlation measured between intraperitoneal tumor load (PCI) and preoperative overall QoL ($\rho = -0.169$, $p = 0.122$). Higher preoperative QoL score was associated with shorter postoperative LoS (days) ($\rho = -0.213$, $p = 0.05$).

4. Discussion

PIPAC had no negative impact on patients' overall QoL and its components or on main symptoms. First and repetitive PIPAC application was equally well tolerated. Baseline QoL was good in patients with peritoneal disease and independent of intraperitoneal tumor load.

Overall QoL at baseline before start of PIPAC treatment was surprisingly high in the present cohort of patients with peritoneal carcinomatosis. As comparison, a control group of 16,151 healthy citizens had a significantly higher QoL score than this cohort (Figure 10) [22]. However, the observed absolute difference between both groups was marginal in terms of clinical relevance according to Osoba et al. [15]. Furthermore, there was no worse QoL in PIPAC patients with high intraperitoneal tumor load (assessed by PCI). The only difference was that patients with better overall QoL scores at baseline had a significant shorter hospital stay.

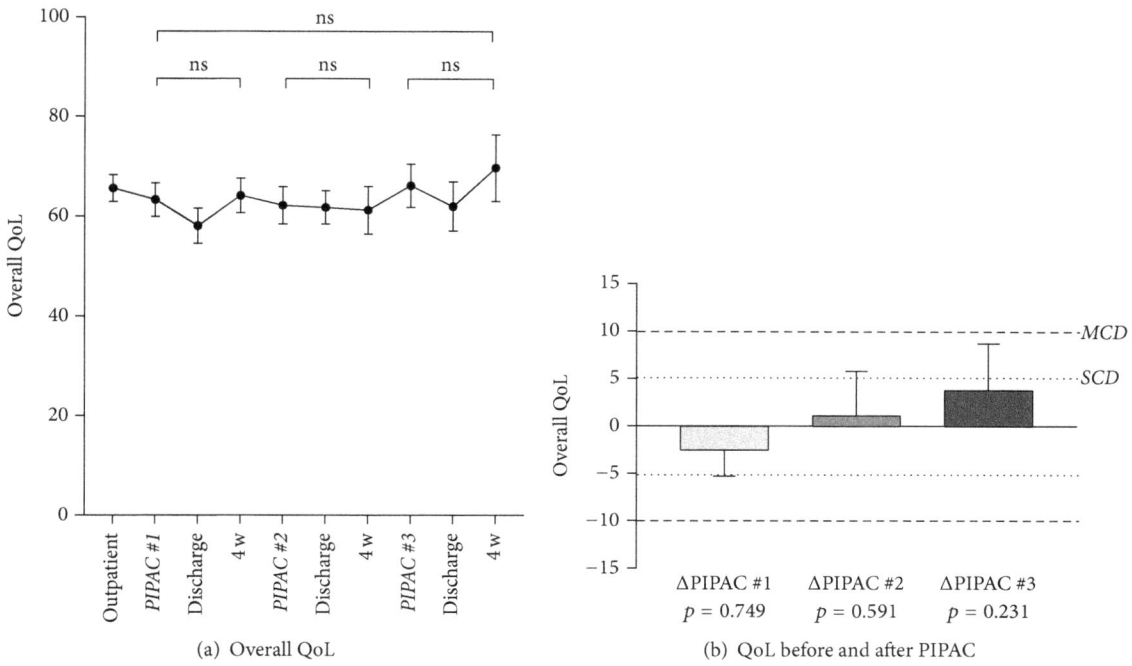

FIGURE 2: Quality of Life (QoL) under Pressurized Intraperitoneal Aerosol Chemotherapy (PIPAC) treatment. Overall Quality of Life (QoL: EORTC QLQ-C30 [14]) under PIPAC treatment is displayed (mean ± SEM). (a) No statistically significant difference ($p < 0.05$) was found when QoL was compared before and after different PIPAC applications (a, b). The dotted lines (b) represent the thresholds for small (SCD) and moderate clinically relevant differences (MCD), respectively [15].

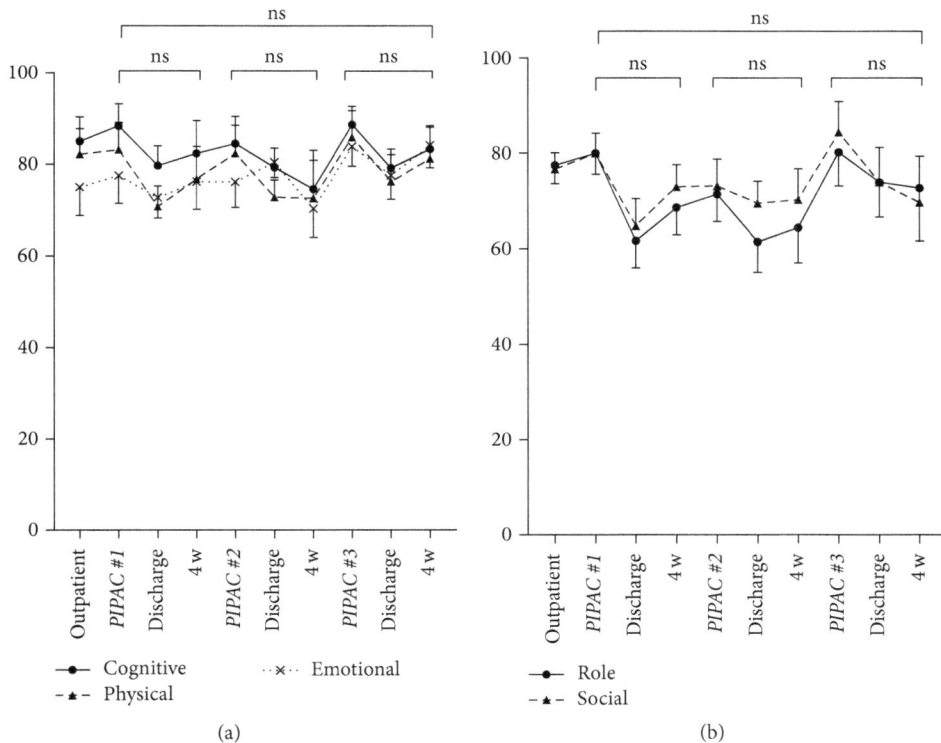

FIGURE 3: Cognitive, physical, emotional, role, and social functioning under Pressurized Intraperitoneal Aerosol Chemotherapy (PIPAC). Quality of Life (QoL: EORTC QLQ-C30 [14]) components under PIPAC treatment (mean ± SEM). No significant difference ($p < 0.05$) was found when QoL was compared before and after different PIPAC applications (ns—not significant).

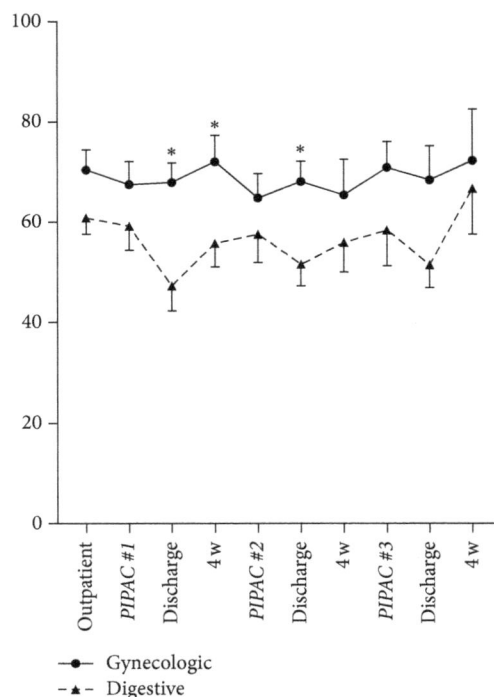

FIGURE 4: Quality of Life (QoL) under Pressurized Intraperitoneal Aerosol Chemotherapy (PIPAC) in patients with gynecological versus digestive malignancies. Overall Quality of Life (QoL: EORTC QLQ-C30 [14]) is displayed as mean ± SEM. * indicates statistical significance ($p < 0.05$).

These findings confirm two reports from the German PIPAC pioneer group. Tempfer reported in a phase II study on ovarian carcinomatosis patients a baseline global physical health score of 52.0 with improvements in QoL scores and symptoms under PIPAC treatment [11]. In the second study, Odendahl et al. assessed QoL and symptoms in a mixed cohort of PIPAC patients [13]. In the 48 reported patients with repeated PIPAC treatment, baseline global physical score was astonishingly high with 82 points. This score was not only higher than the baseline score of our own cohort but compared also favorably with the benchmark QoL scores of the general population cited above [22]. Under PIPAC treatment, QoL and symptoms remained unchanged in the Odendahl et al. study [13] as it was the case in our present series. There are two important differences between the two studies. First, 66 out of 114 eligible patients of the German cohort had to be excluded for missing QoL questionnaires [13]. QoL and symptoms of over the half of their cohort remain therefore unknown, while QoL assessment was complete in our present series. Second, QoL assessment was done only the day before surgery in the two German studies [11, 13]. Therefore, transitory deterioration might have been missed given the long washout period of about 6 weeks between PIPAC applications. For these reasons, in the present study, it was decided to add more time points to measure QoL and symptoms in between applications, namely, immediately at discharge day and 4 weeks after discharge. As suspected, some worsening of QoL and symptoms was observed at discharge

(Figures 2(a) and 3), which was in most patients only 2-3 days after PIPAC treatment. However, those deviations from baseline were minimal and transitory.

It is important to assess QoL and symptoms under oncological treatment because both disease and treatment may have negative impact. A recent prospective multicenter longitudinal study evaluated results of systemic palliative chemotherapy in end-stage cancer patients. The authors observed no survival benefit and no improvements of QoL for patients with moderate and poor performance status (ECOG = 2, 3) at baseline. In patients with good baseline performance status (ECOG = 1), QoL was even significantly worse under systemic palliative chemotherapy [6]. In a secondary analysis, the authors compared patients receiving palliative chemotherapy versus best supportive care employing propensity score weighted adjustment. Patients under palliative systemic chemotherapy had a higher risk for cardiopulmonary resuscitation, invasive ventilation, and late hospice referrals. Patients without treatment had the same survival times but a significantly higher chance of dying in their preferred place instead of in the intensive care unit [23].

In the management of peritoneal carcinomatosis, HIPEC has a curative intent while PIPAC is considered palliation, since no data on long-term outcome after PIPAC is available so far. Therefore, their respective indications are different. In this context, it is important to weigh the expected survival benefits against morbid-mortality and impact on QoL. Two

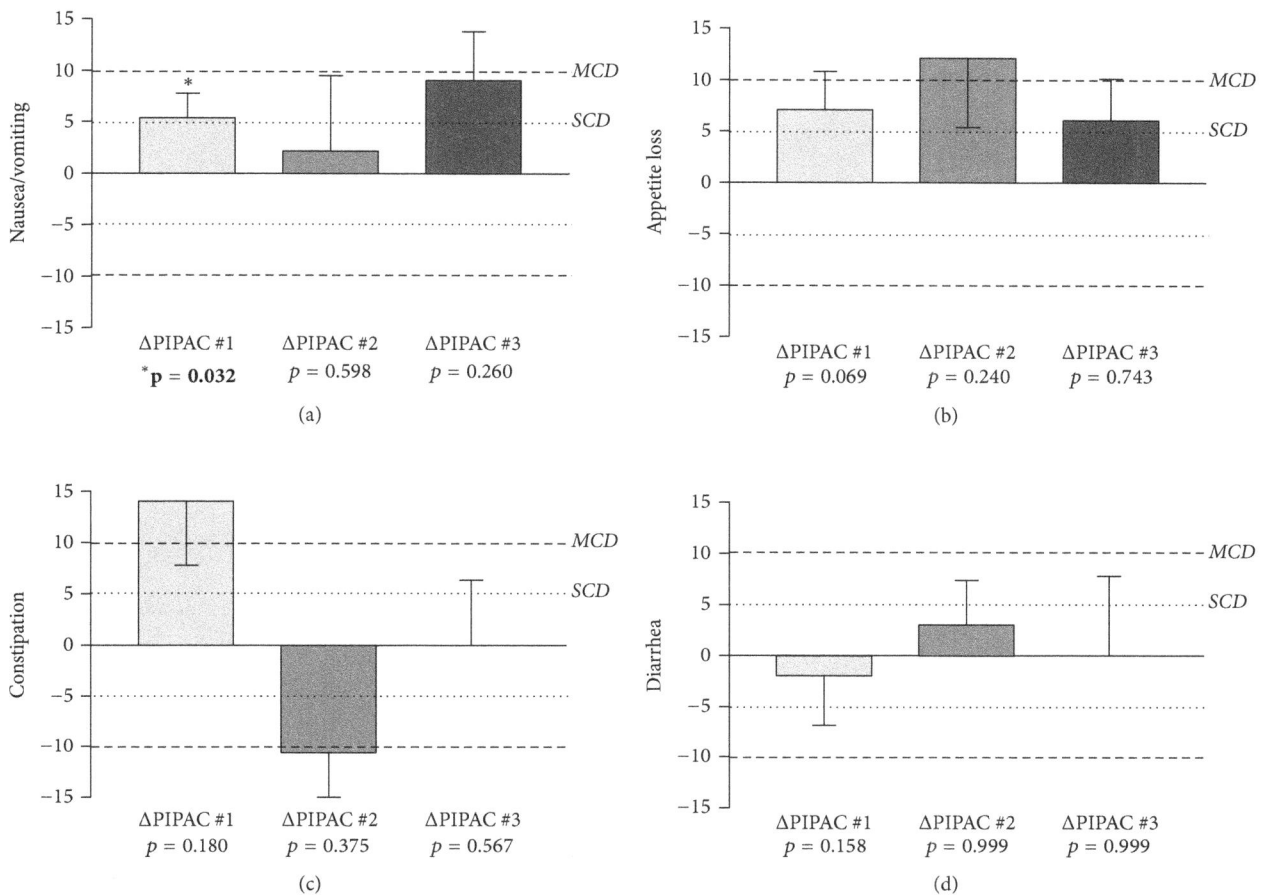

FIGURE 5: Digestive symptoms under Pressurized Intraperitoneal Aerosol Chemotherapy (PIPAC). Digestive symptoms were assessed by use of EORTC QLQ-C30 [14] and displayed as difference (Δ before − after). Statistical significance ($p < 0.05$) is highlighted (bold) and small (SCD) and modest (MCD) clinically relevant differences [15] are illustrated by dashed lines.

recent studies reported decreased QoL and increased symptoms 6–12 months after HIPEC treatment. And this was also observed in patients without postoperative complications [24, 25].

Good tolerance profile and QoL under PIPAC treatment allowed assessing bidirectional regimens combining systemic and intraperitoneal PIPAC treatment. Safety, tolerance, and QoL were still acceptable under bidirectional treatment that might offer a chance for downstaging and secondary CRS + HIPEC in selected patients [12, 26–28].

Concerning efficacy, first results of the pioneer center from Herne, Germany, were encouraging, but longer follow-up periods are required for assessment of oncological outcomes [11, 12, 28]. Furthermore, independent confirmation of histological regression under PIPAC treatment in a standardized way is needed. Future prospective studies should present histological results in a systematic way using a recently published tumor regression score [29].

Main limitations of this study are its small and heterogeneous patient cohort and its retrospective design. On the other hand, QoL assessment was prospectively performed in all consecutive patients from the beginning of the PIPAC program and no patient was excluded from this analysis. Furthermore, PIPAC procedure and treatment algorithms were standardized.

In summary, this study suggests that PIPAC had no negative impact on QoL in patients with peritoneal carcinomatosis. Digestive and nondigestive symptoms remained unchanged after a first PIPAC application but also after repeated treatments. Prospective evaluation of histological response rates and survival times under PIPAC treatment is underway.

Abbreviations

PC: Peritoneal carcinomatosis
QoL: Quality of Life
PIPAC: Pressurized Intraperitoneal Aerosol
        Chemotherapy
PCI: Peritoneal Carcinomatosis Index.

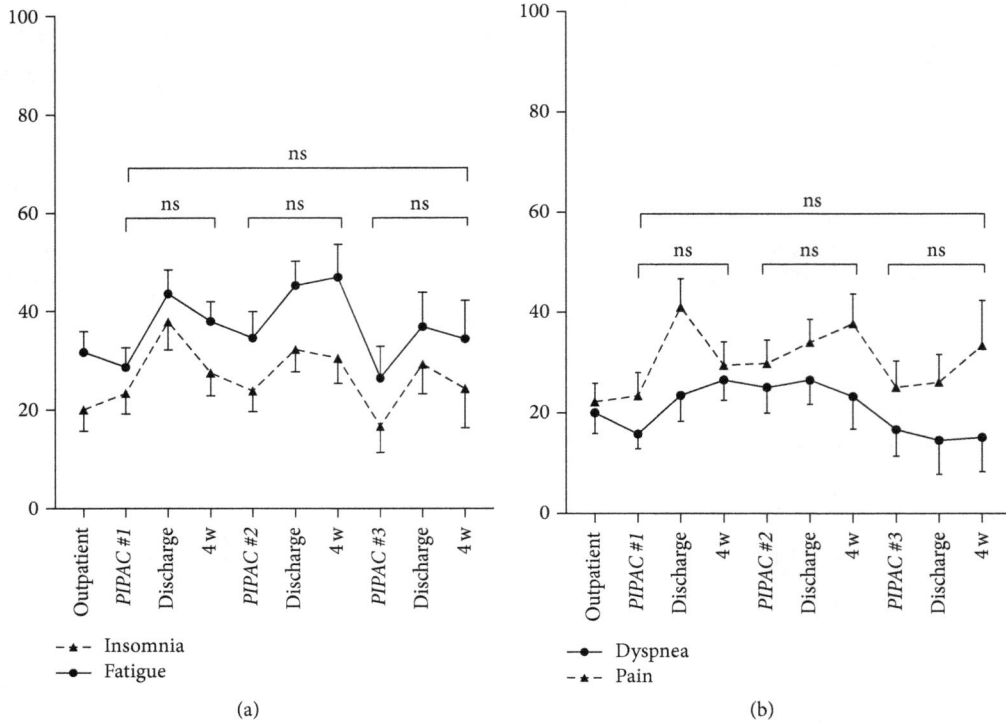

(a)   (b)

FIGURE 6: Nondigestive symptoms under Pressurized Intraperitoneal Aerosol Chemotherapy (PIPAC). Nondigestive symptoms (QoL: EORTC QLQ-C30 [14]) under PIPAC treatment (mean ± SEM). No significant difference ($p < 0.05$) was found when QoL was compared before and after different PIPAC applications (ns—not significant).

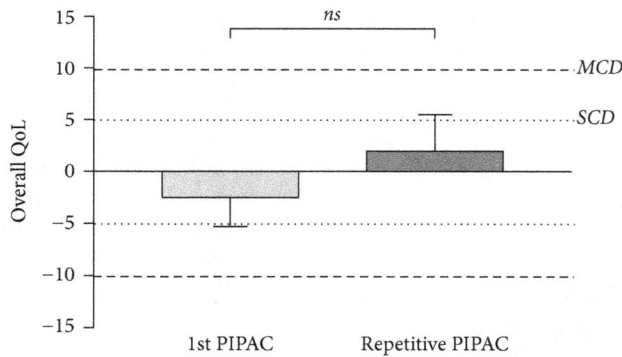

FIGURE 7: Quality of Life (QoL) change after Pressurized Intraperitoneal Aerosol Chemotherapy (PIPAC): 1st application versus repeated procedures. Quality of Life (QoL: EORTC QLQ-C30 [14]) as Δ before – after was compared for PIPAC#1 versus repeated procedures. Statistical significance: $p < 0.05$. ns—not significant. SCD: small clinically relevant difference, MCD: modest MCD clinically relevant difference [15].

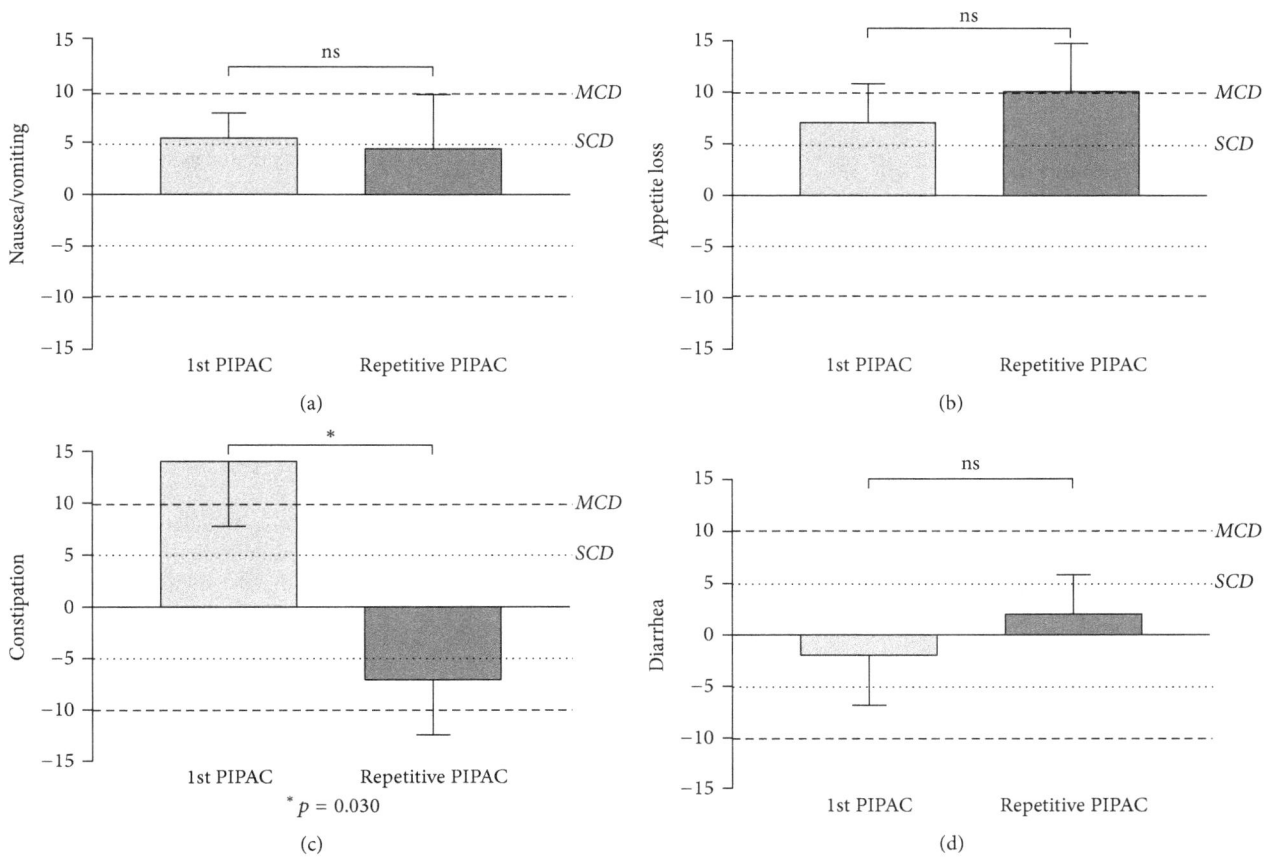

FIGURE 8: Symptom change after Pressurized Intraperitoneal Aerosol Chemotherapy (PIPAC): 1st application versus repeated procedures. Digestive symptoms were assessed by use of EORTC QLQ-C30 [14] and displayed as difference (Δ before − after). *Statistical significance ($p < 0.05$). SCD: small clinically relevant difference, MCD: moderate clinically relevant difference [15].

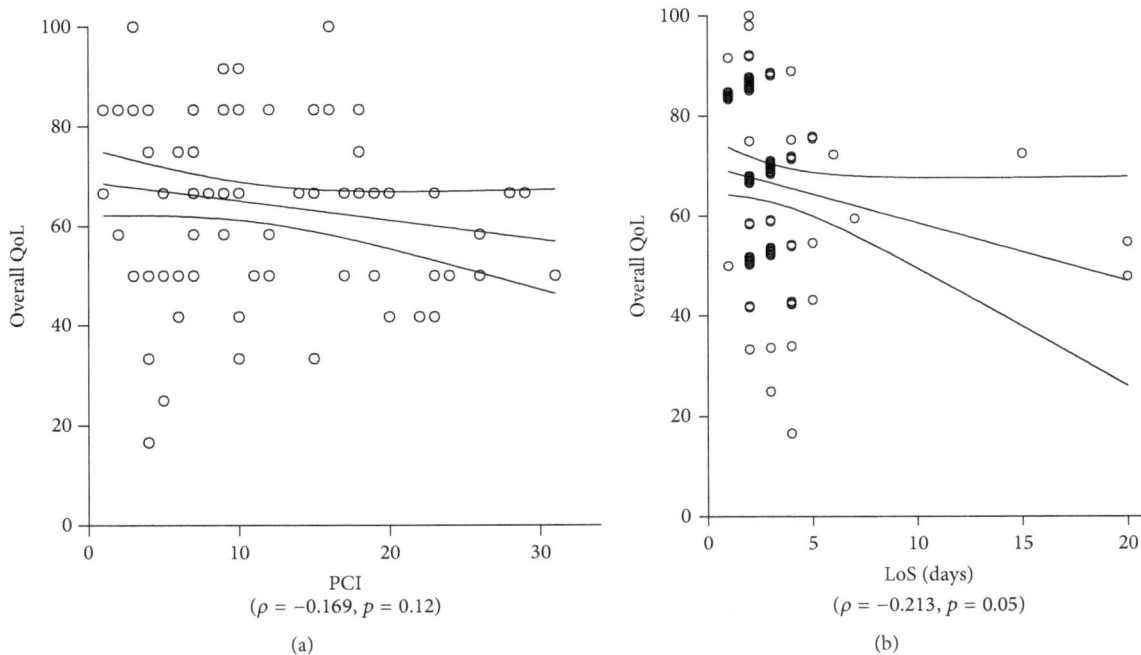

FIGURE 9: Quality of Life, tumor load, and hospital stay. Overall QoL was plotted against the extent of peritoneal disease (measured by the Peritoneal Cancer Index (PCI) [16]) (a) and length of hospital stay (LoS) (b).

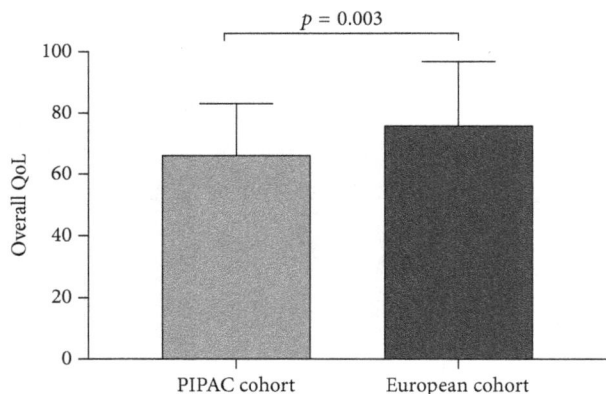

FIGURE 10: Overall Quality of Life (QoL) in PIPAC patients (Lausanne cohort) as compared with the general population. Overall QoL was compared by use of EORTC QLQ-C30 [14] for the Lausanne PIPAC cohort versus a European cohort of 16,151 healthy citizens (general population). The control group had a slightly better QoL score that was statistically significant but of small clinical relevance (<10%) according to Osoba et al. [15].

Disclosure

This study was presented as oral communication to the Swiss Surgical Society, June 1–3, 2016, Lugano, Switzerland, and as poster presentation at the ESCP Congress, September 28–30, 2016, in Milano, Italy.

Competing Interests

The authors declare that they have no competing interests.

References

[1] V. E. Lemmens, Y. L. Klaver, V. J. Verwaal, H. J. Rutten, J. W. W. Coebergh, and I. H. De Hingh, "Predictors and survival of synchronous peritoneal carcinomatosis of colorectal origin: A population-based study," *International Journal of Cancer*, vol. 128, no. 11, pp. 2717–2725, 2011.

[2] Y. L. B. Klaver, V. E. P. P. Lemmens, G. J. Creemers, H. J. T. Rutten, S. W. Nienhuijs, and I. H. J. T. de Hingh, "Population-based survival of patients with peritoneal carcinomatosis from colorectal origin in the era of increasing use of palliative chemotherapy," *Annals of Oncology*, vol. 22, no. 10, pp. 2250–2256, 2011.

[3] A. I. Minchinton and I. F. Tannock, "Drug penetration in solid tumours," *Nature Reviews Cancer*, vol. 6, no. 8, pp. 583–592, 2006.

[4] W. P. Ceelen, L. Påhlman, and H. Mahteme, "Pharmacodynamic aspects of intraperitoneal cytotoxic therapy," *Cancer Treatment and Research*, vol. 134, pp. 195–214, 2007.

[5] R. L. Dedrick and M. F. Flessner, "Pharmacokinetic problems in peritoneal drug administration: tissue penetration and surface exposure," *Journal of the National Cancer Institute*, vol. 89, no. 7, pp. 480–487, 1997.

[6] H. G. Prigerson, Y. Bao, M. A. Shah et al., "Chemotherapy use, performance status, and quality of life at the end of life," *JAMA Oncology*, vol. 1, no. 6, pp. 778–784, 2015.

[7] W. Solaß, A. Hetzel, G. Nadiradze, E. Sagynaliev, and M. A. Reymond, "Description of a novel approach for intraperitoneal drug delivery and the related device," *Surgical Endoscopy*, vol. 26, no. 7, pp. 1849–1855, 2012.

[8] W. Solass, R. Kerb, T. Mürdter et al., "Intraperitoneal chemotherapy of peritoneal carcinomatosis using pressurized aerosol as an alternative to liquid solution: first evidence for efficacy," *Annals of Surgical Oncology*, vol. 21, no. 2, pp. 553–559, 2014.

[9] W. Solaß, U. Giger-Pabst, J. Zieren, and M. A. Reymond, "Pressurized intraperitoneal aerosol chemotherapy (PIPAC): occupational health and safety aspects," *Annals of Surgical Oncology*, vol. 20, no. 11, pp. 3504–3511, 2013.

[10] C. B. Tempfer, G. A. Rezniczek, P. Ende, W. Solass, and M.-A. Reymond, "Pressurized intraperitoneal aerosol chemotherapy with cisplatin and doxorubicin in women with peritoneal carcinomatosis: a cohort study," *Anticancer research*, vol. 35, no. 12, pp. 6723–6729, 2015.

[11] C. B. Tempfer, G. Winnekendonk, W. Solass et al., "Pressurized intraperitoneal aerosol chemotherapy in women with recurrent ovarian cancer: a phase 2 study," *Gynecologic Oncology*, vol. 137, no. 2, pp. 223–228, 2015.

[12] G. Nadiradze, U. Giger-Pabst, J. Zieren, D. Strumberg, W. Solass, and M.-A. Reymond, "Pressurized intraperitoneal aerosol chemotherapy (PIPAC) with low-dose cisplatin and doxorubicin in gastric peritoneal metastasis," *Journal of Gastrointestinal Surgery*, vol. 20, no. 2, pp. 367–373, 2016.

[13] K. Odendahl, W. Solass, C. Demtröder et al., "Quality of life of patients with end-stage peritoneal metastasis treated with Pressurized IntraPeritoneal Aerosol Chemotherapy (PIPAC)," *European Journal of Surgical Oncology*, vol. 41, no. 10, pp. 1379–1385, 2015.

[14] N. K. Aaronson, S. Ahmedzai, B. Bergman et al., "The European organization for research and treatment of cancer QLQ-C30: a quality-of-life instrument for use in international clinical trials in oncology," *Journal of the National Cancer Institute*, vol. 85, no. 5, pp. 365–376, 1993.

[15] D. Osoba, G. Rodrigues, J. Myles, B. Zee, and J. Pater, "Interpreting the significance of changes in health-related quality-of-life scores," *Journal of Clinical Oncology*, vol. 16, no. 1, pp. 139–144, 1998.

[16] P. Jacquet and P. H. Sugarbaker, "Clinical research methodologies in diagnosis and staging of patients with peritoneal carcinomatosis," *Cancer Treatment and Research*, vol. 82, pp. 359–374, 1996.

[17] A. Blanco, U. Giger-Pabst, W. Solass, J. Zieren, and M. A. Reymond, "Renal and hepatic toxicities after pressurized intraperitoneal aerosol chemotherapy (PIPAC)," *Annals of Surgical Oncology*, vol. 20, no. 7, pp. 2311–2316, 2013.

[18] M. Groenvold, M. C. Klee, M. A. G. Sprangers, and N. K. Aaronson, "Validation of the EORTC QLQ-C30 quality of life questionnaire through combined qualitative and quantitative assessment of patient-observer agreement," *Journal of Clinical Epidemiology*, vol. 50, no. 4, pp. 441–450, 1997.

[19] P. M. Fayers, N. K. Aaronson, K. Bjordal et al., *The EORTC QLQ-C30 Scoring Manual*, European Organization for Research and Treatment of Cancer, Brussels, Belgium, 3rd edition, 2001.

[20] M. M. Oken, R. H. Creech, and T. E. Davis, "Toxicity and response criteria of the Eastern Cooperative Oncology Group," *American Journal of Clinical Oncology*, vol. 5, no. 6, pp. 649–655, 1982.

Impact of Pressurized Intraperitoneal Aerosol Chemotherapy on Quality of Life and Symptoms in Patients...

197

[21] D. Dindo, N. Demartines, and P.-A. Clavien, "Classification of surgical complications: a new proposal with evaluation in a cohort of 6336 patients and results of a survey," *Annals of Surgery*, vol. 240, no. 2, pp. 205–213, 2004.

[22] A. Hinz, S. Singer, and E. Brähler, "European reference values for the quality of life questionnaire EORTC QLQ-C30: results of a German investigation and a summarizing analysis of six European general population normative studies," *Acta Oncologica*, vol. 53, no. 7, pp. 958–965, 2014.

[23] A. A. Wright, B. Zhang, N. L. Keating, J. C. Weeks, and H. G. Prigerson, "Associations between palliative chemotherapy and adult cancer patients' end of life care and place of death: prospective cohort study," *BMJ*, vol. 348, Article ID g1219, 2014.

[24] T. D. Hamilton, E. L. Taylor, A. J. Cannell, J. A. McCart, and A. Govindarajan, "Impact of major complications on patients' quality of life after cytoreductive surgery and hyperthermic intraperitoneal chemotherapy," *Annals of Surgical Oncology*, vol. 23, no. 9, pp. 2946–2952, 2016.

[25] C. S. Chia, G. H. C. Tan, C. Lim, K. C. Soo, and M. C. C. Teo, "Prospective quality of life study for colorectal cancer patients with peritoneal carcinomatosis undergoing cytoreductive surgery and hyperthermic intraperitoneal chemotherapy," *Annals of Surgical Oncology*, vol. 23, no. 9, pp. 2905–2913, 2016.

[26] R. Girshally, C. Demtröder, N. Albayrak, J. Zieren, C. Tempfer, and M. A. Reymond, "Pressurized intraperitoneal aerosol chemotherapy (PIPAC) as a neoadjuvant therapy before cytoreductive surgery and hyperthermic intraperitoneal chemotherapy," *World Journal of Surgical Oncology*, vol. 14, no. 1, article no. 253, 2016.

[27] M. Robella, M. Vaira, and M. De Simone, "Safety and feasibility of pressurized intraperitoneal aerosol chemotherapy (PIPAC) associated with systemic chemotherapy: an innovative approach to treat peritoneal carcinomatosis," *World Journal of Surgical Oncology*, vol. 14, article 128, 2016.

[28] C. Demtröder, W. Solass, J. Zieren, D. Strumberg, U. Giger-Pabst, and M.-A. Reymond, "Pressurized intraperitoneal aerosol chemotherapy with oxaliplatin in colorectal peritoneal metastasis," *Colorectal Disease*, vol. 18, no. 4, pp. 364–371, 2016.

[29] W. Solass, C. Sempoux, S. Detlefsen, N. J. Carr, and F. Bibeau, "Peritoneal sampling and histological assessment of therapeutic response in peritoneal metastasis: proposal of the Peritoneal Regression Grading Score (PRGS)," *Pleura and Peritoneum*, vol. 1, no. 2, pp. 99–107, 2016.

24

Clinical Significance of UCA1 to Predict Metastasis and Poor Prognosis of Digestive System Malignancies

Xiao-Dong Sun,[1] Chen Huan,[2] Wei Qiu,[1] Da-Wei Sun,[1] Xiao-Ju Shi,[1] Chuan-Lei Wang,[1] Chao Jiang,[1] Guang-Yi Wang,[1] and Guo-Yue Lv[1]

[1]*Department of Hepatobiliary and Pancreatic Surgery, The First Hospital of Jilin University, Changchun, Jilin Province 130021, China*
[2]*Institute of Virology and AIDS Research, The First Hospital of Jilin University, Changchun, Jilin Province 130021, China*

Correspondence should be addressed to Guang-Yi Wang; wgymd@sina.com and Guo-Yue Lv; lvguoyue@sina.com

Academic Editor: Stephen Fink

Purpose. Urothelial carcinoma-associated 1 (UCA1) has been reported to be overexpressed and correlated with progression in various cancers. However, the association between UCA1 expression and some clinicopathological features of digestive system malignancies, such as metastasis and survival, remains inconclusive. Therefore, a meta-analysis was performed to investigate the clinical significance of UCA1 in digestive system malignancies. *Methods.* Relevant literatures were searched in PubMed, Web of Science, Cochrane Library, and Embase databases updated to May 2016. *Results.* A total of 1089 patients from 10 studies were included in this meta-analysis. Meta-analysis results showed that digestive system malignancy patients with UCA1 overexpression were significantly more susceptible to developing lymph node metastasis (LNM) (OR = 1.85, 95% CI: 1.28–2.67) and distant metastasis (DM) (OR = 3.14, 95% CI: 1.77–5.58) and suffer from poor overall survival (OS) (HR = 2.31, 95% CI: 1.89–2.82, univariate analysis; HR = 2.24, 95% CI: 1.69–2.98, multivariate analysis) and poor disease-free survival (DFS) (HR = 2.65, 95% CI: 1.59–4.43, univariate analysis; HR = 2.50, 95% CI: 1.62–3.86, multivariate analysis). *Conclusion.* UCA1 overexpression was correlated with LNM, DM, poor OS, and poor DFS. UCA1 may serve as an indicator for metastasis and poor prognosis in digestive system malignancies.

1. Introduction

Digestive system malignancies have threatened human health seriously. According to the GLOBOCAN estimates, there were about 3.4 million new cases and 2.9 million deaths caused by digestive system malignancies in 2012 worldwide [1]. Although great achievements have been made in therapeutic approaches, such as surgery and chemotherapy, the outcome of digestive system malignancies remains poor. Nowadays, advantage of biomarkers in diagnosis and prognosis of cancers has been suggested, which might provide more precise information for individualized treatment and disease monitoring [2, 3].

Long noncoding RNAs (lncRNAs) are a class of RNAs longer than 200 nt that lack protein-coding capacity [4]. Despite the fact that they used to be regarded as "junk" of genome, increasing number of studies have suggested the contribution of lncRNAs to various biological processes via transcriptional and posttranscriptional regulation [5, 6]. In particular, role of lncRNA in carcinogenesis has been highlighted recently [7]. LncRNAs were found to be dysregulated and function as oncogene or tumor suppressor in various cancers. Furthermore, a growing body of evidence has demonstrated that there was significant association between the expression of lncRNA and the progression of cancer, including clinical-pathological features and survival, indicating that lncRNA can serve as biomarker for cancers. Some lncRNAs, such as HOX transcript antisense RNA (HOTAIR) and metastasis associated lung adenocarcinoma transcript 1 (MALAT1), have been illustrated to potentially predict metastasis and prognosis of digestive system malignancies through meta-analysis [8–10].

Recently, lncRNA urothelial carcinoma-associated 1 (UCA1) has attracted great attention due to its involvement in diverse cancers. UCA1, which was also called cancer upregulated drug resistant (CUDR), was originally identified in bladder transitional cell carcinoma in 2008 and suggested to promote cell proliferation and transformation [11, 12]. So far, the overexpression of UCA1 has been reported in other cancers, especially in digestive system malignancies, including hepatocellular carcinoma [13, 14], gastric cancer [15, 16], colorectal cancer [17–20], pancreatic cancer [21], and esophageal squamous cell carcinoma [22]. Although the association between UCA1 expression and cancer progression was a particular concern for these studies, these results were limited by small sample sizes or inconsistent conclusions. For instance, the patients with high UCA1 level in cancerous tissues were suggested to suffer from elevated lymph node metastasis (LNM) and distant metastasis (DM) rate in numerous cancers [13, 18, 19, 22]; nevertheless, this association has not been detected in other studies [15, 17]. Moreover, the issue of whether the overexpression of UCA1 could predict poor prognosis [16, 20] or not [14] also needs to be clarified. Therefore, to investigate the clinical value of UCA1, we performed this quantitative meta-analysis to assess the correlation of UCA1 expression with metastasis and prognosis in digestive system malignancies.

2. Material and Methods

2.1. Literature Search Strategy. All literatures investigating the association of lncRNA UCA1 with metastasis and prognosis of digestive system malignancies were searched in PubMed, Web of Science, Cochrane Library, and Embase databases updated to May 2016. Search terms are as follows: "UCA1" or "urothelial carcinoma-associated 1" or "CUDR" or "cancer up-regulated drug resistant", "cancer" or "carcinoma" or "tumor" or "neoplasm", and "survival" or "prognosis" or "prognostic" or "progression" or "recurrence" or "outcome" or "metastasis" or "clinicopathological". The searching strategy used in PubMed was "((((((UCA1 [Title/Abstract]) OR urothelial carcinoma-associated 1 [Title/Abstract]) OR CUDR [Title/Abstract]) OR cancer up-regulated drug resistant [Title/Abstract])) AND ((((cancer) OR carcinoma) OR tumor) OR neoplasma)) AND (((((((survival) OR prognosis) OR prognositic) OR progression) OR recurrence) OR outcome) OR metastasis) OR clinicopathological)". In addition, the references in retrieved articles were screened manually for potential relevant studies.

2.2. Selection and Exclusion Criteria. The articles collected were considered eligible if they met the inclusion criteria: (1) articles were investigating the association of UCA1 with progression of digestive system malignancies; (2) the expression levels of UCA1 in primary cancerous tissues were measured; (3) patients were grouped according to the expression levels of UCA1; (4) related clinicopathological parameters were described. Exclusion criteria are the following: (1) duplicate publications; (2) reviews, letters, comments, and conference articles; (3) studies focusing on UCA1 in other types of cancers, rather than digestive system malignancies; (4) studies using cells lines or animals, rather than cancer patients; (5) studies without usable data. Regarding multiple publications

from the same medical center, only the most recent or the most complete study was included in the meta-analysis.

2.3. Data Extract. Two investigators (Xiao-Dong Sun, Chen Huan) extracted data from the eligible studies independently, according to the inclusion and exclusion criteria. For disagreements, a consensus was achieved by a third investigator (Wei Qiu). The following information was collected from each eligible study: first author, publication year, region of patients, cancer type, total number of patients, detecting method of UCA1 expression, cut-off value of grouping, number of patients in high/low UCA1 expression group, number of patients with LNM and DM in each group, follow-up time, study endpoint, survival analysis method (multivariate or univariate), and hazard ratio (HR) with 95% confidence interval (CI) for overall survival (OS) or disease-free survival (DFS). When the HRs and their 95% CIs were given in the articles, these data were extracted directly. If the prognosis was plotted as Kaplan–Meier curve, data was digitized by the software Engauge Digitizer version 4.1 (http://digitizer.sourceforge.net/) and calculated as described [23].

2.4. Quality Assessment. Quality assessment of the included studies was performed according to the Newcastle-Ottawa Scale (NOS) criteria [24]. The NOS criteria is scored based on three aspects (subject selection, comparability of subject, and clinical outcome) with the final scores ranging from 0 to 9, and a score ≥6 indicates a high quality.

2.5. Data Analysis. To assess the heterogeneity among the included studies, χ^2-based Q test and I^2 statistics were used. When heterogeneity was significant ($I^2 > 50\%$ or $P < 0.10$ for χ^2), a random effects model was used; otherwise, fixed effects model was adopted. The potential publication bias was evaluated using a "funnel plot" as well as Begg's and Egger's test.

The meta-analysis was performed through using Stata SE12.0 (Stata Corporation). All P values were two-sided, and $P < 0.05$ was considered statistically significant.

3. Results

3.1. Literature Information. A total of 156 records were retrieved by searching the databases of PubMed, Web of Science, Cochrane Library, and Embase. After screening the title and abstract, 125 articles were excluded because they were either duplication or reviews or about other lncRNAs. For the thirty-one articles remaining, full text was assessed carefully and 21 were excluded for their insufficient data, or for they focused on the level of UCA1 from other cancers rather than digestive system malignancies. Finally, 10 articles comprising 1089 patients were identified as eligible and included in the present meta-analysis. The flow diagram was shown in Figure 1.

3.2. Study Characteristics. The baseline characteristics of the included studies were summarized in Table 1. The articles

TABLE 1: Characteristics of included studies in this meta-analysis.

First author [ref.]	Year	Cancer	Country	Sample size	Methods for UCA1 detecting	Cut-off value for UCA1	UCA1 expression						Study endpoints	(HR, 95% CI)	Data source	Follow-up time (months)
							High expression	High with LNM	High with DM	Low expression	Low with LNM	Low with DM				
Han [17]	2014	CRC	China	80	qRT-PCR	Mean value	37	17	7	43	18	7	OS	OS (U), 3.02 (1.19–7.68)	Curve	Mean 42.6
Li [22]	2014	ESCC	China	90	qRT-PCR	Mean value	41	22	NA	49	12	NA.	OS	OS (U), 2.93 (1.72–6.21) — Direct; OS (M), 2.63 (1.42–5.87) — Direct		Median 43
Wang [13]	2015	HCC	China	98	qRT-PCR	Median value	49	NA	30	49	NA	11	OS	OS (U), 2.69 (1.56–4.64) — Direct; OS (M), 1.86 (1.08–3.21) — Direct		Up to 60
Zheng [15]	2015	GC	China	112	qRT-PCR	Median value	56	35	NA	56	37	NA	OS, DFS	OS (U), 2.35 (1.40–4.51) — Direct; OS (M), 2.35 (1.22–4.52) — Direct; DFS (U), 2.90 (1.51–5.80) — Direct; DFS (M), 2.55 (1.33–4.97) — Direct		Up to 60
Yang [14]	2015	HCC	Korea	240	Illumina expression beadchip	Median value	120	NA	NA	120	NA	NA	OS, DFS	OS (U), 1.99 (0.84–4.69) — Direct; DFS (U), 2.35 (1.07–5.17) — Direct; DFS (M), 2.40 (1.09–5.27) — Direct		Up to 120
Ni [18]	2015	CRC	China	54	qRT-PCR	Median value	27	12	6	27	5	1	OS	OS (U), 5.07 (1.25–20.54) — Available data; OS (M), 3.14 (1.17–8.41) — Available data		Up to 50
Chen [21]	2015	PDAC	USA	63	Affymetrix 2.0 microarray	NA	NA	NA	NA	NA	NA	NA	OS	OS (U), 2.76 (1.15–6.61) — Available data		Median 21

TABLE 1: Continued.

First author [ref.]	Year	Cancer	Country	Sample size	Methods for UCA1 detecting	Cut-off value for UCA1	UCA1 expression						Study endpoints	(HR, 95% CI)	Data source	Follow-up time (months)
							High expression	High with LNM	High with DM	Low expression	Low with LNM	Low with DM				
Tao [19]	2015	CRC	China	80	qRT-PCR	Fourth quartile	20	13	NA	60	21	NA	OS	OS (U), 2.46 (1.26–4.78)	Direct	Up to 72
														OS (M), 2.00 (1.01–2.98)	Direct	
Bian [20]*	2016	CRC	China	90[a]	qRT-PCR	Median value	45	30	8	45	23	4	OS	OS (U), 3.27 (1.44–7.41)	Direct	Up to 80
														OS (M), 2.40 (1.04–5.50)	Direct	
				105[b]			NA	NA	NA	NA	NA	NA	OS	OS (U), 1.71 (1.21–2.40)	Curve	Up to 120
Shang [16]	2016	GC	China	77	qRT-PCR	NA	NA	NA	NA	NA	NA	NA	DFS	DFS (M), 2.54 (1.09–5.92)	Direct	Up to 72

NA, not available; qRT-PCR, quantitative reverse transcription-polymerase chain reaction; LNM, lymph node metastasis; DM, distant metastasis; OS, overall survival; DFS, disease-free survival; U, univariate analysis; M, multivariate analysis; Curve, Kaplan–Meier curve; * this study included two cohorts of CRC patients; we named them Bian et al.[a] and Bian et al.[b], respectively, in the following analysis.

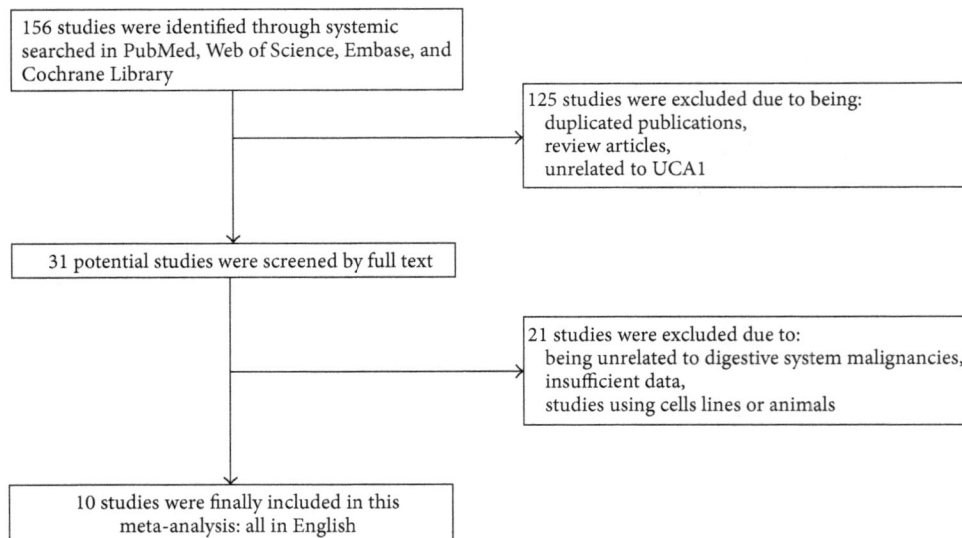

FIGURE 1: Flow diagram of searching relevant studies used in this meta-analysis.

were published between 2014 and 2016 with sample sizes ranging from 54 to 240. Nearly all of them were conducted in Asia, 8 studies in China, 1 study in Korea, and 1 in USA. To detect the UCA1 expression, quantitative reverse transcription-polymerase chain reaction (RT-PCR) was used in 8 studies, Illumina expression beadchip was used in 1 study, and Affymetrix 2.0 microarray was used in 1 study. The cut-off value for UCA1 expression was unavailable in 2 studies, and the remaining 8 were based on median value of UCA1 level (in 5 studies), mean value of UCA1 level (in 2 studies), and fourth quartile of UCA1 level (in 1 study). According to the NOS criteria, all of the included studies got 7 scores or more, indicating their high methodological quality (Table 2).

3.3. Meta-Analysis for OS

3.3.1. Association between UCA1 and Metastasis. In total 6 studies including 506 cases reported the association of UCA1 with LNM of digestive system malignancies. Since there was no significant heterogeneity among these studies ($I^2 = 45.9\%$ and $P = 0.100$), the fixed model was adopted. The pooled OR with 95% CI indicated that digestive system malignancy patients with high UCA1 level in tumor tissues were more susceptible to developing LNM (OR = 1.85, 95% CI: 1.28–2.67, $P = 0.001$) (Figure 2(a)).

Moreover, there were four studies comprising 322 patients that investigated correlation of UCA1 expression and the occurrence of DM in digestive system malignancies. There was also no significant heterogeneity among these studies ($I^2 = 40.5\%$ and $P = 0.169$), so the fixed model was applied to calculate the pooled OR and its 95% CI. The result showed that increased UCA1 expression was significantly correlated with DM (OR = 3.14, 95% CI: 1.77–5.58, $P = 0.000$) (Figure 2(b)).

Taken together, the results above showed that UCA1 overexpression was significantly correlated with LNM and

DM in digestive system cancer patients, suggesting that UCA1 may serve as an indicator for metastasis of digestive system malignancies.

3.3.2. Association between UCA1 and OS. On one hand, 9 studies with a total number of 1012 patients investigated the association between UCA1 expression and OS through univariate analysis. The fixed model was used to assess the pooled HR and its 95% CI since no significant heterogeneity was found among these studies ($I^2 = 0\%$, $P = 0.707$). We found that high UCA1 level was significantly associated with poor OS (HR = 2.31, 95% CI: 1.89–2.82, $P = 0.000$) (Figure 3(a)). On the other hand, 6 studies with a total number of 524 patients investigated the association between UCA1 expression and OS through multivariate analysis. Since there was no significant heterogeneity among these studies ($I^2 = 0\%$, $P = 0.940$), the fixed model was used to assess the pooled HR and its 95% CI. We found that UCA1 overexpression was also significantly associated with poor OS (HR = 2.24, 95% CI: 1.69–2.98, $P = 0.000$) (Figure 3(b)).

Results from the above analysis indicated that high expression of UCA1 was significantly correlated with poor OS in digestive system cancer patients, suggesting that UCA1 was an indicator of decreased survival rate in digestive system malignancies.

3.3.3. Association between UCA1 and DFS. Totally, there were 3 studies including 429 patients investigating the prognostic value of UCA1 on DFS in the form of either univariate or multivariate analysis. Since no significant heterogeneity was found among these studies ($I^2 = 0.0\%$, $P = 0.691$, univariate analysis; $I^2 = 0.0\%$, $P = 0.992$, multivariate analysis), fixed-effect model was adopted to calculate the pooled HRs and their 95% CIs. The results showed that increased UCA1 expression was also significantly associated with poor DFS

TABLE 2: Newcastle-Ottawa quality for included studies in this meta-analysis.

First author and year [ref.]	Selection (score)				Comparability (score)		Outcome (score)			Total score
	Representativeness of exposed	Selection of nonexposed	Ascertainment of exposure	No interest before study	Study design (cohort study)	Control for other confounding factors	Assessment of outcome	Follow-up time long enough (>5 years)	Adequacy number of follow-ups (>80%)	
Han 2014 [17]	1	1	1	0	1	0	1	1	1	7
Li 2014 [22]	1	1	1	0	1	1	1	1	1	8
Wang 2015 [13]	1	1	1	1	1	1	1	1	1	9
Zheng 2015 [15]	1	1	1	0	1	1	1	1	1	8
Yang 2015 [14]	1	1	1	0	1	1	1	1	1	8
Ni 2015 [18]	1	1	1	0	1	1	1	0	1	7
Chen 2015 [21]	1	1	1	0	1	1	1	1	1	8
Tao 2015 [19]	1	1	1	0	1	1	1	1	1	8
Bian 2016 [20]	1	1	1	0	1	1	1	1	1	8
Shang 2016 [16]	1	1	1	0	1	1	1	1	1	8

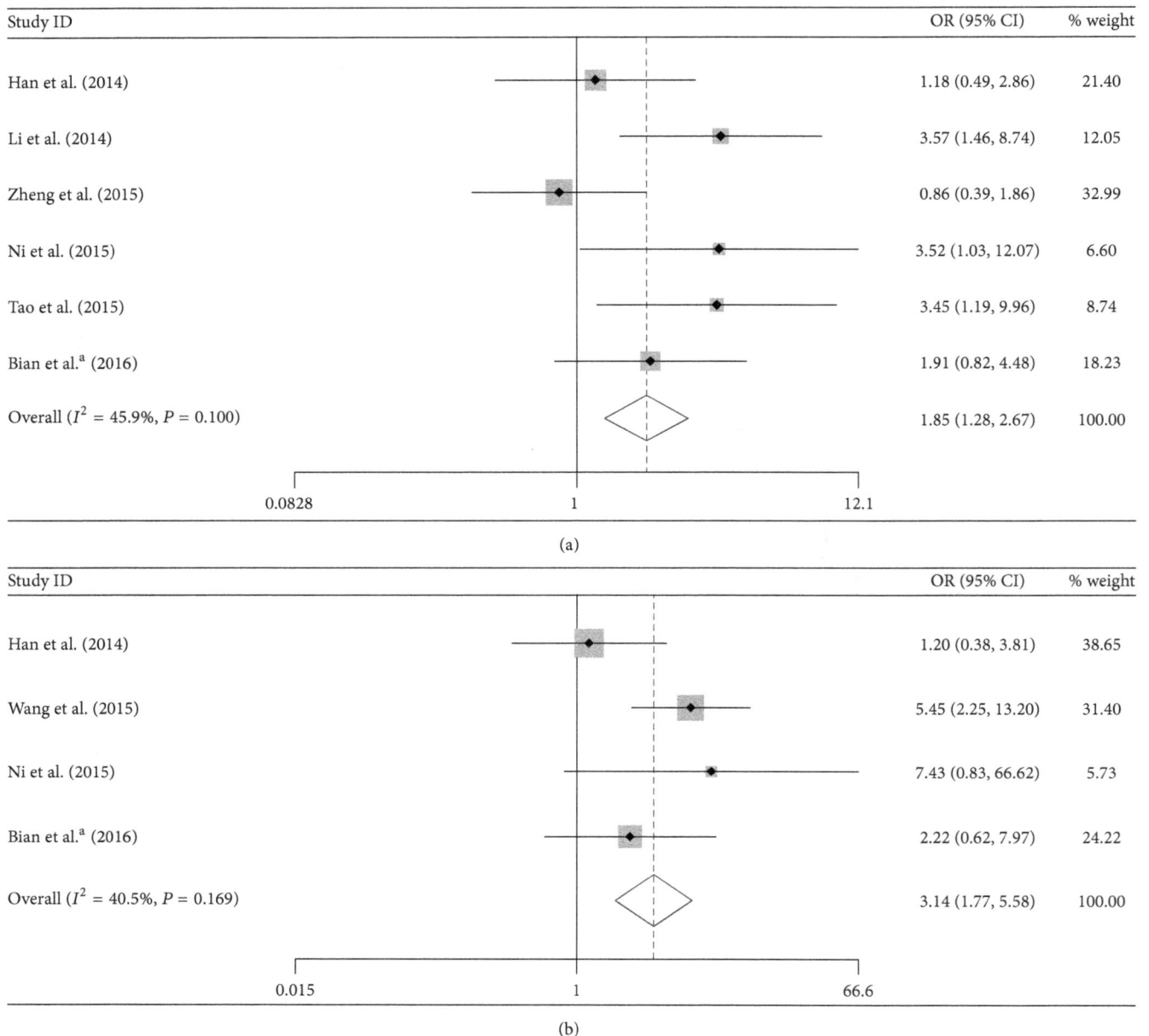

FIGURE 2: Forest plots of odds ratios (ORs) for the association between UCA1 expression and lymph node metastasis (LNM) (a) and distant metastasis (DM) (b).

(HR = 2.65, 95% CI: 1.59–4.43, $P = 0.000$, univariate analysis; HR = 2.50, 95% CI: 1.62–3.86, $P = 0.000$, multivariate analysis) (Figures 4(a) and 4(b)), indicating that increased UCA1 expression was an indicator of early tumor recurrence in digestive system cancer patients.

3.4. Publication Bias. In this meta-analysis, both Begg's and Egger's P value tests were used to assess the potential publication bias. No publication bias was found in the studies with LNM ($P = 0.188, 0.109$), DM ($P = 1.000, 0.949$), or OS ($P = 0.128$ for Begg's test, univariate analysis) or DFS ($P = 0.602, 0.746$, multivariate analysis). However, publication bias

was found in the studies with OS ($P = 0.003$ for Egger's test, univariate analysis; $P = 0.039, 0.035$, multivariate analysis). Besides, the funnel plots for LNM (Figure 5(a)), DM (Figure 5(b)), OS from multivariate analysis (Figure 5(c)), and DFS from multivariate analysis (Figure 5(d)) were largely symmetrical. Therefore, we speculate that most of our meta-analysis results are reliable.

4. Discussion

Digestive system malignancies constitute a major part of human cancers [1]. Their rapid progression and poor outcome

Study ID		HR (95% CI)	% weight
Han et al. (2014)		3.02 (1.19, 7.68)	4.55
Li et al. (2014)		2.93 (1.72, 6.21)	9.59
Wang et al. (2015)		2.69 (1.56, 4.64)	13.30
Zheng et al. (2015)		2.35 (1.40, 4.51)	11.55
Yang et al. (2015)		1.99 (0.84, 4.69)	5.34
Ni et al. (2015)		5.07 (1.25, 20.54)	2.02
Chen et al. (2015)		2.76 (1.15, 6.62)	5.16
Tao et al. (2015)		2.46 (1.26, 4.78)	8.89
Bian et al.[a] (2016)		3.27 (1.44, 7.41)	5.89
Bian et al.[b] (2016)		1.71 (1.21, 2.40)	33.70
Overall ($I^2 = 0.0\%$, $P = 0.707$)		2.31 (1.89, 2.82)	100.00

0.0487   1   20.5

(a)

Study ID		HR (95% CI)	% weight
Li et al. (2014)		2.63 (1.42, 5.87)	16.16
Wang et al. (2015)		1.86 (1.08, 3.21)	27.44
Zheng et al. (2015)		2.35 (1.22, 4.52)	18.98
Ni et al. (2015)		3.14 (1.17, 8.41)	8.37
Tao et al. (2015)		2.00 (1.01, 3.98)	17.31
Bian et al.[a] (2016)		2.40 (1.04, 5.50)	11.74
Overall ($I^2 = 0.0\%$, $P = 0.940$)		2.24 (1.69, 2.98)	100.00

0.119   1   8.41

(b)

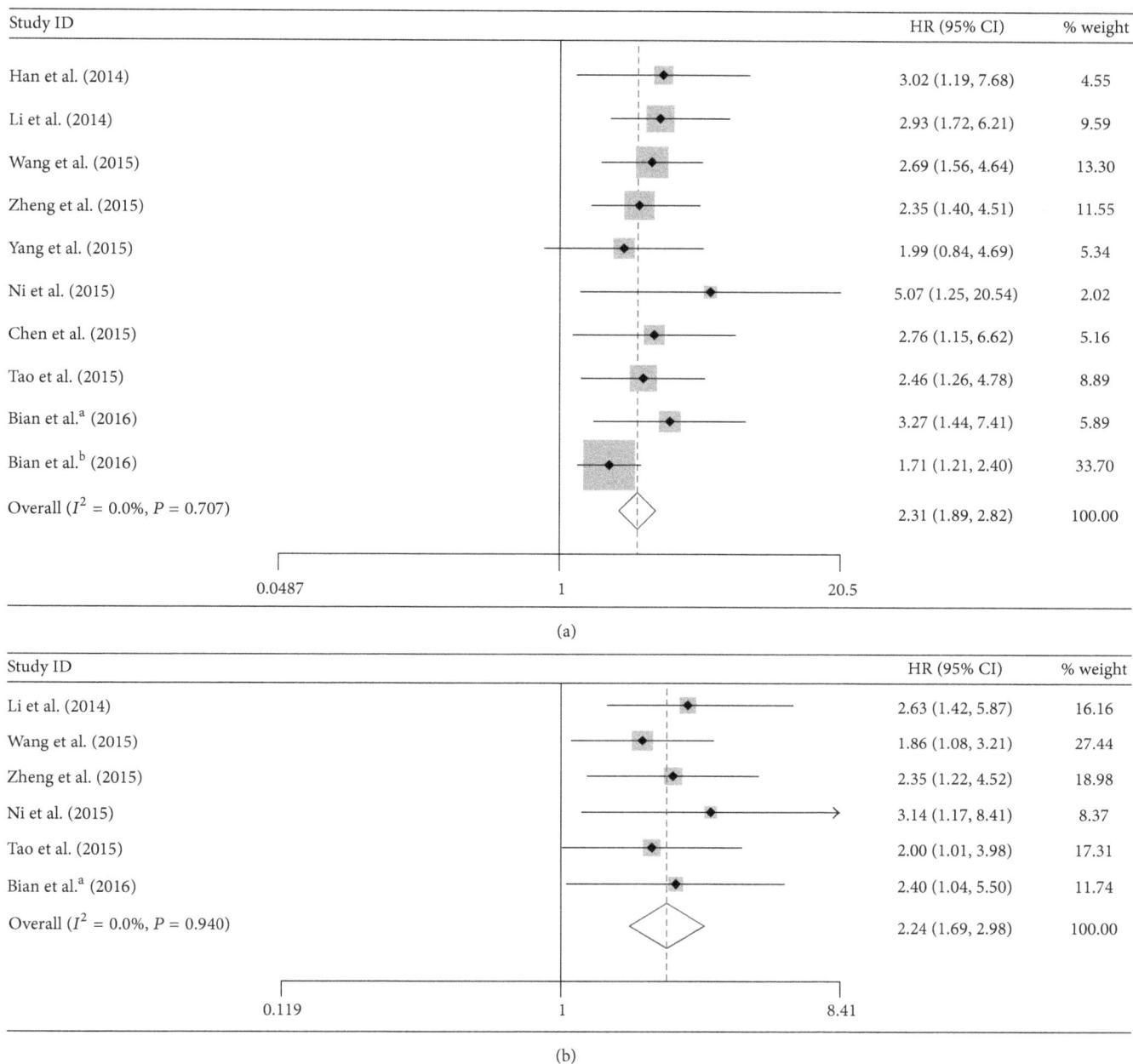

FIGURE 3: Forest plots of hazard ratios (HRs) for the association between UCA1 expression with overall survival (OS) from univariate analysis results (a) and OS from multivariate analysis results (b).

make it necessary and essential to identify biomarkers, which could improve the diagnosis and therapy by providing more precise and valuable information. UCA1, a lncRNA located at 19p13.12, has been found to be upregulated and exert oncogenic function in digestive system malignancies. In colorectal carcinoma, for example, overexpression of UCA1 was illustrated to promote proliferation and cell cycle progression and inhibit apoptosis, whereas suppression of UCA1 inhibited cell proliferation and cell cycle progression and facilitated

apoptosis [17]. Regarding the mechanism, UCA1 can act as a competing endogenous RNA (ceRNA) by directly binding to microRNAs (miRNAs). In hepatocellular carcinoma, upregulated UCA1 contributes to the progression of cancer by counteracting the inhibitory effect of miR-216b and activating the FGFR1/ERK signaling pathway [13]. In colorectal cancer, UCA1 was found to function as an endogenous sponge by directly binding to miR-204-5p and promote the expression of a new target of miR-204-5p, CREB1 [20]. The results

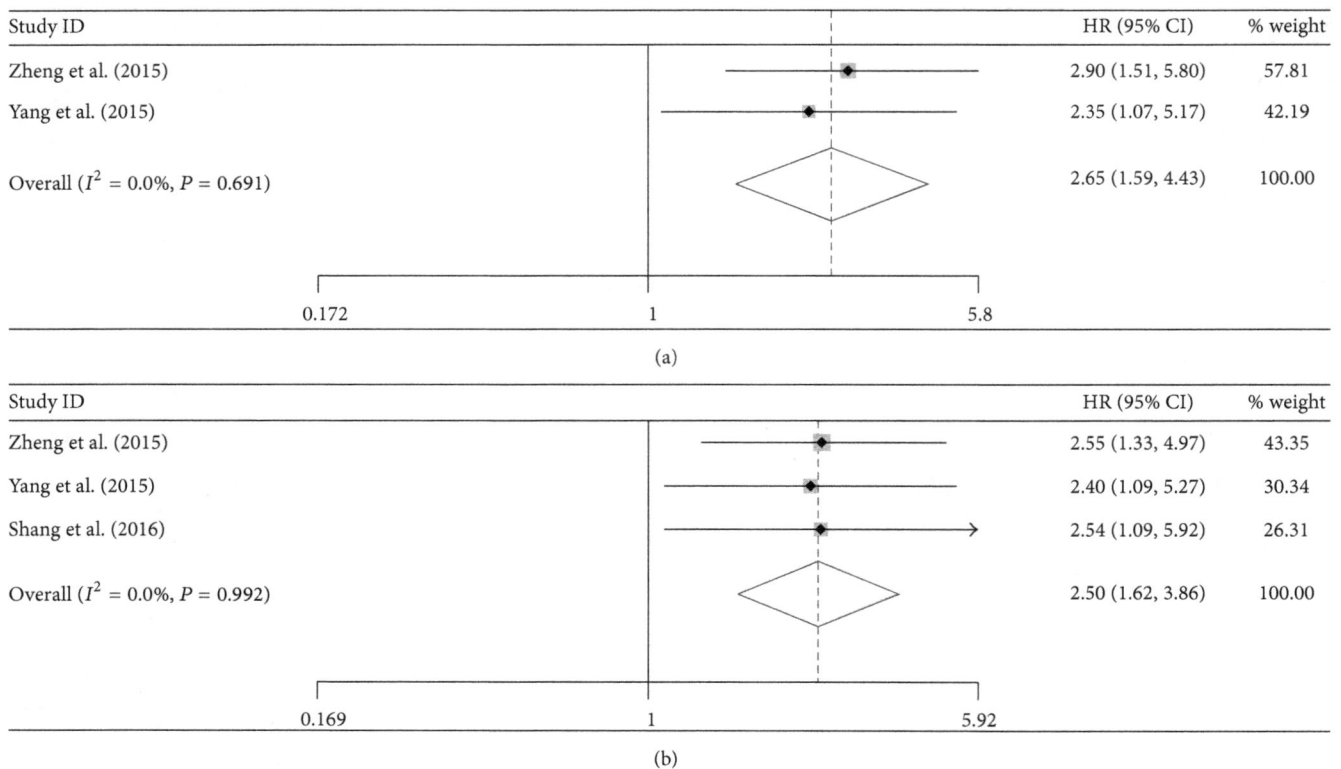

FIGURE 4: Forest plots of hazard ratios (HRs) for the association between UCA1 expression with disease-free survival (DFS) from univariate analysis results (a) and DFS from multivariate analysis results (b).

above suggested that UCA1 plays an important role during the carcinogenesis and may serve as a potential target for treatment of digestive system malignancies. Recently, several studies have investigated the clinicopathological value of UCA1 expression in digestive system malignancies. However, the sample sizes in most studies are small. Besides, it is inconclusive about the association between UCA1 expression and progression of digestive system malignancies, such as metastasis and survival. Therefore, we conducted this meta-analysis with the aim of clarifying the clinical significance of UCA1 expression in digestive system malignancies.

To the best of our knowledge, this is the first meta-analysis to investigate the association of UCA1 expression with the metastasis and prognosis of digestive system malignancy patients. We included 10 studies with a total of 1089 patients. The pooled ORs with their 95% CIs showed that high UCA1 expression was significantly associated with LNM and DM, indicating that UCA1 was an indicator for metastasis of digestive system malignancies. Moreover, the pooled HRs with their 95% CIs showed that UCA1 overexpression was also significantly correlated with both poor OS and poor DFS, indicating that UCA1 overexpression may serve as an indicator of poor survival rate and high recurrence rate of digestive system malignancies, respectively. What is more, as the lncRNA can be secreted by cancer cells or released into the circulation from dead cancer cells, it has been

reported that UCA1 level in plasma significantly decreased 14 days after surgery of colon cancer [19]. To some extent, it demonstrated the correlation between UCA1 overexpression and the aggressive behavior of digestive system malignancies, which was concordant with our conclusion. Taken together, UCA1 could serve as a promising biomarker for monitoring the progression of digestive system malignancies.

Nevertheless, there are several limitations in this meta-analysis. Firstly, most of the included studies were performed in the population from Asian countries rather than worldwide population; our results should be substantiated by additional studies in other races. Secondly, publication bias was observed in the studies with OS, which may be due to the fact that some studies were not included in this meta-analysis for their insufficient data or that some studies reported the correlation in one analytic method. Thirdly, the included studies were of small sample size as well as different cut-off value of UCA1 expression, which may generate errors by variation. Based on these limitations, the pooled ORs and HRs with their 95% CIs calculated in this meta-analysis may be just estimations.

5. Conclusion

In conclusion, our meta-analysis showed that UCA1 overexpression was correlated with LNM, DM, poor OS, and

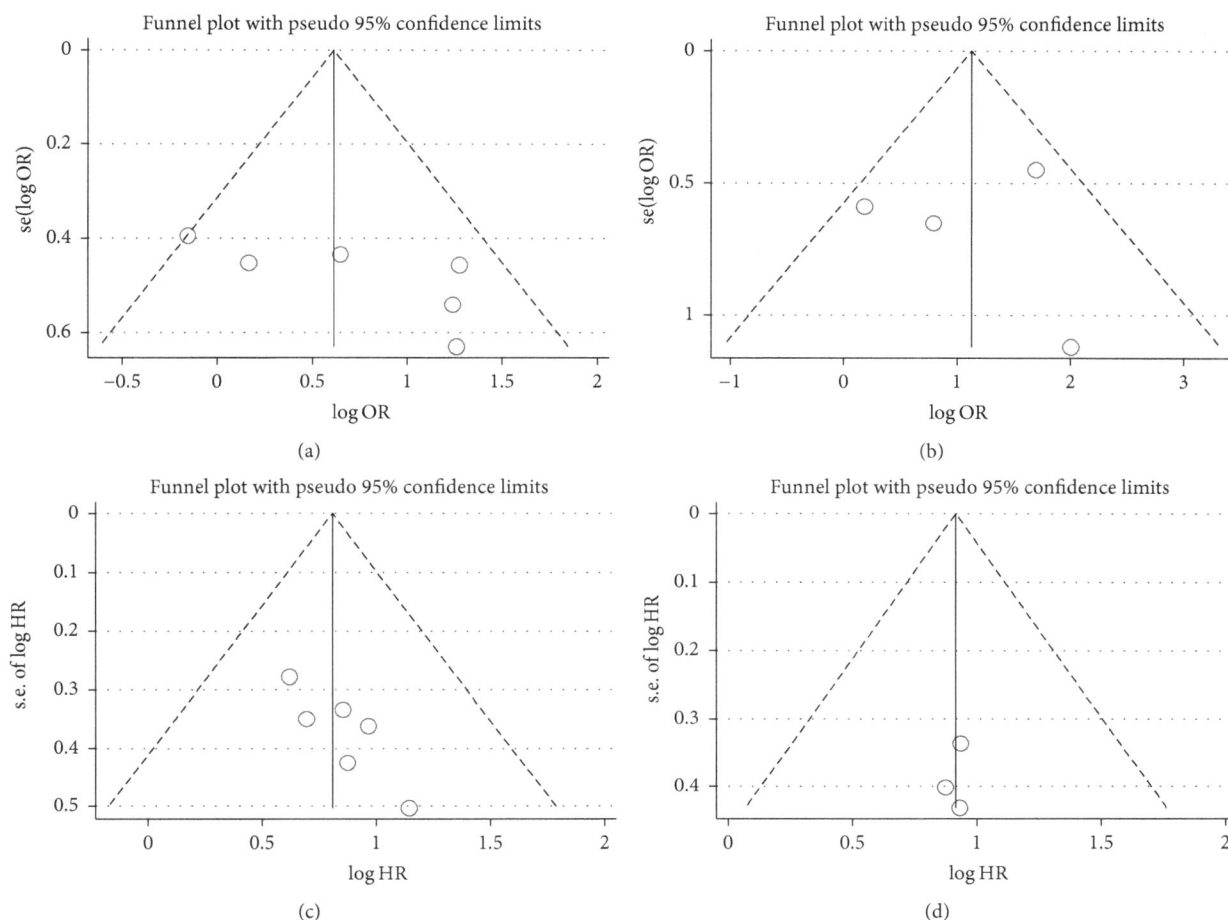

FIGURE 5: Funnel plots for the meta-analysis with lymph node metastasis (LNM) (a), distant metastasis (DM) (b), overall survival (OS) from multivariate analysis results (c), and disease-free survival (DFS) from multivariate analysis results (d).

poor DFS in digestive system malignancy patients. Therefore, UCA1 may serve as an indicator of metastasis and prognosis in digestive system malignancies.

Competing Interests

The authors declare that they have no competing interests.

Authors' Contributions

Xiao-Dong Sun and Chen Huan have contributed equally to this work.

References

[1] L. A. Torre, F. Bray, R. L. Siegel, J. Ferlay, J. Lortet-Tieulent, and A. Jemal, "Global cancer statistics, 2012," *CA: A Cancer Journal for Clinicians*, vol. 65, no. 2, pp. 87–108, 2015.

[2] Z. Cui, Y. Chen, Z. Xiao et al., "Long noncoding RNAs as auxiliary biomarkers for gastric cancer screening: a pooled analysis of individual studies," *Oncotarget*, vol. 7, no. 18, pp. 25791–25800, 2016.

[3] J. Hou, Y. Zhou, Y. Zheng et al., "Hepatic RIG-I predicts survival and interferon-alpha therapeutic response in hepatocellular carcinoma," *Cancer Cell*, vol. 25, no. 1, pp. 49–63, 2014.

[4] P. Johnsson, L. Lipovich, D. Grandér, and K. V. Morris, "Evolutionary conservation of long non-coding RNAs; sequence, structure, function," *Biochimica et Biophysica Acta (BBA)— General Subjects*, vol. 1840, no. 3, pp. 1063–1071, 2014.

[5] T. R. Mercer, M. E. Dinger, and J. S. Mattick, "Long non-coding RNAs: insights into functions," *Nature Reviews Genetics*, vol. 10, no. 3, pp. 155–159, 2009.

[6] J. Zhang, A. Zhang, Y. Wang et al., "New insights into the roles of ncRNA in the STAT3 pathway," *Future Oncology*, vol. 8, no. 6, pp. 723–730, 2012.

[7] H. Zhang, Z. Chen, X. Wang, Z. Huang, Z. He, and Y. Chen, "Long non-coding RNA: a new player in cancer," *Journal of Hematology and Oncology*, vol. 6, no. 1, article 37, 2013.

[8] S. Wang and Z. Wang, "Prognostic value of long noncoding RNA HOTAIR in digestive system malignancies," *Journal of Gastroenterology and Hepatology*, vol. 30, no. 7, pp. 1123–1133, 2015.

[9] H. Zhai, X.-M. Li, A. Maimaiti et al., "Prognostic value of long noncoding RNA MALAT1 in digestive system malignancies," *International Journal of Clinical and Experimental Medicine*, vol. 8, no. 10, pp. 18099–18106, 2015.

[10] G. Ma, Q. Wang, C. Lv et al., "The prognostic significance of HOTAIR for predicting clinical outcome in patients with digestive system tumors," *Journal of Cancer Research and Clinical Oncology*, vol. 141, no. 12, pp. 2139–2145, 2015.

[11] F. Wang, X. Li, X. Xie, L. Zhao, and W. Chen, "UCA1, a non-protein-coding RNA up-regulated in bladder carcinoma and embryo, influencing cell growth and promoting invasion," *FEBS Letters*, vol. 582, no. 13, pp. 1919–1927, 2008.

[12] Y. Fan, B. Shen, M. Tan et al., "Long non-coding RNA UCA1 increases chemoresistance of bladder cancer cells by regulating Wnt signaling," *The FEBS Journal*, vol. 281, no. 7, pp. 1750–1758, 2014.

[13] F. Wang, H.-Q. Ying, B.-S. He et al., "Upregulated lncRNA-UCA1 contributes to progression of hepatocellular carcinoma through inhibition of miR-216b and activation of FGFR1/ERK signaling pathway," *Oncotarget*, vol. 6, no. 10, pp. 7899–7917, 2015.

[14] Z. Yang, Y. Lu, Q. Xu, B. Tang, C.-K. Park, and X. Chen, "HULC and H19 played different roles in overall and disease-free survival from hepatocellular carcinoma after curative hepatectomy: a preliminary analysis from gene expression omnibus," *Disease Markers*, vol. 2015, Article ID 191029, 9 pages, 2015.

[15] Q. Zheng, F. Wu, W.-Y. Dai et al., "Aberrant expression of UCA1 in gastric cancer and its clinical significance," *Clinical and Translational Oncology*, vol. 17, no. 8, pp. 640–646, 2015.

[16] C. Shang, Y. Guo, J. Zhang, and B. Huang, "Silence of long noncoding RNA UCA1 inhibits malignant proliferation and chemotherapy resistance to adriamycin in gastric cancer," *Cancer Chemotherapy and Pharmacology*, vol. 77, no. 5, pp. 1061–1067, 2016.

[17] Y. Han, Y.-N. Yang, H.-H. Yuan et al., "UCA1, a long non-coding RNA up-regulated in colorectal cancer influences cell proliferation, apoptosis and cell cycle distribution," *Pathology*, vol. 46, no. 5, pp. 396–401, 2014.

[18] B. Ni, X. Yu, X. Guo et al., "Increased urothelial cancer associated 1 is associated with tumor proliferation and metastasis and predicts poor prognosis in colorectal cancer," *International Journal of Oncology*, vol. 47, no. 4, pp. 1329–1338, 2015.

[19] K. Tao, J. Yang, Y. Hu et al., "Clinical significance of urothelial carcinoma associated 1 in colon cancer," *International Journal of Clinical and Experimental Medicine*, vol. 8, no. 11, pp. 21854–21860, 2015.

[20] Z. Bian, L. Jin, J. Zhang et al., "LncRNA—UCA1 enhances cell proliferation and 5-fluorouracil resistance in colorectal cancer by inhibiting miR-204-5p," *Scientific Reports*, vol. 6, article 23892, 2016.

[21] D.-T. Chen, A. H. Davis-Yadley, P.-Y. Huang et al., "Prognostic fifteen-gene signature for early stage pancreatic ductal adenocarcinoma," *PLoS ONE*, vol. 10, no. 8, article e0133562, 2015.

[22] J.-Y. Li, X. Ma, and C.-B. Zhang, "Overexpression of long noncoding RNA UCA1 predicts a poor prognosis in patients with esophageal squamous cell carcinoma," *International Journal of Clinical and Experimental Pathology*, vol. 7, no. 11, pp. 7938–7944, 2014.

[23] J. F. Tierney, L. A. Stewart, D. Ghersi, S. Burdett, and M. R. Sydes, "Practical methods for incorporating summary time-to-event data into meta-analysis," *Trials*, vol. 8, article 16, 2007.

[24] A. Stang, "Critical evaluation of the Newcastle-Ottawa scale for the assessment of the quality of nonrandomized studies in meta-analyses," *European Journal of Epidemiology*, vol. 25, no. 9, pp. 603–605, 2010.

Permissions

All chapters in this book were first published in GRAP, by Hindawi Publishing Corporation; hereby published with permission under the Creative Commons Attribution License or equivalent. Every chapter published in this book has been scrutinized by our experts. Their significance has been extensively debated. The topics covered herein carry significant findings which will fuel the growth of the discipline. They may even be implemented as practical applications or may be referred to as a beginning point for another development.

The contributors of this book come from diverse backgrounds, making this book a truly international effort. This book will bring forth new frontiers with its revolutionizing research information and detailed analysis of the nascent developments around the world.

We would like to thank all the contributing authors for lending their expertise to make the book truly unique. They have played a crucial role in the development of this book. Without their invaluable contributions this book wouldn't have been possible. They have made vital efforts to compile up to date information on the varied aspects of this subject to make this book a valuable addition to the collection of many professionals and students.

This book was conceptualized with the vision of imparting up-to-date information and advanced data in this field. To ensure the same, a matchless editorial board was set up. Every individual on the board went through rigorous rounds of assessment to prove their worth. After which they invested a large part of their time researching and compiling the most relevant data for our readers.

The editorial board has been involved in producing this book since its inception. They have spent rigorous hours researching and exploring the diverse topics which have resulted in the successful publishing of this book. They have passed on their knowledge of decades through this book. To expedite this challenging task, the publisher supported the team at every step. A small team of assistant editors was also appointed to further simplify the editing procedure and attain best results for the readers.

Apart from the editorial board, the designing team has also invested a significant amount of their time in understanding the subject and creating the most relevant covers. They scrutinized every image to scout for the most suitable representation of the subject and create an appropriate cover for the book.

The publishing team has been an ardent support to the editorial, designing and production team. Their endless efforts to recruit the best for this project, has resulted in the accomplishment of this book. They are a veteran in the field of academics and their pool of knowledge is as vast as their experience in printing. Their expertise and guidance has proved useful at every step. Their uncompromising quality standards have made this book an exceptional effort. Their encouragement from time to time has been an inspiration for everyone.

The publisher and the editorial board hope that this book will prove to be a valuable piece of knowledge for researchers, students, practitioners and scholars across the globe.

List of Contributors

Cristina Alvarez-Urturi, Inés Ana Ibáñez, Josep Maria Dedeu, Xavier Bessa, Luis Barranco and Montserrat Andreu
Department of Gastroenterology, Hospital del Mar, UAB, Parc de Salut Mar, Barcelona, Catalonia, Spain

Gloria Fernández-Esparrach, Cristina Rodríguez DeMiguel, Henry Córdova, Isis K. Araujo, Maria Pellisé, Francesc Balaguer, Angels Ginés, Josep Llach, Antoni Castells and Begoña González-Suarez
Gastroenterology Department, Endoscopy Unit, ICMDiM, Hospital Clinic, CIBEREHD, IDIBAPS, University of Barcelona, Catalonia, Spain

Shengyang Qiu and Francesca Fiorentino
Department of Surgery and Cancer, Imperial College London, Chelsea & Westminster Hospital Campus, London, UK

Gianluca Pellino, Shahnawaz Rasheed and Ara Darzi
Department of Colorectal Surgery, The Royal Marsden Hospital, Chelsea, London, UK

Paris Tekkis and Christos Kontovounisios
Department of Surgery and Cancer, Imperial College London, Chelsea & Westminster Hospital Campus, London, UK
Department of Colorectal Surgery, The Royal Marsden Hospital, Chelsea, London, UK

Penglei Ge, Huayu Yang, Wenjun Liao, Shunda Du, Haifeng Xu, Haitao Zhao, Xin Lu, Xinting Sang, Shouxian Zhong, Jiefu Huang and Yilei Mao
Department of Liver Surgery, Peking Union Medical College (PUMC) Hospital, Chinese Academy of Medical Sciences and PUMC, Beijing, China

Jingfen Lu and Yingli Xu
State Key Laboratory of Natural and Biomimetic Drugs, School of Pharmaceutical Sciences, Peking University, Beijing, China

Dae Hyun Tak, Hee Seok Moon, Sun Hyung Kang, Jae Kyu Sung and Hyun Yong Jeong
Division of Gastroenterology, Departments of Internal Medicine, Chungnam National University School of Medicine, Daejeon, Republic of Korea

Alexander F. Hagel, Heinz Albrecht, Andreas Nägel, Francesco Vitali, Marcel Vetter and Markus F. Neurath
Department of Gastroenterology, University of Erlangen, Ulmenweg 18, 91054 Erlangen, Germany

Christine Dauth
Institute for Employment Research, Regensburger Straße 104, 90478 Nuremberg, Germany

Martin Raithel
Department of Gastroenterology, Waldkrankenhaus St. Marien, Rathsberger Str. 57, 91054 Erlangen, Germany

Tabea Pang, Sergio B. Sesia, Stefan Holland-Cunz and Johannes Mayr
Department of Pediatric Surgery, University Children's Hospital Basel, Spitalstrasse 33, 4056 Basel, Switzerland

Dawei Gong, Lili Wang, Xinjuan Yu and Quanjiang Dong
Department of Central Laboratories and Gastroenterology, Qingdao Municipal Hospital, School of Medicine, Qingdao University, Qingdao 266071, China

Xiaojie Gong
Department of Emergency Surgery,The Fifth People's Hospital of Ji'nan, Ji'nan 250022, China

Raffaella Liccardo, Marina De Rosa and Francesca Duraturo
Department of Molecular Medicine and Medical Biotechnology, University of Naples "Federico II", 80131 Naples, Italy

Paola Izzo
Department of Molecular Medicine and Medical Biotechnology, University of Naples "Federico II", 80131 Naples, Italy
CEINGE Biotecnologie Avanzate, University of Naples "Federico II", 80131 Naples, Italy

W. Lv, A. Jiao, B. C. Zhao, Y. Shi, B. M. Chen and J. L. Zhang
Department of Hepatobiliary and Transplantation Surgery,The First Hospital of China Medical University, Shenyang, Liaoning Province, China

G. Q. Zhang
Department of Hepatobiliary and Transplantation Surgery,The First Hospital of China Medical University, Shenyang, Liaoning Province, China
Department of Clinical Medicine, First Affiliated Hospital of Zhengzhou University, Zhengzhou, Henan Province, China

Fang Zhang, Luyi Wu, Jimeng Zhao, Tingting Lv, Zhijun Weng, HuanganWu and Huirong Liu
Shanghai Research Institute of Acupuncture and Meridian, Shanghai 200030, China

Zhihai Hu and Shuoshuo Wang
Shanghai TCM-Integrated Hospital, Shanghai University of Traditional Chinese Medicine, Shanghai 200082, China

Shaobo Mo and Guoxiang Cai
Department of Colorectal Surgery, Fudan University Shanghai Cancer Center, Shanghai 200032, China
Department of Oncology, Shanghai Medical College, Fudan University, Shanghai 200032, China

Rong Zhang and Shizan Xu
Department of Gastroenterology, Shanghai Tenth People's Hospital, Tongji University, School of Medicine, Shanghai 200072, China
The First Clinical Medical College of Nanjing Medical University, Nanjing 210029, China

Keran Cheng, Yuqing Zhou, Shunfeng Zhou, Rui Kong and Linqiang Li
Department of Gastroenterology, Shanghai Tenth People's Hospital, Tongji University, School of Medicine, Shanghai 200072, China
The School of Medicine of Soochow University, Suzhou 215006, China

Sainan Li, Jingjing Li, Jiao Feng, LiweiWu, Tong Liu, Yujing Xia, Jie Lu, Chuanyong Guo and Yingqun Zhou
Department of Gastroenterology, Shanghai Tenth People's Hospital, Tongji University, School of Medicine, Shanghai 200072, China

Gi Jun Kim, Sung Min Park, Joon Sung Kim, Jeong Seon Ji, Byung Wook Kim and Hwang Choi
Division of Gastroenterology, Department of Internal Medicine, College of Medicine, The Catholic University of Korea, Seoul, Republic of Korea

Liping Guo, Lu Zhou, Baoru Deng and Bangmao Wang
Department of Gastroenterology and Hepatology, Tianjin Medical University General Hospital, Tianjin 300052, China

Na Zhang
Department of Rheumatology, Tianjin Medical University General Hospital, Tianjin 300052, China

Khaled Abdeljawad and Emad Qayed
Department of Medicine, Division of Digestive Diseases, Emory University School of Medicine, Atlanta, GA, USA

Antonios Wehbeh
Department of Medicine, Emory University School of Medicine, Atlanta, GA, USA

Shi Chen, Jun Xiang and Jun-Sheng Peng
The 6th Affiliated Hospital, Sun Yat-sen University, No. 26, Yuancun Erheng Road, Tianhe District, 510655 Guangzhou, China

Li-Ying Ou-Yang
Department of Intensive Care Unit, Sun Yat-sen University Cancer Center, 651 Dongfeng East Road, 510060 Guangzhou, China

Run-Cong Nie, Yuan-Fang Li, Zhi-Wei Zhou and Ying-Bo Chen
Department of Gastropancreatic Surgery, Sun Yat-sen University Cancer Center, 651 Dongfeng East Road, 510060 Guangzhou, China

Hironori Konuma, TakashiMorimoto and AkihisaMiyazaki
Department of Gastroenterology, Juntendo Nerima Hospital, Tokyo, Japan

Kenshi Matsumoto, Hiroya Ueyama, Hiroyuki Komori, Yoichi Akazawa, Misuzu Ueyama, Yuta Nakagawa, Tsutomu Takeda, KoheiMatsumoto, Daisuke Asaoka, Mariko Hojo and Sumio Watanabe
Department of Gastroenterology, Juntendo University School of Medicine, Tokyo, Japan

Akihito Nagahara
Department of Gastroenterology, Juntendo Sizuoka Hospital, Sizuoka, Japan

Takashi Yao
Department of Human Pathology, Juntendo University School of Medicine, Tokyo, Japan

Valentina Beltrame, Gioia Pozza, Enrico Dalla Bona, Michele Valmasoni and Cosimo Spert
Department of Surgery, Oncology and Gastroenterology, 3rd Surgical Clinic, University of Padua, Via Giustiniani 2, 35128 Padua, Italy

Alberto Fantin
GastroenterologyUnit, University of Padua, Via Giustiniani 2, 35128 Padua, Italy

Xiaoquan Huang and Shiyao Chen
Endoscopy Center and Endoscopy Research Institute, Zhongshan Hospital, Fudan University, Shanghai 200032, China
Department of Gastroenterology, Zhongshan Hospital, Fudan University, Shanghai 200032, China

Lili Ma
Endoscopy Center and Endoscopy Research Institute, Zhongshan Hospital, Fudan University, Shanghai 200032, China

Xiaoqing Zeng, Jian Wang and Jie Chen
Department of Gastroenterology, Zhongshan Hospital, Fudan University, Shanghai 200032, China

Nina Nayara FerreiraMartins, Kelly Cristina da Silva Oliveira, Geraldo Ishak, Paulo Pimentel Assumpção, and Danielle Queiroz Calcagno
Núcleo de Pesquisas em Oncologia, Universidade Federal do Pará, Belém, PA, Brazil

Amanda Braga Bona and Rommel Rodríguez Burbano
Laboratório de Citogenética Humana, Instituto de Ciências Biológicas, Universidade Federal do Pará, Belém, PA, Brazil

Marília de Arruda Cardoso Smith
Universidade Federal de São Paulo, São Paulo, SP, Brazil

Duc Trong Quach and Mai Ngoc Luu
Department of Internal Medicine, University of Medicine and Pharmacy, Ho Chi Minh, Vietnam
Department of Gastroenterology, Gia Dinh People's Hospital, Ho Chi Minh City, Vietnam

Toru Hiyama
Health Service Center, Hiroshima University, Higashihiroshima, Japan

Thuy-HuongThi To, Quy Nhuan Bui, Tuan Anh Tran and Binh Duy Tran
Department of Endoscopy, Gia Dinh People's Hospital, Ho Chi Minh City, Vietnam

Minh-Cong Hong Vo
Department of Gastroenterology, Gia Dinh People's Hospital, Ho Chi Minh City, Vietnam

Shinji Tanaka
Department of Endoscopy, Hiroshima University Hospital, Hiroshima, Japan

Naomi Uemura
Department of Gastroenterology and Hepatology, National Center for Global Health and Medicine, Ichikawa, Japan

Yuan-Lung Cheng
Taipei Municipal Gan-Dau Hospital, Taipei, Taiwan
Faculty of Medicine, School of Medicine, National Yang-Ming University, Taipei, Taiwan

Yuan-Jen Wang
Faculty of Medicine, School of Medicine, National Yang-Ming University, Taipei, Taiwan
Healthcare Center, Taipei Veterans General Hospital, Taipei, Taiwan

Keng-Hsin Lan
Faculty of Medicine, School of Medicine, National Yang-Ming University, Taipei, Taiwan
Division of Gastroenterology and Hepatology, Department of Medicine, Taipei Veterans General Hospital, Taipei, Taiwan
Department and Institute of Pharmacology, National Yang-Ming University, Taipei, Taiwan

Teh-Ia Huo
Division of Gastroenterology and Hepatology, Department of Medicine, Taipei Veterans General Hospital, Taipei, Taiwan
Department and Institute of Pharmacology, National Yang-Ming University, Taipei, Taiwan

Yi-Hsiang Huang
Division of Gastroenterology and Hepatology, Department of Medicine, Taipei Veterans General Hospital, Taipei, Taiwan
Institute of Clinical Medicine, School of Medicine, National Yang-Ming University, Taipei, Taiwan

Chien-Wei Su, Ming-Chih Hou, Han-Chieh Lin and Fa-Yauh Lee
Faculty of Medicine, School of Medicine, National Yang-Ming University, Taipei, Taiwan
Division of Gastroenterology and Hepatology, Department of Medicine, Taipei Veterans General Hospital, Taipei, Taiwan

Wei-Yao Hsieh
Division of Gastroenterology and Hepatology, Department of Medicine, Taipei Veterans General Hospital, Taipei, Taiwan

Jaw-ChingWu
Institute of Clinical Medicine, School of Medicine, National Yang-Ming University, Taipei, Taiwan
Division of Translational Research, Department of Medical Research, Taipei Veterans General Hospital, Taipei, Taiwan

Shou-Dong Lee
Faculty of Medicine, School of Medicine, National Yang-Ming University, Taipei, Taiwan
Division of Gastroenterology, Department of Medicine, Cheng Hsin General Hospital, Taipei, Taiwan

Hugo Teixeira Farinha, Fabian Grass, Amaniel Kefleyesus, Nicolas Demartines and Martin Hübner
Department of Visceral Surgery, University Hospital of Lausanne (CHUV), Lausanne, Switzerland

Chahin Achtari
Department of Gynecology, University Hospital of Lausanne (CHUV), Lausanne, Switzerland

Benoit Romain
Department of Visceral Surgery, University Hospital of Lausanne (CHUV), Lausanne, Switzerland
Department of Digestive Surgery, Strasbourg University, Strasbourg, France

MichaelMontemurro
Department of Oncology, University Hospital of Lausanne (CHUV), Lausanne, Switzerland

Xiao-Dong Sun, Wei Qiu, Da-Wei Sun, Xiao-Ju Shi, Chuan-LeiWang,
Chao Jiang, Guang-YiWang and Guo-Yue Lv
Department of Hepatobiliary and Pancreatic Surgery,The First Hospital of Jilin University, Changchun, Jilin Province 130021, China

Chen Huan
Institute of Virology and AIDS Research,The First Hospital of Jilin University, Changchun, Jilin Province 130021, China

Index

www.ingramcontent.com/pod-product-compliance
Lightning Source LLC
Chambersburg PA
CBHW080632200326
41458CB00013B/4599

9781632425331